50% OFF RNC-NIC Test Prep Course!

By Mometrix

Dear Customer,

We consider it an honor and a privilege that you chose our RNC-NIC Study Guide. As a way of showing our appreciation and to help us better serve you, we are offering **50% off our online RNC-NIC Prep Course.** Many Neonatal Intensive Care Nurse courses are needlessly expensive and don't deliver enough value. With our course, you get access to the best RNC-NIC prep material, and **you only pay half price.**

We have structured our online course to perfectly complement your printed study guide. The RNC-NIC Test Prep Course contains **in-depth lessons** that cover all the most important topics, over **500 practice questions** to ensure you feel prepared, more than **500 flashcards** for studying on the go, and over **20 instructional videos.**

Online RNC-NIC Prep Course

Topics Covered:

- General Assessment
  - Problems in Labor
  - Clinical Laboratory Tests
- General Management
  - Resuscitation and Stabilization
  - Infection and Immunology
- Assess and Manage Pathophysiologic States
  - Cardiovascular
  - Neurological/Neuromuscular
- Psychosocial Support
  - Discharge Planning and Parent Teaching
  - Maternal and Family Grief
- Professional Issues
  - Evidence Based Practice
  - Patient Safety
- And More!

Course Features:

- RNC-NIC Study Guide
  - Get access to content from the best reviewed study guide available.
- Track Your Progress
  - Our customized course allows you to check off content you have studied or feel confident with.
- 3 Full-Length Practice Tests
  - With 500+ practice questions and lesson reviews, you can test yourself again and again to build confidence.
- RNC-NIC Flashcards
  - Our course includes a flashcard mode consisting of over 500 content cards to help you study.

To receive this discount, visit us at mometrix.com/university/rncnic/ or simply scan this QR code with your smartphone. At the checkout page, enter the discount code: **RNCNIC50OFF**

If you have any questions or concerns, please contact us at support@mometrix.com.

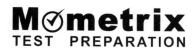

FREE Study Skills Videos/DVD Offer

Dear Customer,

Thank you for your purchase from Mometrix! We consider it an honor and a privilege that you have purchased our product and we want to ensure your satisfaction.

As part of our ongoing effort to meet the needs of test takers, we have developed a set of Study Skills Videos that we would like to give you for <u>FREE</u>. These videos cover our *best practices* for getting ready for your exam, from how to use our study materials to how to best prepare for the day of the test.

All that we ask is that you email us with feedback that would describe your experience so far with our product. Good, bad, or indifferent, we want to know what you think!

To get your FREE Study Skills Videos, you can use the **QR code** below, or send us an **email** at studyvideos@mometrix.com with *FREE VIDEOS* in the subject line and the following information in the body of the email:

- The name of the product you purchased.
- Your product rating on a scale of 1-5, with 5 being the highest rating.
- Your feedback. It can be long, short, or anything in between. We just want to know your impressions and experience so far with our product. (Good feedback might include how our study material met your needs and ways we might be able to make it even better. You could highlight features that you found helpful or features that you think we should add.)

If you have any questions or concerns, please don't hesitate to contact me directly.

Thanks again!

Sincerely,

Jay Willis
Vice President
jay.willis@mometrix.com
1-800-673-8175

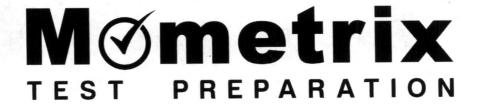

Neonatal Intensive Care Nurse Exam
SECRETS

Study Guide
Your Key to Exam Success

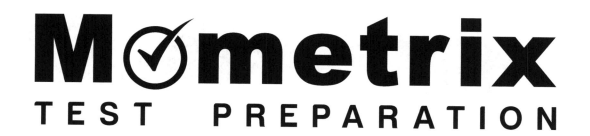

Written and edited by the Mometrix Nursing Certification Test Team

Printed in the United States of America

This paper meets the requirements of ANSI/NISO Z39.48-1992 (Permanence of Paper).

Mometrix offers volume discount pricing to institutions. For more information or a price quote, please contact our sales department at sales@mometrix.com or 888-248-1219.

Mometrix Media LLC is not affiliated with or endorsed by any official testing organization. All organizational and test names are trademarks of their respective owners.

Paperback
ISBN 13: 978-1-61072-251-3
ISBN 10: 1-61072-251-5

Ebook
ISBN 13: 978-1-5167-0639-6
ISBN 10: 1-5167-0639-0

DEAR FUTURE EXAM SUCCESS STORY

First of all, **THANK YOU** for purchasing Mometrix study materials!

Second, congratulations! You are one of the few determined test-takers who are committed to doing whatever it takes to excel on your exam. **You have come to the right place.** We developed these study materials with one goal in mind: to deliver you the information you need in a format that's concise and easy to use.

In addition to optimizing your guide for the content of the test, we've outlined our recommended steps for breaking down the preparation process into small, attainable goals so you can make sure you stay on track.

We've also analyzed the entire test-taking process, identifying the most common pitfalls and showing how you can overcome them and be ready for any curveball the test throws you.

Standardized testing is one of the biggest obstacles on your road to success, which only increases the importance of doing well in the high-pressure, high-stakes environment of test day. Your results on this test could have a significant impact on your future, and this guide provides the information and practical advice to help you achieve your full potential on test day.

Your success is our success

We would love to hear from you! If you would like to share the story of your exam success or if you have any questions or comments in regard to our products, please contact us at **800-673-8175** or **support@mometrix.com**.

Thanks again for your business and we wish you continued success!

Sincerely,
The Mometrix Test Preparation Team

> **Need more help? Check out our flashcards at:**
> **http://mometrixflashcards.com/Neonatal**

TABLE OF CONTENTS

Introduction

Thank you for purchasing this resource! You have made the choice to prepare yourself for a test that could have a huge impact on your future, and this guide is designed to help you be fully ready for test day. Obviously, it's important to have a solid understanding of the test material, but you also need to be prepared for the unique environment and stressors of the test, so that you can perform to the best of your abilities.

For this purpose, the first section that appears in this guide is the **Secret Keys**. We've devoted countless hours to meticulously researching what works and what doesn't, and we've boiled down our findings to the five most impactful steps you can take to improve your performance on the test. We start at the beginning with study planning and move through the preparation process, all the way to the testing strategies that will help you get the most out of what you know when you're finally sitting in front of the test.

We recommend that you start preparing for your test as far in advance as possible. However, if you've bought this guide as a last-minute study resource and only have a few days before your test, we recommend that you skip over the first two Secret Keys since they address a long-term study plan.

If you struggle with **test anxiety**, we strongly encourage you to check out our recommendations for how you can overcome it. Test anxiety is a formidable foe, but it can be beaten, and we want to make sure you have the tools you need to defeat it.

Secret Key #1 – Plan Big, Study Small

There's a lot riding on your performance. If you want to ace this test, you're going to need to keep your skills sharp and the material fresh in your mind. You need a plan that lets you review everything you need to know while still fitting in your schedule. We'll break this strategy down into three categories.

Information Organization

Start with the information you already have: the official test outline. From this, you can make a complete list of all the concepts you need to cover before the test. Organize these concepts into groups that can be studied together, and create a list of any related vocabulary you need to learn so you can brush up on any difficult terms. You'll want to keep this vocabulary list handy once you actually start studying since you may need to add to it along the way.

Time Management

Once you have your set of study concepts, decide how to spread them out over the time you have left before the test. Break your study plan into small, clear goals so you have a manageable task for each day and know exactly what you're doing. Then just focus on one small step at a time. When you manage your time this way, you don't need to spend hours at a time studying. Studying a small block of content for a short period each day helps you retain information better and avoid stressing over how much you have left to do. You can relax knowing that you have a plan to cover everything in time. In order for this strategy to be effective though, you have to start studying early and stick to your schedule. Avoid the exhaustion and futility that comes from last-minute cramming!

Study Environment

The environment you study in has a big impact on your learning. Studying in a coffee shop, while probably more enjoyable, is not likely to be as fruitful as studying in a quiet room. It's important to keep distractions to a minimum. You're only planning to study for a short block of time, so make the most of it. Don't pause to check your phone or get up to find a snack. It's also important to **avoid multitasking**. Research has consistently shown that multitasking will make your studying dramatically less effective. Your study area should also be comfortable and well-lit so you don't have the distraction of straining your eyes or sitting on an uncomfortable chair.

 The time of day you study is also important. You want to be rested and alert. Don't wait until just before bedtime. Study when you'll be most likely to comprehend and remember. Even better, if you know what time of day your test will be, set that time aside for study. That way your brain will be used to working on that subject at that specific time and you'll have a better chance of recalling information.

Finally, it can be helpful to team up with others who are studying for the same test. Your actual studying should be done in as isolated an environment as possible, but the work of organizing the information and setting up the study plan can be divided up. In between study sessions, you can discuss with your teammates the concepts that you're all studying and quiz each other on the details. Just be sure that your teammates are as serious about the test as you are. If you find that your study time is being replaced with social time, you might need to find a new team.

Secret Key #2 – Make Your Studying Count

You're devoting a lot of time and effort to preparing for this test, so you want to be absolutely certain it will pay off. This means doing more than just reading the content and hoping you can remember it on test day. It's important to make every minute of study count. There are two main areas you can focus on to make your studying count.

Retention

It doesn't matter how much time you study if you can't remember the material. You need to make sure you are retaining the concepts. To check your retention of the information you're learning, try recalling it at later times with minimal prompting. Try carrying around flashcards and glance at one or two from time to time or ask a friend who's also studying for the test to quiz you.

To enhance your retention, look for ways to put the information into practice so that you can apply it rather than simply recalling it. If you're using the information in practical ways, it will be much easier to remember. Similarly, it helps to solidify a concept in your mind if you're not only reading it to yourself but also explaining it to someone else. Ask a friend to let you teach them about a concept you're a little shaky on (or speak aloud to an imaginary audience if necessary). As you try to summarize, define, give examples, and answer your friend's questions, you'll understand the concepts better and they will stay with you longer. Finally, step back for a big picture view and ask yourself how each piece of information fits with the whole subject. When you link the different concepts together and see them working together as a whole, it's easier to remember the individual components.

Finally, practice showing your work on any multi-step problems, even if you're just studying. Writing out each step you take to solve a problem will help solidify the process in your mind, and you'll be more likely to remember it during the test.

Modality

Modality simply refers to the means or method by which you study. Choosing a study modality that fits your own individual learning style is crucial. No two people learn best in exactly the same way, so it's important to know your strengths and use them to your advantage.

For example, if you learn best by visualization, focus on visualizing a concept in your mind and draw an image or a diagram. Try color-coding your notes, illustrating them, or creating symbols that will trigger your mind to recall a learned concept. If you learn best by hearing or discussing information, find a study partner who learns the same way or read aloud to yourself. Think about how to put the information in your own words. Imagine that you are giving a lecture on the topic and record yourself so you can listen to it later.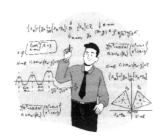

For any learning style, flashcards can be helpful. Organize the information so you can take advantage of spare moments to review. Underline key words or phrases. Use different colors for different categories. Mnemonic devices (such as creating a short list in which every item starts with the same letter) can also help with retention. Find what works best for you and use it to store the information in your mind most effectively and easily.

Secret Key #3 – Practice the Right Way

Your success on test day depends not only on how many hours you put into preparing, but also on whether you prepared the right way. It's good to check along the way to see if your studying is paying off. One of the most effective ways to do this is by taking practice tests to evaluate your progress. Practice tests are useful because they show exactly where you need to improve. Every time you take a practice test, pay special attention to these three groups of questions:

- The questions you got wrong
- The questions you had to guess on, even if you guessed right
- The questions you found difficult or slow to work through

This will show you exactly what your weak areas are, and where you need to devote more study time. Ask yourself why each of these questions gave you trouble. Was it because you didn't understand the material? Was it because you didn't remember the vocabulary? Do you need more repetitions on this type of question to build speed and confidence? Dig into those questions and figure out how you can strengthen your weak areas as you go back to review the material.

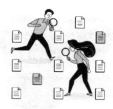 Additionally, many practice tests have a section explaining the answer choices. It can be tempting to read the explanation and think that you now have a good understanding of the concept. However, an explanation likely only covers part of the question's broader context. Even if the explanation makes perfect sense, **go back and investigate** every concept related to the question until you're positive you have a thorough understanding.

As you go along, keep in mind that the practice test is just that: practice. Memorizing these questions and answers will not be very helpful on the actual test because it is unlikely to have any of the same exact questions. If you only know the right answers to the sample questions, you won't be prepared for the real thing. **Study the concepts** until you understand them fully, and then you'll be able to answer any question that shows up on the test.

It's important to wait on the practice tests until you're ready. If you take a test on your first day of study, you may be overwhelmed by the amount of material covered and how much you need to learn. Work up to it gradually.

On test day, you'll need to be prepared for answering questions, managing your time, and using the test-taking strategies you've learned. It's a lot to balance, like a mental marathon that will have a big impact on your future. Like training for a marathon, you'll need to start slowly and work your way up. When test day arrives, you'll be ready.

Start with the strategies you've read in the first two Secret Keys—plan your course and study in the way that works best for you. If you have time, consider using multiple study resources to get different approaches to the same concepts. It can be helpful to see difficult concepts from more than one angle. Then find a good source for practice tests. Many times, the test website will suggest potential study resources or provide sample tests.

Practice Test Strategy

If you're able to find at least three practice tests, we recommend this strategy:

UNTIMED AND OPEN-BOOK PRACTICE

Take the first test with no time constraints and with your notes and study guide handy. Take your time and focus on applying the strategies you've learned.

TIMED AND OPEN-BOOK PRACTICE

Take the second practice test open-book as well, but set a timer and practice pacing yourself to finish in time.

TIMED AND CLOSED-BOOK PRACTICE

Take any other practice tests as if it were test day. Set a timer and put away your study materials. Sit at a table or desk in a quiet room, imagine yourself at the testing center, and answer questions as quickly and accurately as possible.

Keep repeating timed and closed-book tests on a regular basis until you run out of practice tests or it's time for the actual test. Your mind will be ready for the schedule and stress of test day, and you'll be able to focus on recalling the material you've learned.

Secret Key #4 – Pace Yourself

Once you're fully prepared for the material on the test, your biggest challenge on test day will be managing your time. Just knowing that the clock is ticking can make you panic even if you have plenty of time left. Work on pacing yourself so you can build confidence against the time constraints of the exam. Pacing is a difficult skill to master, especially in a high-pressure environment, so **practice is vital**.

Set time expectations for your pace based on how much time is available. For example, if a section has 60 questions and the time limit is 30 minutes, you know you have to average 30 seconds or less per question in order to answer them all. Although 30 seconds is the hard limit, set 25 seconds per question as your goal, so you reserve extra time to spend on harder questions. When you budget extra time for the harder questions, you no longer have any reason to stress when those questions take longer to answer.

Don't let this time expectation distract you from working through the test at a calm, steady pace, but keep it in mind so you don't spend too much time on any one question. Recognize that taking extra time on one question you don't understand may keep you from answering two that you do understand later in the test. If your time limit for a question is up and you're still not sure of the answer, mark it and move on, and come back to it later if the time and the test format allow. If the testing format doesn't allow you to return to earlier questions, just make an educated guess; then put it out of your mind and move on.

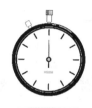

On the easier questions, be careful not to rush. It may seem wise to hurry through them so you have more time for the challenging ones, but it's not worth missing one if you know the concept and just didn't take the time to read the question fully. Work efficiently but make sure you understand the question and have looked at all of the answer choices, since more than one may seem right at first.

Even if you're paying attention to the time, you may find yourself a little behind at some point. You should speed up to get back on track, but do so wisely. Don't panic; just take a few seconds less on each question until you're caught up. Don't guess without thinking, but do look through the answer choices and eliminate any you know are wrong. If you can get down to two choices, it is often worthwhile to guess from those. Once you've chosen an answer, move on and don't dwell on any that you skipped or had to hurry through. If a question was taking too long, chances are it was one of the harder ones, so you weren't as likely to get it right anyway.

On the other hand, if you find yourself getting ahead of schedule, it may be beneficial to slow down a little. The more quickly you work, the more likely you are to make a careless mistake that will affect your score. You've budgeted time for each question, so don't be afraid to spend that time. Practice an efficient but careful pace to get the most out of the time you have.

Secret Key #5 – Have a Plan for Guessing

When you're taking the test, you may find yourself stuck on a question. Some of the answer choices seem better than others, but you don't see the one answer choice that is obviously correct. What do you do?

The scenario described above is very common, yet most test takers have not effectively prepared for it. Developing and practicing a plan for guessing may be one of the single most effective uses of your time as you get ready for the exam.

In developing your plan for guessing, there are three questions to address:

- When should you start the guessing process?
- How should you narrow down the choices?
- Which answer should you choose?

When to Start the Guessing Process

Unless your plan for guessing is to select C every time (which, despite its merits, is not what we recommend), you need to leave yourself enough time to apply your answer elimination strategies. Since you have a limited amount of time for each question, that means that if you're going to give yourself the best shot at guessing correctly, you have to decide quickly whether or not you will guess.

Of course, the best-case scenario is that you don't have to guess at all, so first, see if you can answer the question based on your knowledge of the subject and basic reasoning skills. Focus on the key words in the question and try to jog your memory of related topics. Give yourself a chance to bring the knowledge to mind, but once you realize that you don't have (or you can't access) the knowledge you need to answer the question, it's time to start the guessing process.

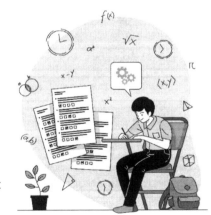

It's almost always better to start the guessing process too early than too late. It only takes a few seconds to remember something and answer the question from knowledge. Carefully eliminating wrong answer choices takes longer. Plus, going through the process of eliminating answer choices can actually help jog your memory.

Summary: Start the guessing process as soon as you decide that you can't answer the question based on your knowledge.

8

How to Narrow Down the Choices

The next chapter in this book (**Test-Taking Strategies**) includes a wide range of strategies for how to approach questions and how to look for answer choices to eliminate. You will definitely want to read those carefully, practice them, and figure out which ones work best for you. Here though, we're going to address a mindset rather than a particular strategy.

Your odds of guessing an answer correctly depend on how many options you are choosing from.

Number of options left	5	4	3	2	1
Odds of guessing correctly	20%	25%	33%	50%	100%

You can see from this chart just how valuable it is to be able to eliminate incorrect answers and make an educated guess, but there are two things that many test takers do that cause them to miss out on the benefits of guessing:

- Accidentally eliminating the correct answer
- Selecting an answer based on an impression

We'll look at the first one here, and the second one in the next section.

To avoid accidentally eliminating the correct answer, we recommend a thought exercise called **the $5 challenge**. In this challenge, you only eliminate an answer choice from contention if you are willing to bet $5 on it being wrong. Why $5? Five dollars is a small but not insignificant amount of money. It's an amount you could afford to lose but wouldn't want to throw away. And while losing

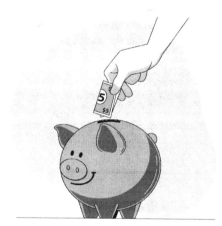

$5 once might not hurt too much, doing it twenty times will set you back $100. In the same way, each small decision you make—eliminating a choice here, guessing on a question there—won't by itself impact your score very much, but when you put them all together, they can make a big difference. By holding each answer choice elimination decision to a higher standard, you can reduce the risk of accidentally eliminating the correct answer.

The $5 challenge can also be applied in a positive sense: If you are willing to bet $5 that an answer choice *is* correct, go ahead and mark it as correct.

Summary: Only eliminate an answer choice if you are willing to bet $5 that it is wrong.

Which Answer to Choose

You're taking the test. You've run into a hard question and decided you'll have to guess. You've eliminated all the answer choices you're willing to bet $5 on. Now you have to pick an answer. Why do we even need to talk about this? Why can't you just pick whichever one you feel like when the time comes?

The answer to these questions is that if you don't come into the test with a plan, you'll rely on your impression to select an answer choice, and if you do that, you risk falling into a trap. The test writers know that everyone who takes their test will be guessing on some of the questions, so they intentionally write wrong answer choices to seem plausible. You still have to pick an answer though, and if the wrong answer choices are designed to look right, how can you ever be sure that you're not falling for their trap? The best solution we've found to this dilemma is to take the decision out of your hands entirely. Here is the process we recommend:

Once you've eliminated any choices that you are confident (willing to bet $5) are wrong, select the first remaining choice as your answer.

Whether you choose to select the first remaining choice, the second, or the last, the important thing is that you use some preselected standard. Using this approach guarantees that you will not be enticed into selecting an answer choice that looks right, because you are not basing your decision on how the answer choices look.

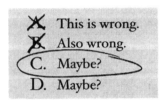

This is not meant to make you question your knowledge. Instead, it is to help you recognize the difference between your knowledge and your impressions. There's a huge difference between thinking an answer is right because of what you know, and thinking an answer is right because it looks or sounds like it should be right.

Summary: To ensure that your selection is appropriately random, make a predetermined selection from among all answer choices you have not eliminated.

Test-Taking Strategies

This section contains a list of test-taking strategies that you may find helpful as you work through the test. By taking what you know and applying logical thought, you can maximize your chances of answering any question correctly!

It is very important to realize that every question is different and every person is different: no single strategy will work on every question, and no single strategy will work for every person. That's why we've included all of them here, so you can try them out and determine which ones work best for different types of questions and which ones work best for you.

Question Strategies

☑ READ CAREFULLY

Read the question and the answer choices carefully. Don't miss the question because you misread the terms. You have plenty of time to read each question thoroughly and make sure you understand what is being asked. Yet a happy medium must be attained, so don't waste too much time. You must read carefully and efficiently.

☑ CONTEXTUAL CLUES

Look for contextual clues. If the question includes a word you are not familiar with, look at the immediate context for some indication of what the word might mean. Contextual clues can often give you all the information you need to decipher the meaning of an unfamiliar word. Even if you can't determine the meaning, you may be able to narrow down the possibilities enough to make a solid guess at the answer to the question.

☑ PREFIXES

If you're having trouble with a word in the question or answer choices, try dissecting it. Take advantage of every clue that the word might include. Prefixes can be a huge help. Usually, they allow you to determine a basic meaning. *Pre-* means before, *post-* means after, *pro-* is positive, *de-* is negative. From prefixes, you can get an idea of the general meaning of the word and try to put it into context.

☑ HEDGE WORDS

Watch out for critical hedge words, such as *likely, may, can, sometimes, often, almost, mostly, usually, generally, rarely,* and *sometimes.* Question writers insert these hedge phrases to cover every possibility. Often an answer choice will be wrong simply because it leaves no room for exception. Be on guard for answer choices that have definitive words such as *exactly* and *always.*

☑ SWITCHBACK WORDS

Stay alert for *switchbacks.* These are the words and phrases frequently used to alert you to shifts in thought. The most common switchback words are *but, although,* and *however.* Others include *nevertheless, on the other hand, even though, while, in spite of, despite,* and *regardless of.* Switchback words are important to catch because they can change the direction of the question or an answer choice.

⦸ FACE VALUE

When in doubt, use common sense. Accept the situation in the problem at face value. Don't read too much into it. These problems will not require you to make wild assumptions. If you have to go beyond creativity and warp time or space in order to have an answer choice fit the question, then you should move on and consider the other answer choices. These are normal problems rooted in reality. The applicable relationship or explanation may not be readily apparent, but it is there for you to figure out. Use your common sense to interpret anything that isn't clear.

Answer Choice Strategies

⦸ ANSWER SELECTION

The most thorough way to pick an answer choice is to identify and eliminate wrong answers until only one is left, then confirm it is the correct answer. Sometimes an answer choice may immediately seem right, but be careful. The test writers will usually put more than one reasonable answer choice on each question, so take a second to read all of them and make sure that the other choices are not equally obvious. As long as you have time left, it is better to read every answer choice than to pick the first one that looks right without checking the others.

⦸ ANSWER CHOICE FAMILIES

An answer choice family consists of two (in rare cases, three) answer choices that are very similar in construction and cannot all be true at the same time. If you see two answer choices that are direct opposites or parallels, one of them is usually the correct answer. For instance, if one answer choice says that quantity x increases and another either says that quantity x decreases (opposite) or says that quantity y increases (parallel), then those answer choices would fall into the same family. An answer choice that doesn't match the construction of the answer choice family is more likely to be incorrect. Most questions will not have answer choice families, but when they do appear, you should be prepared to recognize them.

⦸ ELIMINATE ANSWERS

Eliminate answer choices as soon as you realize they are wrong, but make sure you consider all possibilities. If you are eliminating answer choices and realize that the last one you are left with is also wrong, don't panic. Start over and consider each choice again. There may be something you missed the first time that you will realize on the second pass.

⦸ AVOID FACT TRAPS

Don't be distracted by an answer choice that is factually true but doesn't answer the question. You are looking for the choice that answers the question. Stay focused on what the question is asking for so you don't accidentally pick an answer that is true but incorrect. Always go back to the question and make sure the answer choice you've selected actually answers the question and is not merely a true statement.

⦸ EXTREME STATEMENTS

In general, you should avoid answers that put forth extreme actions as standard practice or proclaim controversial ideas as established fact. An answer choice that states the "process should be used in certain situations, if..." is much more likely to be correct than one that states the "process should be discontinued completely." The first is a calm rational statement and doesn't even make a definitive, uncompromising stance, using a hedge word *if* to provide wiggle room, whereas the second choice is far more extreme.

⊘ BENCHMARK

As you read through the answer choices and you come across one that seems to answer the question well, mentally select that answer choice. This is not your final answer, but it's the one that will help you evaluate the other answer choices. The one that you selected is your benchmark or standard for judging each of the other answer choices. Every other answer choice must be compared to your benchmark. That choice is correct until proven otherwise by another answer choice beating it. If you find a better answer, then that one becomes your new benchmark. Once you've decided that no other choice answers the question as well as your benchmark, you have your final answer.

⊘ PREDICT THE ANSWER

Before you even start looking at the answer choices, it is often best to try to predict the answer. When you come up with the answer on your own, it is easier to avoid distractions and traps because you will know exactly what to look for. The right answer choice is unlikely to be word-for-word what you came up with, but it should be a close match. Even if you are confident that you have the right answer, you should still take the time to read each option before moving on.

General Strategies

⊘ TOUGH QUESTIONS

If you are stumped on a problem or it appears too hard or too difficult, don't waste time. Move on! Remember though, if you can quickly check for obviously incorrect answer choices, your chances of guessing correctly are greatly improved. Before you completely give up, at least try to knock out a couple of possible answers. Eliminate what you can and then guess at the remaining answer choices before moving on.

⊘ CHECK YOUR WORK

Since you will probably not know every term listed and the answer to every question, it is important that you get credit for the ones that you do know. Don't miss any questions through careless mistakes. If at all possible, try to take a second to look back over your answer selection and make sure you've selected the correct answer choice and haven't made a costly careless mistake (such as marking an answer choice that you didn't mean to mark). This quick double check should more than pay for itself in caught mistakes for the time it costs.

⊘ PACE YOURSELF

It's easy to be overwhelmed when you're looking at a page full of questions; your mind is confused and full of random thoughts, and the clock is ticking down faster than you would like. Calm down and maintain the pace that you have set for yourself. Especially as you get down to the last few minutes of the test, don't let the small numbers on the clock make you panic. As long as you are on track by monitoring your pace, you are guaranteed to have time for each question.

⊘ DON'T RUSH

It is very easy to make errors when you are in a hurry. Maintaining a fast pace in answering questions is pointless if it makes you miss questions that you would have gotten right otherwise. Test writers like to include distracting information and wrong answers that seem right. Taking a little extra time to avoid careless mistakes can make all the difference in your test score. Find a pace that allows you to be confident in the answers that you select.

13

⊘ Keep Moving

Panicking will not help you pass the test, so do your best to stay calm and keep moving. Taking deep breaths and going through the answer elimination steps you practiced can help to break through a stress barrier and keep your pace.

Final Notes

The combination of a solid foundation of content knowledge and the confidence that comes from practicing your plan for applying that knowledge is the key to maximizing your performance on test day. As your foundation of content knowledge is built up and strengthened, you'll find that the strategies included in this chapter become more and more effective in helping you quickly sift through the distractions and traps of the test to isolate the correct answer.

Now that you're preparing to move forward into the test content chapters of this book, be sure to keep your goal in mind. As you read, think about how you will be able to apply this information on the test. If you've already seen sample questions for the test and you have an idea of the question format and style, try to come up with questions of your own that you can answer based on what you're reading. This will give you valuable practice applying your knowledge in the same ways you can expect to on test day.

Good luck and good studying!

General Assessment

Effects of Maternal Medical Complications

PREECLAMPSIA AND ECLAMPSIA

Preeclampsia is a disorder that develops in approximately 5% of all pregnancies. It is defined as a new onset of elevated blood pressure of at least 140/90 on two occasions at least 4 hours apart. In addition to elevated BP, diagnosis requires one or more of the following complications after the 20th week of pregnancy: proteinuria, new-onset headaches or visual disturbances, thrombocytopenia, impaired liver or kidney function, or pulmonary edema. Proteinuria is a common feature of preeclampsia, but diagnostically, it is possible to have preeclampsia without proteinuria when there is evidence of significant end-organ dysfunction. Preeclampsia is more commonly seen after 34 weeks gestation. Delivery is the only cure for preeclampsia. If it is not severe, patients are often induced after 37 weeks gestation. In patients with severe features, induction should be considered after 34 weeks gestation. Antihypertensive treatment, such as thiazide, hydralazine, propranolol, labetalol, nifedipine, and methyldopa, is recommended for severe hypertension, as well as anticonvulsants if seizures occur. Magnesium sulfate is given prophylactically for severe preeclampsia and for treatment of seizures. **Eclampsia** is a complication of severe preeclampsia in which seizures occur. The main detrimental effect on the fetus occurs when longstanding hypertension leads to uteroplacental vascular insufficiency, which impairs the transfer of nutrients and oxygen to the fetus, resulting in intrauterine growth restriction (IUGR). Placental abruption also occurs more frequently. The IUGR is usually asymmetric (fetal head size is normal for gestational age). Infants who are born with IUGR and/or prematurity have increased morbidity and mortality.

HELLP SYNDROME

HELLP syndrome occurs in 4-12% of those with preeclampsia, most often during weeks 27-37, but it may develop within 24 hours postpartum. It is characterized by the following:

- **H**—hemolysis
- **EL**—elevated liver enzymes
- **LP**—low platelet count

HELLP syndrome is most common in older multiparous mothers. Hypertension may be less pronounced than in others with preeclampsia. Pain in the right upper quadrant related to liver dysfunction may be misdiagnosed as gastrointestinal upset or gall bladder disease. Mothers often present with flu-like nonspecific symptoms, including headache, nausea and vomiting, and visual disturbances. Prompt diagnosis and treatment are necessary because of high mortality. Platelet transfusions are given if platelet counts are <20,000/mm³ before vaginal delivery or <50,000/mm³ before Cesarean section. The primary treatment is immediate delivery of the fetus as the mother may develop hepatic hemorrhage or permanent liver damage. Both the mother and the fetus are at risk. Neonates are at increased risk and may require mechanical ventilation. Complications include abruptio placentae, DIC, and postpartum hemorrhage.

CLASSES I TO IV CARDIAC DISEASE IN PREGNANCY

Maternal heart disease complicates approximately one percent of all pregnancies, with congenital heart disease accounting for more than half of the cases. Pre-pregnancy cardiac function is an excellent predictor of cardiac complications in pregnancy and is based on the New York Heart Association classification:

> I. No cardiac insufficiency or activity limitations
> II. Slight activity limitations: symptoms present with ordinary physical activity
> III. Marked activity limitations: mild activity causes symptoms
> IV. Inability to carry out physical activities without severe symptoms

The **maternal classification** affects the fetus. There is minimal danger to the fetus for mothers in Class I or Class II, but increased risk to both the mother and the fetus for Classes III and IV. Most medications cross the placenta, and the degree of safety during pregnancy has not been established for all of these. The most common drugs—heparin, digitalis glycosides, antiarrhythmics, thiazide, and loop diuretics—are not **teratogenic**. For Classes III and IV, delivery may be facilitated by low forceps or vacuum assistance, and Cesarean may be done if the mother or the fetus is in danger. Labor and delivery are particularly dangerous to the fetus because of inadequate oxygen and blood supply, so continuous fetal monitoring is essential.

PREGNANCY WITH CONGENITAL HEART DEFECTS

With improved surgical repair techniques for **congenital heart defects,** many women survive to childbearing age. These are common **maternal defects**:

- Tetralogy of Fallot
- Ventricular and atrial septal defects
- Patent ductus arteriosus
- Coarctation of the aorta

If surgical correction was successful, there is no added **fetal risk,** but if the condition has not been completely repaired or involves cyanosis, pregnancy can put the fetus at risk because of inadequate oxygen supply. Mothers with cardiac disease have a 5-10% increased risk of having a baby with cardiac anomalies. Fetal echocardiography is recommended in pregnancy to evaluate the structure and function of the fetus' heart.

Marfan syndrome poses severe risks to the mother, with mortality rates of 25-50% because of possible rupture of the aorta, which also puts the fetus at risk. Additionally, because this is an autosomal dominant disorder, there is a 50% chance that an infant will inherit the syndrome.

Mitral valve prolapse usually does not pose a risk to the fetus.

Severe maternal cardiopulmonary disorders can result in death of the mother and/or fetus. However, the most common fetal complications are premature labor/birth and a fetus that is small for gestational age.

INFANTS OF A DIABETIC MOTHER (IDM)

Infants of a diabetic mother (IDM) suffer from increased morbidity and mortality. Glucose crosses the placenta, so when the mother has elevated blood glucose, the infant also has elevated blood glucose. Insulin does not cross the placenta. The pancreas of the fetus begins to produce insulin at about 20 weeks of gestation. Prior to the fetus producing insulin, the infant is exposed to elevated levels of glucose that restrict fetal growth. After week 20, the fetus responds to hyperglycemia with elevated production of insulin. The combination of elevated blood glucose and elevated insulin triggers rapid fetal growth, with increased fat and glycogen stores, hepatosplenomegaly, cardiomegaly, and increased head size. Sudden withdrawal from the consistent maternal source of glucose after birth, combined with the continued production of insulin by the newborn, result in hypoglycemia shortly after birth.

MATERNAL SICKLE CELL ANEMIA

Sickle cell disease is a recessive genetic disorder of chromosome 11, causing hemoglobin to be defective so that red blood cells (RBCs) are sickle-shaped and inflexible, resulting in their accumulating in small vessels and causing painful blockage. There are 5 variations of sickle cell disease, with **sickle cell anemia** the most severe. Pregnant women with sickle cell anemia are at risk for urinary and pulmonary infections, congestive heart failure, and acute renal failure, all of which can trigger a vaso-occlusive crises that puts the fetus at risk. Perinatal mortality rates are about 18%, caused by sickling in the placenta. Neonates are at increased risk for prematurity and intrauterine growth restriction. Maternal infections must be treated promptly to avoid dehydration and/or fever that can trigger sickling. Steps to shorten the second stage of labor (oxytocin, forceps, episiotomy) may be necessary to protect the fetus if sickling occurs during labor.

> **Review Video: What is Sickle Cell Disease?**
> Visit mometrix.com/academy and enter code: 603869

PREGNANCY AND IRON-DEFICIENCY ANEMIA

Iron is necessary for the development of red blood cells. During pregnancy, the mother's plasma volume increases by about 50% but red cell mass increases less, so the **hematocrit** drops from a normal of 38-47% to as low as 30% (physiologic/iron deficiency anemia of pregnancy). Because the fetus takes iron from the mother, the mother's iron intake must compensate for this loss. When **hemoglobin** falls <10 g/dL, the mother is at increased risk of infection, preeclampsia, and postpartal hemorrhage, with associated dangers to the fetus. If hemoglobin falls <6 g/dL, the mother may suffer cardiac failure, and the fetus is at high risk, with increased rates of miscarriage, stillbirth, low birth weight, and neonatal death. Initial symptoms of iron deficiency include pallor, glossitis, headache, and pica, progressing to weakness, lethargy, confusion, ataxia, and cardiovascular abnormalities. Recommended treatment for iron-deficiency anemia is 60-120 mg daily of elemental iron. To promote absorption, it is best to avoid caffeine and dairy products within an hour of taking the iron supplement and to take some source of vitamin C with the iron. Pregnancy and Folate/Folic Acid Deficiency Anemia

Folate/folic acid deficiency can result in megaloblastic anemia. Folate is the naturally occurring form of vitamin B9 and is necessary for DNA synthesis and the formation and maturation of red blood cells. Folic acid is the synthetic form of vitamin B9, used in supplements and added to processed foods. Causes of folate deficiency include inadequate diet, malabsorption syndromes (especially of the small intestine), medications that interfere with absorption (oral contraceptives, methotrexate, phenobarbital, and diphenylhydantoin), anorexia, alcoholism, and dialysis. Diagnostic findings include decreased hemoglobin, hematocrit, and folate (normal value is 3-25 mg/mL), as well as increased MCV and MCHV. Cobalamin level is normal and gastric analysis is positive for hydrochloric acid. Other blood studies are usually within normal range. RBCs are macrocytic and normochromic. Folate deficiency is associated with **neural tube defects**, such as myelomeningocele, spina bifida, and anencephaly in the fetus.

Signs and symptoms include:

- Asymptomatic (initially)
- GI disturbances, such as indigestion, anorexia, and weight loss
- Red, beefy-appearing tongue
- Pallor
- Weakness, fatigue
- Forgetfulness, impaired concentration

Treatment:

- Diet high in folate: green leafy vegetables, liver, citrus fruits, legumes, nuts, and grains
- Oral supplementation: L-Methylfolate 600-1000 mcg daily or folic acid 1-5 mg per day

MATERNAL ACIDOSIS

Maternal pH directly impacts the pH of the fetus, particularly in the case of **metabolic acidosis**. Because the fetus is extremely vulnerable to even minor changes in pH, this can be a very threatening condition. Maternal acidosis is linked with decreased fetal pH (fetal acidosis), resulting in lower Apgar scores for these neonates. Maternal causes of acidosis include uncontrolled diabetes (leading to diabetic ketoacidosis), renal dysfunction, and severe diarrhea. Fetal acid-base balance should be closely monitored in mothers with these conditions. Should the fetus show signs of distress (FHR abnormalities, decreased fetal movement, etc.) and acidosis in the fetus be suspected, the mother should immediately be tested in the case that fetal acidosis is secondary to maternal acidosis.

ACUTE FATTY LIVER PREGNANCY (AFLP)

Acute fatty liver of pregnancy (AFLP) (the most common cause of liver failure during pregnancy) is characterized by micro-vesicular fat deposits throughout the liver that crowd out hepatocytes and interfere with liver function. AFLP, which is associated with genetic mutations, occurs in the third trimester or postpartal period. Women may exhibit nausea and vomiting, upper GI hemorrhage, coagulopathy, pancreatitis, hypoglycemia, hepatic encephalopathy (with confusion and altered mental status), hypertension, jaundice, general malaise, and renal and hepatic failure. Neonates may exhibit fatty acid oxidation defects that affect multiple body systems: cardiomyopathy, liver failure, myopathy, neuropathy, and hypoglycemia (nonketotic). Some may die *in utero* and 15% die after birth. The key to treatment of AFLP is immediate delivery of the fetus through labor induction or Cesarean (although coagulopathy may pose risks). Supportive care may include IV fluids, blood products, coagulation factors, and/or plasma exchange or plasmapheresis with continuous renal replacement therapy. Some women may require liver transplantation.

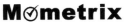

MATERNAL SYSTEMIC LUPUS ERYTHEMATOSUS (SLE)

Systemic lupus erythematosus (SLE), a systemic reaction to collagen or connective tissue in the body, is believed to be triggered by an antibody-antigen immune response to an environmental agent, resulting in widespread damage of vessels and organs, primarily in females. Symptoms may include: malar and discoid rash; photosensitivity; oral ulcers; arthritis; serositis; and renal (proteinuria/nephritis), neurological (seizures, psychosis), and immunological disorders. Pregnant women with SLE have high rates of hypertension (up to 30%) and preeclampsia, especially with lupus nephritis, so they may need to continue immunosuppressive drugs during pregnancy. Women must be monitored carefully during pregnancy for flare-ups of SLE. Impaired circulation to the fetus may result from maternal decidual vasculopathy with placental infarction. Fetal risks include preterm delivery, fetal growth restriction, spontaneous abortion, and stillbirths. The newborn may inherit neonatal lupus, with symptoms appearing up to 4 weeks after birth. Indications include congenital heart block, autoimmune hemolysis, thrombocytopenia, and lupus dermatitis.

CHOLELITHIASIS AND CHOLECYSTITIS

Pregnancy increases the risk of a woman developing **cholelithiasis** and **cholecystitis** because of increased levels of estrogen and increased biliary sludge (forerunner to gallstones). Symptoms occur when stones block the bile duct and may include RUQ pain, nausea, vomiting, low-grade fever, and mildly elevated white blood cell count. Some may have clay-colored stools and jaundice. Medical management has been most common in the first and third trimesters and surgical repair in the second trimester (when it is safest). However, early cholecystitis often recurs later in the pregnancy, increasing the risk of pre-term delivery and making surgery more difficult because of the size of the uterus, so some authorities advise against conservative treatment. Surgical procedures include laparoscopic cholecystectomy and endoscopic retrograde cholangiopancreatography for stones in the common bile duct. The fetus is usually unimpaired if the blockage is resolved.

MATERNAL HYPOTHYROIDISM AND HYPERTHYROIDISM

Maternal hypothyroidism threatens the development of the fetal brain and spinal cord. T4 is needed for proper development, and the fetus is not capable of T4 production during the critical period of growth. Decreased mental capacity or fetal death can occur.

Hyperthyroidism is difficult to detect since symptoms mimic normal pregnancy problems. The pregnant woman may have temporary hyperthyroidism in early pregnancy but levels should return to normal by the beginning of the second trimester. Continued high levels can cause thyroid crisis and result in fetal death or premature birth.

MATERNAL TRAUMA

Maternal trauma can occur at any time during the pregnancy. Motor vehicle accidents are the leading cause of trauma to the pregnant woman. Maternal falls and trauma to the abdomen from domestic abuse are other common causes. Trauma to the abdomen by blunt force can result in abruptio placentae, placental injury, injury to the fetus, or uterine rupture causing fetal death by hemorrhage and hypoxia. Maternal hemorrhage and shock from traumatic injuries can result in both fetal and maternal death from hypoxia. Any trauma that compromises respiration will also cause hypoxia to the mother-fetal unit. Neurological trauma that results in shock, hemorrhage, or damage to the brain will also compromise the fetus when maternal vital functions deteriorate.

CHEAP TORCHES

CHEAP TORCHES is the acronym used to recall common causes of congenital and neonatal infections. Many congenital infections are present for at least a month prior to birth and remain present at birth:

C	Chickenpox (varicella)
H	Hepatitis (B, C, & E)
E	Enterovirus (RNA viruses, including coxsackievirus, echovirus, and poliovirus)
A	AIDS (HIV)
P	Parvovirus (B 19)
T	Toxoplasmosis
O	Other (Group B streptococcus, *Candida*, *Listeria*, TB, lymphocytic choriomeningitis)
R	Rubella (measles)
C	Cytomegalovirus
H	Herpes simplex virus
E	Every other STI (*Chlamydia*, gonorrhea, *Ureaplasma*, papillomavirus
S	Syphilis

Exposure to these pathogens *in utero* may cause a miscarriage or congenital defect, especially if the exposure was during the first trimester.

> **Review Video: Infant TORCH Syndrome**
> Visit mometrix.com/academy and enter code: 502502

CONGENITAL VARICELLA SYNDROME

Varicella infection (chickenpox) in the mother can affect the fetus in different ways, depending upon the time of exposure. **Congenital varicella syndrome** is characterized by many abnormalities, including eye abnormalities (cataracts, microphthalmia, pendular nystagmus, and retinal scarring), skin abnormalities (hypertrophy and cicatrix scarring), malformation of limbs, hypoplasia of digits, restricted growth, microcephalus, abnormalities of the brain and autonomic nervous system, developmental delay, and intellectual disability. Mortality rates are high (≥50%) for those with severe defects:

- First trimester: 1% risk of congenital varicella syndrome.
- Weeks 23-20: 2% risk of congenital varicella syndrome.
- 5 days before delivery to 2 days after delivery: Neonate may develop congenital varicella (20-25%).
- 6-12 days after delivery: Neonate may contract congenital varicella but, if breast-feeding, the child may receive the mother's antibodies, so the disease will be milder.

FETAL EXPOSURE TO HEPATITIS

Routine screening of all pregnant women and all newborns helps to identify those infected with the **hepatitis B virus**. Infants are routinely immunized at discharge from hospital, at 2 months, and at 6 months of age. In the case of a premature infant, the immunization schedule is started when the infant weighs 2 kg or is 2 months old. If the mother is HVB-positive, surface antigen treatment of that infant should include careful bathing (wearing gloves) to remove all maternal blood and body fluids. The infant should also receive an IM injection of the hepatitis B immunoglobulin within 12 hours of birth. This immunoglobulin treatment is up to 95% effective in preventing the development of the disease in the infant.

Hepatitis C is rarely transmitted to the fetus, and of those infected, about 75% clear the infection by 2 years.

Hepatitis E poses the greatest risk to the mother, with a mortality of about 20% during pregnancy and an increased risk of fetal complications and death.

FETAL EXPOSURE TO TUBERCULOSIS

Tuberculosis (TB), infection with *Mycobacterium tuberculosis,* does not appear to worsen with pregnancy and responds to treatment. The risk of transmission to the fetus is low. However, the fetus may acquire the infection directly from the mother's blood or from swallowing amniotic fluid, although most transmission occurs postpartum through maternal contact, so mothers with active disease should not have contact with a neonate until they are noninfectious. Fetal infection may cause death of the fetus, increased risk of miscarriage, or neonatal infection. If the mother's TB is untreated, the fetal death rate is 30-40%, so treating the mother during pregnancy is very important. Isoniazid (INH), rifampin, and ethambutol cross the placenta but do not appear to be teratogenic, and the need for treatment outweighs risks. Streptomycin should be avoided as it may result in sensorineural deafness in the neonate. Mothers with inactive disease taking medications may breastfeed.

FETAL EXPOSURE TO AIDS/HIV

Most children infected with AIDS/HIV acquire the infection from their mothers (vertical transmission). The perinatal transmission rate is 30% in untreated HIV positive mothers, usually acquired during delivery. Neonates are usually asymptomatic but are at risk for prematurity, low birth weight, and small for gestational age (SGA). Infants may show failure to thrive, hepatomegaly, interstitial lymphocytic pneumonia, recurrent infections, and CNS abnormalities. Optimal treatment reduces the perinatal transmission rate to as low as 1-2%:

- **Antiviral therapy during the pregnancy**: A reduced viral load in the mother lessens the likelihood of prenatal transmission.
- **Elective Cesarean**: Elective C-section before the amniotic membranes rupture is especially recommended for women with a viral load >1000 copies/mL and is associated with reduced rates of vertical transmission. Emergency Cesarean, rupture of membranes longer than 4 hours, and the need for an episiotomy all increase the likelihood of infection during delivery.
- **Antiviral medications for the neonate for the first 6 weeks of life**: The first dose should be given within 12 hours of delivery.
- **Avoiding breastfeeding**: The risk of HIV transmission with breastfeeding is 0.7% per month of breastfeeding.

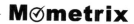

FETAL EXPOSURE TO PARVOVIRUS B19

Parvovirus B19 is a DNA virus that is very common and causes fever, malaise, and depression of progenitor cells in the bone marrow with a drop in reticulocyte count that can lead to anemia in those with preexisting low blood count. Most people are asymptomatic, although they can develop generalized rash and arthralgia/arthritis. Most mothers (≥50%) are seropositive with parvovirus before pregnancy and can become reinfected during pregnancy. Most infections do not adversely affect the fetus, but about 1-2% of maternal infections may cause spontaneous abortion or nonimmune hydrops fetalis. Hydrops fetalis is characterized by marked anemia, cardiac failure, and extramedullary hematopoiesis. A Parvovirus congenital infection syndrome may also occur with rash, anemia, and enlargement of the heart and liver.

FETAL EXPOSURE TO TOXOPLASMOSIS

Toxoplasmosis, caused by a protozoal infection with *Toxoplasma gondii,* is a common disease. About 38% of pregnant women have antibodies from a previous infection, but about 1 in 1000 pregnant women become infected during pregnancy, primarily from eating undercooked meat, drinking unpasteurized goat's milk, or contacting infected cat feces, putting the fetus at risk. Risk to the fetus is greatest if the disease occurs during the first trimester, often causing severe fetal abnormalities, such as microcephaly and hydrocephalus, or miscarriage. However, risk of fetal transmission is greatest during the 3rd trimester, although 70% are born without indications of infection. Mild infection may manifest as retinochoroiditis at birth (with other symptoms delayed). Severe infection may result in convulsions and coma from CNS abnormalities, and the child may die in the neonatal period. Children who survive with severe infection may suffer blindness, deafness, and marked intellectual disability. If a diagnosis of fetal infection is made during pregnancy, the mother should be treated aggressively.

FETAL EXPOSURE TO GBS

Group B *Streptococcus* (GBS) is the most common neonatal bacterial infection. Many women are asymptomatic carriers. Screening of all pregnant women occurs between 37+0 and 37+6 weeks of gestation followed by antibiotic treatment of the mother during labor to prevent neonatal infection. A mother needs at least 4 hours' worth of antibiotic treatment for the infant to benefit. If an infant is born and the mother has not received the recommended treatment, the infant will often be treated with IV ampicillin and gentamicin for 10-14 days. If treatment is ineffective or impossible, the infant with a GBS infection that manifests in the first 24 hours after birth may develop pneumonia and/or meningitis, respiratory distress, floppiness, poor feeding, tachycardia, shock, and seizures. An infant may be asymptomatic at birth but have late-onset infection occurring at around 7 to 10 days old. Late-onset infections (usually meningitis) are generally more serious than earlier onset, and survivors often have serious damage, such as intellectual disability, quadriplegia, blindness, deafness, uncontrollable seizures, and hydrocephalus.

FETAL EXPOSURE TO RUBELLA

Women should always be vaccinated for rubella before becoming pregnant, as exposure to the virus has devastating effects on the newborn. The mother may not experience any symptoms of the disease or only mild symptoms like mild respiratory problems or rash. If the rubella exposure is during the first 4-5 months of pregnancy, the consequences for the infant are greater. Infants exposed to this virus *in utero* can develop a set of symptoms known as congenital rubella syndrome. This syndrome includes all or some of the following signs and symptoms:

- Intrauterine growth restriction (IUGR)
- Deafness
- Cataracts
- Jaundice
- Purpura
- Hepatosplenomegaly
- Microcephaly
- Chronic encephalitis
- Cardiac defects

FETAL EXPOSURE TO CYTOMEGALOVIRUS

Cytomegalovirus, a member of the herpes simplex virus group, can cause asymptomatic infection in women. Over 50% of women are seropositive and may have chronic infections that persist for years. Cytomegalovirus is the most common intrauterine viral infection. Cytomegalovirus can be transmitted placentally or cervically during delivery (infecting ≤2.5% of neonates) and can put the fetus at high risk with death rates of 20-30% among infants born with symptoms. About 90% of survivors have neurological disorders, such as microcephaly, hydrocephalus, cerebral palsy, and/or intellectual disability. In less severe infections, symptoms (intellectual disability, hearing deficits, learning disabilities) may be delayed. Commonly, the neonate is small for gestational age (SGA). The brain and liver are commonly affected, but all organs can be infected. Multiple blood abnormalities can occur: anemia, hyperbilirubinemia, thrombocytopenia, and hepatosplenomegaly.

FETAL EXPOSURE TO HERPES SIMPLEX VIRUS

Most pregnant women infected with herpes simplex virus (HSV) are asymptomatic and unaware of the infection. Most vertical transmissions occur when the neonate travels through a colonized birth canal. The risk of transmitting HSV during the birth process varies greatly, depending on if the infection is a new infection (primary) or a secondary outbreak. The transmission rate from women with a primary HSV infection is approximately 50%, while the transmission rate is 1-2% if the infection is a recurrence of HSV. Signs of a neonatal infection with HSV include:

- Skin, eye, and mucous membrane blistering at 10-12 days of life.
- Disseminated disease may spread to multiple organs, leading to pneumonitis, hepatitis, and intravascular coagulation.
- Encephalitis may be the only presentation, with signs of lethargy, irritability, poor feeding, and seizures.

A mother with active herpes should deliver by Cesarean section within 4-6 hours after membranes rupture. An infant that is inadvertently exposed to an active lesion should be treated with acyclovir.

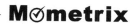

FETAL EXPOSURE TO CHLAMYDIA

Chlamydia is the most common sexually transmitted infection in the United States and can be passed on at the time of birth if the infant is delivered vaginally and comes into contact with contaminated vaginal secretions. The organism responsible for this infection is *Chlamydia trachomatis*. Because the mother infected with this organism is usually asymptomatic, preventive care for the newborn is essential. The usual infection site for the newborn is the eye, in the form of conjunctivitis. States now require all newborns to be given a prophylactic dose of either erythromycin or tetracycline ointment in the eyes at birth to prevent this infection. While the antibiotic ointment stops the eye infection, a few infants exposed to the pathogen will develop pneumonitis and/or ear infection.

FETAL EXPOSURE TO SYPHILIS

An infant can be exposed to the syphilis organism, *Treponema pallidum,* during gestation and become infected *in utero* starting with the 10th-15th week of gestation. Many infected fetuses abort spontaneously or are stillborn. An infant born infected with syphilis can be asymptomatic at birth or can have a full multi-system infection. An infant who is symptomatic may have non-viral hepatitis with jaundice, hepatosplenomegaly, pseudoparalysis, pneumonitis, bone marrow failure, myocarditis, meningitis, anemia, edema associated with nephritic syndrome, and a rash on the palms of the hands and soles of the feet. Other symptoms, such as interstitial keratitis and dental and facial abnormalities, may occur as the child develops. Treatment involves an aggressive regimen of penicillin administration with frequent follow-up until blood tests are negative.

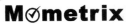

Problems Associated with Amniotic Fluid and Membranes

AFI, OLIGOHYDRAMNIOS, AND POLYHYDRAMNIOS

The **AFI** is determined by measuring the biggest pockets of amniotic fluid in all four of the uterine quadrants and adding the measurements together. The **normal index** is 5-24 cm, depending on which week of gestation the measurements are taken. Amniotic fluid volume increases during pregnancy to 1,000 mL by 36 weeks of gestation, then slowly decreases over the next 4 weeks.

- **Oligohydramnios** is defined by an AFI of 5 cm or less. It is linked with fetal urinary tract anomalies. The fetus is threatened by the risk of amnion adhesions that can cause amputation of body parts and pressure that can cause deformities of the musculoskeletal system, especially club foot. Cord compression and fetal distress can occur during labor and delivery.
- **Polyhydramnios** is defined by an AFI over 24 cm. It can occur acutely or over time. One-third of these cases are associated with fetal anomalies of the CNS or GI systems, maternal diabetes, or multifetal gestation. More severe polyhydramnios increases the risk of perinatal death.

AMNIOTIC FLUID EMBOLISM

Amniotic fluid embolism (AKA anaphylactoid syndrome of pregnancy) occurs when amniotic fluid enters the mother's circulatory system, such as may occur during cesareans and labor and delivery, during which small tears in the lower uterine segment or cervix allow amniotic fluid to enter maternal circulation. In most mothers, this poses no problem, but some mothers have an anaphylactoid response that can include hypotension, pulmonary edema, cyanosis, coagulopathy, dyspnea, seizures, and cardiac arrest for the mother as well as fetal distress.

- The **initial phase** usually includes cardiovascular collapse with severe pulmonary vasoconstriction, which results in inability of the heart to transfer blood from the right to the left and marked oxygen desaturation with neurological injury. Uterine hypertonus and lack of blood flow to the uterus occurs.
- The **second phase**, if the mother survives the first, usually includes lung injury and coagulopathy.

Treatment includes immediate CPR, circulatory support, and blood and blood components as needed. If undelivered, emergent delivery is critical to save the infant.

COMPLICATIONS REGARDING RUPTURE OF MEMBRANES

There are various complications in regards to the rupture of membranes:

- **Premature rupture of membranes (PROM):** The chorioamniotic membrane breaks, ideally at term (40 weeks), prior to onset of labor. Rupture of membranes is premature if labor fails to begin within an hour. About 80% of women go into labor within 24 hours. If labor doesn't begin in 12-24 hours, the patient must be frequently monitored to ensure that adequate amniotic fluid remains, or labor may be induced or augmented to prevent infection if the child is at term.
- **Spontaneous rupture (SROM)** usually occurs in the early stage of labor during an intense contraction, causing the fluid to gush out of the vagina.
- **Preterm premature rupture of membranes (PPROM)** occurs in a woman <37 weeks of gestation and prior to the onset of labor. The patient is monitored, as with premature rupture. It is one of the leading causes of premature birth.
- **Prolonged rupture of membranes**: Prolonged PROM persists for greater than 18-24 hours prior to the onset of labor. It is associated with increased risk of infection in the neonate.

PRETERM PREMATURE RUPTURE OF MEMBRANES CAUSES AND FETAL VIABILITY

There are numerous **causes for PPROM**, including infections and digital pelvic exams. When a woman presents in labor, the estimated date of delivery should be obtained by determining the date of the last menstrual period (LMP) and using a gestation calculator wheel or estimating with Naegele's rule: first day LMP minus 3 months plus 7 days equals estimated date of delivery.

Fetal viability is very low before 23 weeks of gestation; by 25 weeks, delaying delivery for 2 days can increase survival rates by 10%. Tocolytic drugs, which have many negative side effects, may be used to delay delivery in order to administer glucocorticoids, such as betamethasone or dexamethasone, to improve fetal lung maturity between weeks 24 and 36.

Significance of Findings

ULTRASOUND

Ultrasound is an imaging technique that uses high-frequency sound waves to create computer images of vessels, tissues, and organs. Newer scans include two-dimensional Doppler readings. Fetal ultrasound can be done at about the fifth week of gestation and is commonly done at 20 weeks for all pregnant women. Ultrasound is typically done **transabdominally** (though it may also be done **transvaginally**) to evaluate the gestational sac and embryo/fetus, providing the most accurate measurement of gestational age.

Trimester	Purpose
First	Estimate gestational age (accuracy ±5-7 days)
	Assess vaginal bleeding
	Determine if multiple fetuses are present
	Examine for indications of birth defects of the brain/spine
Second	Estimate gestational age (accuracy ±7-10 days)
	Determine size and position of placenta, fetus, and umbilical cord
	Examine for indications of major birth defects (cardiovascular/neural tube)
Third	Estimate gestational age (accuracy ±21-30 days)
	Assess fetal viability
	Determine size and position of placenta, fetus, and umbilical cord
	Estimate volume of amniotic fluid

CVS

Chorionic villus sampling (CVS) is performed by inserting a catheter into the uterus to obtain placental villi for testing. The tissue may also be obtained through the abdominal wall if needed to safely reach the placenta. Chromosomal, DNA, and enzymatic analysis is done on the tissue. This test is best performed at 10-13 weeks of gestation. This test provides results during early pregnancy to either reassure parents or to provide information needed to decide whether to continue the pregnancy. There is a small risk of fetal injury resulting in death during the procedure.

AMNIOCENTESIS

Amniocentesis is done at 15-20 weeks to evaluate for genetic disease and at 30-35 weeks to determine fetal lung maturity. Ultrasound locates the placenta and fetus and identifies an area with adequate amniotic fluid. The needle is then inserted carefully to avoid major structures, the fetus, and arteries. A local anesthetic may be administered before insertion of a 22-gauge spinal needle into the uterine cavity. The first drops of fluid are discarded and a syringe attached. About 15-20 mL of amniotic fluid are withdrawn and placed in tubes, brown-tinted to shield the fluid from light that might break down bilirubin or other pigments. Ultrasound is again used to monitor removal of the needle, and the insertion point is checked for streaming (leakage of fluid). If the mother is Rh-negative, she is given Rh immune globulin immediately, unless already sensitized. The fetal heart rate is monitored. Miscarriage occurs in about 1 in 1600 amniocenteses. If the procedure is performed at 11-14 weeks, there is increased risk to the fetus. Infection of the placenta (chorioamnionitis) is a rare complication.

BIOPHYSICAL PROFILE (BPP)

The fetal biophysical profile is a noninvasive antepartum test that uses ultrasound to evaluate four biophysical parameters: fetal respirations, fetal movement, fetal tone, and amniotic fluid volume. A separate nonstress test (NST) can also be performed to assess the fetal heart rate.

Measure	Discussion	Normal (2)	Abnormal (0)
Fetal Heart Rate	Measures fetal heart rate and acceleration with movement as measured by the NST	≥2 FHR accelerations of 15 bmp above baseline for ≥15 seconds in a 20-40-minute period (Reactive)	0-1 FHR accelerations in 40 minutes (Nonreactive)
Fetal Respirations	Assessed by ultrasound	≥1 episode of rhythmic breathing for ≥30 seconds in a 30-minute period	≤30 seconds of rhythmic breathing in 30 minutes
Fetal Movement	Assessed by ultrasound and tocodynamometer	≥3 separate movements in 30 minutes	≤2 movements in 30 minutes
Fetal Tone	Assessed by ultrasound	≥2 episodes of extension and flexion of arm/leg (or opening/closing of a hand)	No extension/flexion
Amniotic Fluid Volume	Assessed by ultrasound and amniotic fluid index	At least one single vertical pocket >2 cm	Largest single vertical pocket is ≤2 cm

Scoring:

- 10/10, 8/8 (NST omitted), or 8/10 (-2 points for either fetal movement, tone, or breathing but not amniotic fluid): Normal test result.
- 6/10 (-4 points for two of movement, tone, or breathing, but +2 points for amniotic fluid): Equivocal result—a significant possibility of developing fetal asphyxia cannot be excluded; test needs to be repeated or fetus needs to be delivered.
- 6/10 or 8/10 with 0 points for amniotic fluid: Abnormal; risk of fetal asphyxia within 1 week is high.
- 0-4/10: Abnormal; risk of fetal asphyxia within one week is high; delivery is usually indicated.

ALPHA-FETOPROTEIN

Alpha-fetoprotein (AFT) is a protein produced by the yolk sac for the first 6 weeks of gestation and then by the fetal liver. Cutoff levels have been established for each week of gestation, with peak levels at about week 15. The test is used primarily to detect neural tube defects (NTDs), which develop in the first trimester. AFT can be measured in amniotic fluid or maternal serum.

Triple screening includes **serum AFT level** done in the second trimester. A positive result (which may be the result of errors in the duration of gestation) is followed by **ultrasound** and **amniocentesis** to check the **amniotic AFT level**. There is increased production of AFT with NTDs as well as abdominal wall defects and congenital nephrosis, so these levels can be used for assessment. (High quality ultrasound may also provide evidence of neural tube defects). The accuracy of tests varies depending upon the week of gestation. The most accurate results are acquired with testing during weeks 15-16. In addition to the serum AFT level, the Triple Screening also includes an examination of serum hCG (produced by the placenta) and estriol (produced by the placenta and the fetus).

QUAD SCREEN

The Quad Screen is done between gestation weeks 16 and 20 to assess for risk of genetic abnormalities and is usually offered to all pregnant women but is especially important for those with the following risk factors: history of birth defects in family, age ≥35, use of teratogenic medications during pregnancy, diabetes mellitus with insulin use, exposure to high-dose radiation, and history of viral infection during pregnancy. The **Quad Screen** includes: (1) Alpha-fetoprotein (AFP), (2) Human chorionic gonadotropin (hCG), (3) Estriol (uE^3), and (4) Inhibin A (INH-A).

Disorder	AFP	hCG	uE^3	INH-A
Neural Tube Defects	High	Normal	Normal	Normal
Trisomy 21	Low	High	Low	High
Trisomy 18	Low	Low	Low	Low
Multiple Gestation	High	High	Normal	Normal

The fourth marker, inhibin A, improves the accuracy of screening for trisomy 21, especially in patients <35 years of age. With abnormal findings, an ultrasound may be used to verify weeks of gestation and an amniocentesis to confirm trisomy 21 or neural tube defects because of possible false positives.

FETAL FIBRONECTIN TEST

Fetal fibronectin (fFN) is a fetal extracellular glycoprotein that can be found in maternal cervical and vaginal secretions for the first 16-20 weeks of gestation, but then it is not found until near term. The fetal fibronectin test is one that is carried out to assess the risk of preterm birth. If an increase in fFN is noted, this may be an indication that preterm labor may start, although this is not always the case. False positives may occur with fetal or maternal infection, cervical manipulation before collection of the specimen, sexual intercourse within 24 hours, lubricating gels, and vaginal bleeding. However, the absence of increased fFN almost always indicates that labor will not begin within the next 7 days. **Contraindications** include cervical dilation of ≥3 cm, suspected placental abruption or previa, vaginal bleeding, membrane rupture, or gestational age <22 weeks or >35 weeks. Special fFN kits are available for sample collection, which is taken with a speculum exam by rotating a swab across the vaginal fornix for 10 seconds and then inserting the swab into the collection tube.

PUBS

Percutaneous umbilical cord blood sampling (PUBS; also called cordocentesis) obtains fetal blood cells. A 22-gauge spinal needle is inserted into the umbilical vein at or very near the place where it joins the placenta while using ultrasound to guide placement. Fetal blood is collected and used to assess red cell and platelet status. Fetal blood cells are also used for genetic analysis with karyotyping available within 24-48 hours. Immunological, hematological, and metabolic studies can be done. The fetal acid-base balance can also be determined. Complications of the procedure include fetal injury or death, fetal bradycardia, amniotic fluid loss, vaginal bleeding, infections, or bleeding into the cord or from the fetus into the mother's circulation. The procedure may be done to verify results from other tests.

IUT

Indications for **intrauterine transfusion** (IUT) include various types of fetal anemia:

- **Erythrocyte alloimmunization**: CDE or other red cell antigens result in hemolytic anemia and lead to fetalis hydrops; antibodies build up with a first pregnancy and alloimmunization occurs with subsequent pregnancies.
- **Platelet alloimmunization**: Mother is alloimmunized against fetal paternal platelet antigens. This may occur with a first pregnancy. IUTs may be given to prevent cerebral hemorrhage but are required weekly and associated with significant morbidity.
- **Fetal-to-maternal hemorrhage**: IUT may be indicated if the hemorrhage is not ongoing, although cerebral hypoperfusion may result in irreversible neurological damage.
- **Infection**: Parvovirus B19 infection results in red cell hypoplasia and severe anemia. The fetus may develop viral myocarditis and, therefore, not respond well to the IUT.
- **Genetic disorders**: Alpha thalassemia major may be treated with IUT to correct the anemia and prevent fetal loss.

Risks associated with intrauterine transfusions include preterm rupture of membranes resulting in preterm delivery, fetal infection, maternal infection, fetal distress leading to cesarean, fetal fluid overload, and fetal/neonatal death.

UMBILICAL ARTERY DOPPLER FLOW STUDY

Umbilical artery Doppler flow studies measure the blood flow waveform from the uterine arteries through the umbilical cord and help to calculate the systolic/diastolic (S/D) ratio. Umbilical artery Doppler flow studies are used during the third trimester for high-risk pregnancies to assess fetal wellbeing, signs of placental insufficiency, and intrauterine growth restriction or preeclampsia. The peak of the systolic waveform shows the maximum velocity of the blood flow when the fetal heart is contracting and the end-diastolic waveform shows the continuing flow of blood in the umbilical artery when the heart is relaxed. As the placenta matures and gestation advances in a normal pregnancy, there is increased flow during diastole and the S/D ratio decreases. However, with growth restriction, end-diastolic flow may be absent or even reversed (indicating the need for immediate delivery). If the absent or reverse end-diastolic flow is associated with maternal preeclampsia, then the fetus is at increased risk of hypoglycemia and polycythemia.

TESTS FOR FETAL LUNG MATURITY

Tests for fetal lung maturity are important for monitoring a fetus if there is an indication for early termination of pregnancy. Pulmonary maturity is often an important factor in neonatal survival, as immaturity can result in respiratory distress syndrome (RDS). Commonly, two tests are used to confirm lung maturity. Tests of amniotic fluid include:

- **Lecithin/sphingomyelin (L/S) ratio:** The ratio of the surfactants lecithin and sphingomyelin changes during pregnancy, with L/S ratio at 0.5:1 early in pregnancy, 1:1 at 30-32 weeks, and 2:1 at 35 weeks. At 2:1, RDS is unlikely, although this finding is not always accurate for infants of diabetic mothers (IDM), as they may show an adequate ratio but still develop RDS. These neonates must be monitored carefully. This test is not accurate if the amniotic fluid contains blood or meconium.
- **Phosphatidylglycerol (PG):** This phospholipid first appears in surfactant at about week 35 in IDM with complications and week 36 in other pregnancies. Its presence is a sign of lung maturity.

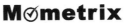

FETOMATERNAL HEMORRHAGE AND KLEIHAUER-BETKE TEST

Fetomaternal hemorrhage (FMH) occurs in many pregnancies without any signs or symptoms. A small amount of fetal blood in the maternal circulation (1-2 mL) has no clinical significance. Massive FMH (blood loss greater than 30 mL) occurs in about 3 of every 1,000 pregnancies, and is a major cause of stillbirths. Neonates' blood volume ranges from 85-100 mL/kg, so 30 mL of blood loss represents 10-12% of the blood volume in a 3 kg neonate. Risk factors for FMH include maternal trauma, placental abruption, placental tumors, third trimester amniocentesis, fetal hydrops, and twinning. One test used to diagnose the presence of FMH is the **Kleihauer-Betke (KB) test**, in which a sample of the mother's blood is examined for the presence of fetal hemoglobin. The KB test estimates the amount of hemorrhage that has taken place.

FETAL SCALP BLOOD SAMPLING

Fetal scalp blood sampling (FBS) can be obtained to check blood gases of the fetus during labor when membranes have already ruptured and there is access to the scalp. The most important parameters used are those of pH and base excess. These results can be affected by many factors, including length of time drawing the sample, exposure to air, improper handling or technique, drawing a sample during a contraction, maternal position, fever, hypertension, and the presence of caput succedaneum. A pH below 7 and base excess below -7 combined with signs of distress on electronic fetal heart monitor tracings will prompt an emergency birth. Fetal blood sampling requires skill and because of many false-positives, it is used infrequently. Scalp stimulation is used more often to determine FHR reactivity as a sign of fetal status.

OBTAINING UMBILICAL CORD BLOOD GASES

Cord blood gases give a picture of the acid base status in the newborn's tissues at the time of birth. After birth, a segment of the umbilical cord is clamped on each end and placed on the delivery table until newborn status is determined. An accurate **pH and blood gas analysis** can be performed on this cord blood for up to 60 minutes after birth. ACOG recommends obtaining arterial and venous cord blood samples after cesarean sections for fetal distress, abnormalities during FHR evaluation in labor, low Apgar scores, growth restriction, maternal hypothyroidism, maternal fever, or multiple fetuses. When done rapidly after birth, the blood gas results can guide the treatment of the compromised neonate.

Fetal Heart Rate Problems

CONTINUOUS FETAL HEART RATE MONITORING

Fetal heart rate (FHR) monitoring is usually done by **electronic fetal monitoring** (EFM), as it provides a continuous tracing. FHR can be assessed by auscultation or ultrasound with an abdominal transducer, but tracings can be poor with an active fetus, maternal movement, and hydramnios. Intermittent monitoring is usually every 15 minutes in the first stage of labor and every 5 minutes in the second. Internal monitoring requires cervical dilation of ≥2 cm so an electrode can be applied to the fetal presenting part (head or buttocks). Internal scalp electrodes should not be used if the mother has a communicable disease, such as HIV, or with preterm infants. Telemetry with ultrasound or fetal ECG transducers and external uterine pressure transducers can also be used to monitor FHR. This type of battery-operated monitoring can be used while the mother ambulates, as it is less invasive. FHR patterns are evaluated against a baseline rate (rate for 10 minutes between contractions), usually 110-160 bpm.

NICHD CATEGORY I, II, AND III FETAL HEART RATE TRACINGS

NICHD Category fetal heart tracings assess acid-base status at the time of observation only, as fetal status may change over time and the fetus's category may change:

- **I (Normal)**: Tracings indicate baseline FHR of 110-160 bpm with only moderate variability. There may be early decelerations but no late or variable decelerations. This category predicts normal acid-base status.
- **II (Indeterminate)**: May include numerous findings inconsistent with category I or III. Variability may be minimal or marked. Variability without recurrent decelerations may be absent. Accelerations after fetal stimulation may be absent. Deceleration may be prolonged, variable, or recurrent late with only moderate variability. Data is insufficient to categorize as normal or to assume abnormal acid-base status.
- **III (Abnormal)**: There is no variability in FHR with recurrent late decelerations, recurrent variable decelerations, or bradycardia. A sinusoidal pattern may be noted. This category predicts abnormal acid-base status.

EXTERNAL FHR MONITORING

External FHR monitoring may be used prior to the rupture of membranes and dilatation of the cervix because it is noninvasive; however, it is not as accurate as internal monitoring. A **transducer** is strapped to the abdomen to pick up the sounds of the fetal heart valves and blood ejection during systole. The resultant FHR is then displayed on the monitor. A gel is used to obtain proper conduction of sound from the fetal heart to the transducer. Leopold maneuvers determine fetal lie; the transducer is then applied over the back or chest of the fetus. A tocodynamometer is used to monitor uterine activity to allow correlation between fetal heart activity and uterine contractions. This method is problematic in the obese patient. It is also affected by maternal position and movement and fetal movement. Fetal heart tones may not be reliably obtained during a contraction.

INTERNAL FETAL HEART MONITOR

An internal fetal heart monitor may be used when the membranes are ruptured and the cervix is dilated to 2-3 cm. A **spiral electrode** is screwed into the fetal scalp. This allows the FHR to be more accurately distinguished from the maternal heartbeat. If fetal death has occurred, the maternal heart beat will be detected by the electrode. A reference electrode is attached to the maternal thigh. An intrauterine pressure monitoring catheter is inserted into the uterus next to the fetus to monitor contractions, allowing direct correlation between fetal heart activity and uterine contractions. Internal monitoring is the most accurate method of monitoring contractions and the FHR.

FETAL HEART RATE ABNORMALITIES

Fetal heart rate usually varies with accelerations and decelerations. Fetal reactivity (accelerated fetal heart rate with fetal activity) begins at about 32 weeks. Heart rate often increases for periods of 20-40 minutes. These are causes for accelerated or decelerated fetal heart rate.

- **Tachycardia:** HR >160 for ≥10 minutes (severe, HR >180). Transient tachycardia occurs <10 minutes and is usually not significant. Tachycardia may result from early fetal hypoxia, prematurity, medications (such as terbutaline), fetal infection, maternal fever, or anxiety.
- **Bradycardia:** HR <120 for ≥10 minutes (severe, HR <80). Bradycardia at 100-119 is usually not significant, but bradycardia may indicate heart block or placentae abruptio. Uterine contractions slow the fetal heart rate because of compression of the head affecting cerebral blood flow, compression of the myometrial vessels of the uterus, and/or occlusion of the umbilical cord causing fetal hypertension or hypoxemia. Epidural anesthesia and medications such as narcotics and oxytocin can also cause decreased heart rate.

> **Review Video: Fetal Heart Rate**
> Visit mometrix.com/academy and enter code: 980576

FETAL HEART RATE VARIABILITY AND ACCELERATIONS

Fetal heart rate **variability** shows sensitivity to oxygenation and acid-base status. Good variability indicates adequate oxygenation of the fetus's central nervous system (CNS). Decreased variability corresponds to fetal hypoxia and acidemia. Fetal heart rate variability is fluctuation in the fetal heart rate of two cycles or more, graded according to the range of amplitude:

- Absent: range not detectable
- Minimal: ≤5 bpm
- Moderate: 6-25 bpm
- Marked: >25 bpm

Short-term variability is a variation in amplitude of 3-8 bpm on a beat-to-beat basis. Long-term variability is an irregular pattern of variability of 3-5 cycles per minute with an amplitude of 5-15 bpm.

FHR **accelerations** are transient increases in fetal heart rate. Non-periodic accelerations relate to fetal movement. Periodic accelerations accompany contractions and/or compression of the umbilical cord and may indicate low amniotic fluid or dangerous cord compression.

FETAL HEART RATE DECELERATIONS

Decelerations are transient decreases in FHR. They are categorized according to contraction cycle and waveform.

- **Early**: Caused by head compression as it descends the birth canal. Waveform is uniform, with onset just before or at the onset of contraction and the lowest level at the midpoint of contraction, inversely mirroring contraction. Range is usually 120-160 bpm. Deceleration may occur once or may repeat.
- **Late**: Caused by compression of vessels and uteroplacental insufficiency. Waveform is uniform, with shape reflecting contraction. Onset is late in the contraction and the lowest point is after the midpoint of the contraction. Range is 120-130 bpm. Deceleration may be occasional, consistent, or repetitive.
- **Variable**: Caused by umbilical cord compression. Waveform is variable with sharp drops and increases. Onset may be abrupt with fetal insult and not related to contraction. The lowest point is around the midpoint. The range is usually outside normal. Deceleration may be variable and occur once or repetitively. Repetitive deceleration may indicate fetal distress.

ARTIFACTS ON FETAL HEART RATE TRACING

Various **artifacts** (misleading fetal heart tracings) can occur when monitoring fetal heart rate, usually related to the maternal heart rate, which results in **signal ambiguity** (maternal heart rate displayed on FHR monitor). Artifacts can result from:

- **Maternal pacemaker interference**: Fetal electrode may record pacemaker firing.
- **Deceased fetus**: The maternal heartbeat may continue to register on the fetal electrode.
- **Superimposition**: The maternal heart rate or QRS complex may be superimposed on the fetal heart tracing.
- **Maternal heart rate tracing** displayed instead of fetal.

Artifacts and signal ambiguity should be suspected when the fetal heart rate continues at a low normal rate, at least 50% of contractions result in accelerations of FHR, and the FHR appears to decelerate to the maternal heart rate and does not return to baseline. If signal ambiguity is expected, the maternal pulse rate should be counted and traced and fetal and maternal tracings compared. To correct this, the FHR should be assessed with ultrasound, the Doppler sensor relocated, or a scalp electrode placed.

UTERINE CONTRACTION ASSESSMENT

Uterine contraction assessment is correlated with the FHR to determine if labor is progressing normally. Contractions can be palpated with the hands. They can also be externally monitored by using a tocodynamometer or internally monitored by inserting an intrauterine pressure catheter after the membranes are ruptured and the cervix is dilated to 2-3 cm. Contractions should be **assessed** for frequency (amount of time from the beginning of one contraction to the beginning of the next), duration (amount of time in seconds from the beginning to the end of the contraction), and intensity (mild, medium, or strong in strength). **Uterine resting tone** between contractions should also be determined. All four characteristics can be determined by palpation but it is a somewhat subjective method. External monitoring can determine the duration and frequency but not the intensity or resting tone. Internal monitoring is most accurate because the amniotic pressure is measured. It can be used to determine all four characteristics.

ABNORMAL PATTERNS OF UTERINE ACTIVITY

The desirable **pattern of uterine activity** during active labor is the presence of contractions every 2-3 minutes. Inadequate or abnormal patterns may develop, especially during oxytocin augmentation.

A pattern of **hyperstimulation** is the persistence of more than 5 contractions in a 10-minute period or contractions that occur within 1 minute of each other. They may be caused by maternal hormones or agents used to ripen the cervix or augment labor. They can cause fetal distress by interfering with uteroplacental blood flow.

Coupling or tripling occurs when contractions occur in groups of 2 or 3 with very little interval between, followed by a rest period of 2-5 minutes. This may occur as a result of incoordination of the uterine pacemakers or a decrease in sensitivity of oxytocin receptor sites in the uterine muscle.

HYPERTONUS AND UTERINE TACHYSYSTOLE

Uterine hypertonus, a state in which the uterine muscle does not relax between contractions, may result from hormonal imbalance, immature genitals, infections, cervical failure, and fibroid tumors. Ineffectual contractions in the latent phase of labor become more frequent but do not result in dilation or effacement. The resting tone of the myometrium increases. The contractions may interfere with uteroplacental exchange, resulting in fetal distress. The pressure on the fetal head may result in cephalhematoma, caput succedaneum, or excessive molding. Oxytocin infusion or amniotomy may be used for treatment after assessment for cephalo-pelvic disproportion (CPD).

Uterine tachysystole is 6 or more contractions in a 10-minute period (averaged over 30 minutes) or a series of 2-minute or greater single contractions. Common causes include infection, dehydration, placental abruption, and induction. While associated with fetal heart decelerations, the fetus does not generally suffer adverse effects unless the uterine tachysystole is associated with hypertonus.

INTRAUTERINE RESUSCITATION

In the case of NICDH Category III FHR patterns (indicating fetal acidosis) that demonstrate a sinusoidal pattern and are not responding to scalp stimulation, **in utero resuscitation** is indicated. The following actions should be taken for effective intrauterine resuscitation:

- **Reposition** the mother laterally (on the right or left side) to relieve any pressure that may be compressing the cord or causing insufficient perfusion of the placenta. Knees to the chest may be effective if the lateral position is not. Apply oxygen to the mother as a precaution (generally 8-10 L/min via nonrebreather mask).
- **Fluid resuscitation** with a bolus of 500-1000 mL Lactated Ringer's or normal saline. This improves placental perfusion and restores volume in the mother in the case of hypovolemia.
- If **uterotonic drugs** are being administered, stop them immediately. Blood flow to the placenta is decreased during contractions. **Tocolytics** (such as terbutaline) may also be administered to enhance uterine relaxation.
- If hypotension is potentially secondary to the epidural dosing, **consult anesthesia** to make changes or compensate for epidural associated hypotension.

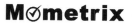

Effects of Maternal Medications on the Neonate

PHARMACOLOGIC CONTROL OF LABOR PAIN

SYSTEMIC ANALGESICS DURING LABOR

Analgesics may be given during labor as needed, but because they cross the placenta and may depress the neonate's breathing, only the minimum amount required for maternal comfort should be given. The neonate's metabolic and excretory processes are immature, so drugs are cleared much more slowly by liver metabolism or urinary excretion once the umbilical cord is cut.

Opioids and sedatives may be given to decrease labor pain, allowing the woman to rest and decrease anxiety. They are usually given only when labor is well established, because they decrease labor contraction frequency and duration and FHR variability. If given too close to birth, CNS depression is increased in the fetus. This depression can persist after delivery, especially in premature infants, affecting Apgar scores. These drugs can also cause maternal respiratory depression and resultant fetal distress. Some drugs, such as morphine and benzodiazepines, are avoided because they can cause excessive fetal depression.

- **Fentanyl** (25-100 µg/hr IV) has a shorter onset (3-10 minutes) with one-hour duration and causes less fetal depression.
- **Butorphanol** (1-2 mg IV or IM every 4 hr) and **nalbuphine** (10-20 mg IV or IM every 3 hr) cause little respiratory effect and provide adequate relief of pain but may result in excessive sedation if given repeatedly.
- **Promethazine** (25-50 mg IM) **or propiomazine hydrochloride** (20-40mg IV or IM) may be given along with narcotics to decrease nausea and vomiting, provide relief of anxiety, and to reduce the dose of opioids.

Nitrous oxide is a weak anesthetic in high concentrations, but in low doses, it is an anxiolytic and an analgesic. While common in countries such as Australia, New Zealand, Canada and Great Britain, the use of **inhaled nitrous oxide** for pain management has only recently become more common in the United States. Nitrous oxide is self-administered by the patient by inhaling the gas through a mask 30-60 seconds prior to an expected contraction (due to its delayed effect). This may be difficult for the mother in later stages of labor. Because nitrous oxide does not accumulate in the lungs, it is safe for both the mother and fetus. It can cause nausea and vomiting or excessive sleepiness, so the mother should be assessed for these side effects.

REGIONAL ANALGESIA USED DURING LABOR

NEURAXIAL ANALGESIA

Neuraxial analgesia techniques, including **epidurals, spinals, and combined epidural-spinal,** have grown in popularity. This is because they have a flexibility and effectiveness that make them ideal for this purpose. They cause less depression of the maternal and fetal CNS. These methods of providing regional anesthesia require skill to provide effective analgesia while retaining as much motor control as possible. A catheter placed in the epidural space delivers an infusion that is intermittent, continuous, or patient-controlled. Local anesthetics used include bupivacaine, lidocaine, and ropivacaine. Narcotics such as fentanyl, sufentanil, alfentanil, and remifentanil are often added to the infusion to lessen the amount of anesthetic used and therefore decrease the amount of motor blockage. The duration and quality of pain relief is also improved. Neuraxial analgesia provides better pain relief than systemic methods.

LUMBAR EPIDURAL

The most common form of regional anesthesia/analgesia for labor and delivery is the **lumbar epidural**. Dilute mixtures of local anesthetic and opioids are combined. The catheter is usually placed early so that it is available when pain relief is needed. At one time, epidurals were delayed until labor was well established, but the current trend is to administer it earlier if the fetus is in no distress, contractions are 3-4 minutes apart and persist for at least 60 seconds, and the fetal head is engaged with 3-4 cm of cervical dilation. The catheter is usually placed with the mother in a sitting position to ensure sacral spread. Placement is usually at L3 to L4 or L4 to L5. If inadvertent spinal placement occurs, spinal anesthesia/analgesia may be given or the catheter removed and replaced at a higher level. Most commonly, bupivacaine or ropivacaine (0.0625-0.125%) is given in combination with fentanyl (2-3 µg/mL) or sufentanil (0.3-0.5 µg/mL). If dilute anesthetic agents are used, the mother may be able to ambulate while receiving the epidural.

INTRATHECAL ANALGESIA WITH OPIOIDS

Intrathecal (spinal) analgesia, injected into the subarachnoid space with only **opioids**, is sometimes used during the **first stage of labor**. Commonly used agents include morphine (0.25-0.5 mg), fentanyl (12.5-15 µg), and sufentanil (10-15 µg, mixed with 10 mL of low dose bupivacaine). Meperidine is the only agent that has local anesthetic characteristics. Higher doses are needed if spinal opioids are used alone, administered as a single dose, or given intermittently per catheter. This can result in higher risk of complications, maternal respiratory depression, and fetal depression. However, if given alone, opioids (except for meperidine) do not provide motor blockade or maternal hypotension, so the mother is able to push. However, the analgesic effect may not be adequate, and side effects (pruritis, nausea, and vomiting) related to the agent may occur. Morphine alone has a slow onset (45-60 minutes), although it provides 4 to 6 hours of analgesia with spinal administration. However, low doses may not provide adequate relief, and high doses increase side effects. Morphine is frequently combined with fentanyl for more rapid onset. Commonly, opioids are combined with local anesthetics.

SPINAL ANESTHESIA (SADDLE BLOCK)

A saddle block, or spinal anesthesia, is usually given just before vaginal delivery to provide rapid **perineal anesthesia**. Spinal blocks are avoided during labor because they interfere with motor function. Because of this, other agents may be used during labor. Prior to receiving the spinal anesthesia, the patient is given a bolus of 500-1000 mL fluid. With the patient in a sitting position, a very small spinal needle (to prevent CSF leakage and post-spinal headache) is inserted into the subarachnoid space. Local anesthetics used include hyperbaric tetracaine, bupivacaine, or lidocaine, often with the addition of fentanyl or sufentanil to potentiate the effect. The agents are administered between contractions over about 30 seconds. The patient remains sitting for 3 minutes and then is placed in lithotomy position with left uterine displacement to prepare for delivery.

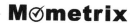

PUDENDAL NERVE BLOCK

Visceral pain occurs in the first stage of labor from contractions and cervical dilation with afferent impulses entering the spinal cord at T10 and T11. However, during the second stage of labor, the stretching of the vagina and perineum caused by the descent of the fetus causes **somatic pain** with impulses carried by the pudendal nerves to the spinal cord at S2 to S4. **Pudendal nerve block** is used during the second stage (sometimes along with perineal infiltration) to reduce **somatic pain** when neuraxial blocks are contraindicated and for episiotomy and relaxation of the pelvic floor for forceps delivery. With the patient in lithotomy position, a transvaginal or transperineal approach is used to block the nerve. For the transvaginal approach (the most common), a Kobak needle or special guide (Iowa trumpet) is used to prevent inadvertent injection into the fetal head. Anesthetic agents include 10 mL of 1% lidocaine or 2% chloroprocaine. The transperineal approach may be used if the head is engaged.

GENERAL ANESTHESIA IN BIRTH PROCESS

General anesthesia is rarely used for vaginal birth but may be used for emergency procedures and Cesarean births if the mother is not a good candidate for epidural or subarachnoid block. Maternal complications can include aspiration of stomach contents, especially if the woman has not been NPO, and this can result in postoperative chemical pneumonitis. Therefore, an oral antacid is sometimes administered prior to anesthesia. A wedge should be placed under the woman's right hip to displace the uterus to the left prior to administration of anesthesia. The woman may experience respiratory depression, and this can affect the oxygenation of the fetus. General anesthesia can also result in relaxation of the uterine muscles, and if this persists in the postoperative period, it increases the risk of postpartum hemorrhage. General anesthesia is contraindicated with a high risk or preterm fetus because of fetal depression. Anesthesia usually affects the fetus within 2 minutes, so rapid delivery reduces risks to the fetus.

TOCOLYTICS

Tocolysis suppresses preterm labor and premature birth, sometimes allowing time to administer betamethasone to accelerate maturity of fetal lungs. Tocolytics (some off-label) include the following:

- **Indomethacin,** an NSAID that inhibits prostaglandin production, can be used up to 32 weeks of gestation. It crosses the placenta and can cause reduction in amniotic fluid, leading to fetal distress, especially >32 weeks. Indomethacin can also cause premature closure of the ductus arteriosus. This medication is the first-line therapy for women 24-32 weeks gestation.
- **Nifedipine**, a calcium channel blocker that reduces muscle contractility, is most commonly used, as it is more effective and safer than many other drugs. It may increase fetal heart rate (FHR). This is second-line therapy for women 24-32 weeks gestation and first-line therapy for women 32-34 weeks gestation.
- **Terbutaline** is a beta-adrenergic asthma drug that also relaxes the uterine muscle. It may increase FHR. It can be used as second-line therapy at 32-34 weeks gestation when nifedipine is used in the 24-32 weeks gestational period.
- **Magnesium sulfate** is similar in action to terbutaline, but it requires close monitoring for maternal adverse effects. It crosses the placenta, and the neonate may suffer respiratory and motor depression.

Concurrent use of tocolytics is discouraged.

Problems in Labor

PRECIPITOUS LABOR/BIRTH

Precipitous labor and birth occurs when onset of labor to birth takes 3 hours or less, often because of strong uterine contractions and low muscle resistance in maternal tissue that promotes rapid dilatation of the cervix (or lacerations) and descent of the fetus. A primigravida may dilate 5 cm per hour; and a multigravida as quickly as 10 cm per hour. The neonate may have a low Apgar score and is at increased risk for aspiration of meconium and intracranial injury, such as subdural/dural tears. The strong uterine contractions may interfere with uterine blood flow and oxygenation of the fetus. Precipitous birth alone, by contrast, is usually an unexpected and sudden birth that takes place outside of the hospital or is unattended by a physician because there is no time to travel or get help. In these cases, the neonate is sometimes expelled into a toilet or onto the floor, causing injury.

PROLONGED LABOR

Prolonged labor results from dysfunctional uterine contractions, accounting for 50% of Cesareans in nulliparous women, but only 5% of Cesareans in multiparous women. Dysfunctional contractions are often irregular, exhibit low amplitude, and result in <1 cm cervical dilatation/hr. In some cases, contractions continue but cervical dilatation is arrested. The **labor patterns** below are associated with prolonged labor:

- **Hypertonic:** Ineffectual contractions in the latent phase of labor become more frequent but do not result in dilatation or effacement. The resting tone of the myometrium increases. The contractions may interfere with uteroplacental exchange, resulting in fetal distress. The pressure on the fetal head may result in cephalohematoma, caput succedaneum, or excessive molding. Oxytocin infusion or amniotomy may be used after assessment for cephalopelvic disproportion (CPD).
- **Hypotonic**: Fewer than 3 contractions occur in 10 minutes during active phase, with less than 1 cm dilatation per hour or arrest of dilatation. Treatment is the same as for hypertonic patterns.

POST-TERM PREGNANCY

Post-term pregnancy (>294 days or 42 weeks past 1st day of last menstrual period) occurs in 3-7% of pregnancies, and is often the result of errors in calculating due date, but true post-term pregnancies, while posing little risk to the mother, can increase the risk to the fetus, and vaginal birth may be facilitated by forceps or vacuum extractor. Increased fetal risks include:

- **Large for gestational age** (LGA), >4500g (about 10 pounds), which may result in prolonged labor, birth trauma with fractures or neurological injury, or Cesarean section.
- **Aspiration of meconium** occurs more frequently because a large fetus is more likely to expel meconium.
- **Post-maturity syndrome** related to restriction of growth in the uterus, often because of restricted blood flow, putting the fetus at risk for respiratory and neurological disorders.

CEPHALOPELVIC/FETOPELVIC DISPROPORTION

Cephalopelvic/fetopelvic disproportion is usually diagnosed when labor does not progress, although in rare cases it may be diagnosed prior to labor. It may relate to pelvic diameters that are too small (most common with android and platypelloid pelvic types) or due to contractures of the pelvic inlet (<10 cm anteroposterior diameter or <12 cm transverse diameter), contracted midpelvis, or contracted outlet (<8 cm interischial tuberous diameter). Rarely is this disproportion caused by excessive fetal size as most fetuses are within normal size and weight limits. Usually, labor is extended and premature rupture of the membranes occurs, increasing danger of cord prolapse. The fetal head is often markedly molded and continued pressure can cause neurological injury or even death of the fetus if the labor continues and the fetus cannot be delivered, but when labor fails to progress, the mother is usually given a Cesarean section (within 2 hours of labor onset) to prevent further injury to the fetus.

FETAL MALPRESENTATION

MILITARY

The head is erect and neck not flexed. This poses little problem because flexion often occurs as the head descends.

BROW

The neck is extended so that the brow presents first. This presentation may relate to SGA, LGA, hydramnios, and uterine or fetal anomalies. Brow presentation, with the largest diameter (about 13.5 cm), increases fetal mortality because of birth trauma, which can include compression of the neck and cerebrum, and tracheal and laryngeal damage. Cesarean delivery or vaginal delivery with episiotomy is usually required.

FACE

The neck is severely extended so that the face presents first (about 9.5 cm diameter). This often prolongs labor and may result in increased edema of the fetus and trauma to the neck and internal structures. The neonate usually has bruising in the facial skin. Cesarean section is generally required.

BREECH

This occurs in 4% of births and is frequently related to early labor and delivery (25% are at 25 to 26 weeks). Frank breech (buttocks presentation with legs extended upward) is most common, but single or double footling breech or complete breech (buttocks presentation with legs flexed) can occur. Breech presentation is most common with placenta previa, hydramnios, fetal anomalies, and multiple gestations. Cord prolapse is more likely. Head trauma may occur because molding does not occur, and the head can become entrapped. Mortality and morbidity are reduced with Cesarean section, especially with low or high fetal weight, hyperextension of neck (>90°), fetal anomalies, and pelvic disproportion. Version may be attempted, in which pressure is placed on the fetus externally, in attempt to move the fetus from breech position to a head-down position. This must be done before contractions begin and the fetal head is engaged. If unsuccessful, Cesarean section is the recommended and safest mode of delivery.

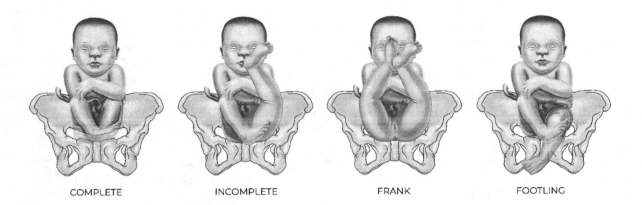

| COMPLETE | INCOMPLETE | FRANK | FOOTLING |

SHOULDER

This transverse lie poses extreme risk of uterine rupture. The fetus cannot be delivered, and Cesarean section is required.

COMPOUND

This is when there are two presenting parts, such as the head and a hand, increasing the chance of laceration. With fetal distress or uterine dysfunction, a Cesarean section is required.

MECONIUM IN AMNIOTIC FLUID

When meconium is present in the amniotic fluid, the following considerations should be taken following birth to avoid meconium aspiration syndrome:

- If the infant is crying and showing no signs of distress (known as being vigorous), current NRP guidelines no longer recommend suctioning. Visible drainage can be wiped away with a cloth.
- If the infant shows signs of respiratory distress in the presence of meconium-stained fluid, NRP guidelines now recommend using a bulb suction as the first attempt to restore ventilation, suctioning the mouth before the nose. Deep suctioning risks the possibility of causing a vagal response that can result in dangerous arrhythmias.
- If respiratory distress continues despite these non-invasive efforts, intubation is indicated. Only if an airway obstruction is suspected (all efforts to ventilate the infant are not resulting in chest rise) should the trachea be suctioned with a large catheter within the endotracheal tube, attached to wall suction.

Once the airway has been adequately suctioned and cleared, the stomach may need to be suctioned as well in order to prevent the regurgitation of the swallowed meconium. Meconium that is swallowed and then regurgitated can be aspirated into the lungs.

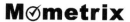

Obstetric Emergencies

PLACENTA PREVIA AND ABRUPTIO PLACENTAE

Placenta previa: Implantation of the placenta is over or near the internal cervical os. Women with placenta previa have increased incidences of hemorrhage in the third trimester. In infants, placenta previa is associated with poor growth, anemia, and increased risk of congenital anomalies in their central nervous systems, heart, respiratory and gastrointestinal tracts. Placenta previa may also cause premature birth with associated neonatal complications of prematurity.

Abruptio placentae: The placenta prematurely detaches, partially or completely, from the uterus. Abruptio placentae is related to maternal hypertension, and incidence increases with cocaine abuse. Partial detachment interferes with the functioning of the placenta, causing intrauterine growth restriction. Severe bleeding occurs with total detachment. Common fetal complications are preterm labor, hypoxia, and anemia. Fetal mortality is about 25% with partial detachment and 100% with complete. Irreversible brain damage may occur with fetal hypoxia, and neurological deficits occur in about 14% of survivors.

VASA PREVIA

Vasa previa is an abnormality where at least one of the fetal blood vessels lies across the internal cervical os. The fetal umbilical vein and arteries lie unprotected on the membrane wall on their way to the placenta. This predisposes the fetus to hemorrhage if one of the vessels is injured during membrane rupture that occurs spontaneously or artificially. The FHR reacts immediately to the vessel damage and death occurs in 56% of all cases. An immediate cesarean section is indicated. Diagnosis may be made prenatally by transvaginal Doppler ultrasound or routine ultrasound that examines placental cord insertion. A planned cesarean increases the fetal survival rate to 97%.

ABNORMAL PLACENTAL IMPLANTATION

Defective decidua basalis is thought to be the cause of abnormal adherence of the placenta to the uterine wall. This is more common when there has been a previous cesarean section or when placenta previa is present. It is diagnosed when manual removal of the placenta fails and surgical intervention is performed. There is a high risk of maternal hemorrhage and hysterectomy may be necessary. Three varieties are recognized:

- **Placenta accreta:** The decidual basalis is absent so the placenta grows directly into the myometrium of the uterine wall. Only a portion or all of the placenta's cotyledons may be adherent to the uterine wall in this way. This is the most common variety.
- **Placenta increta:** Trophoblastic cells invade the myometrium of the uterine wall.
- **Placenta percreta:** Trophoblastic cells penetrate through the uterine wall and invade other organs in the vicinity such as the bladder.

UTERINE RUPTURE AND DEHISCENCE

The uterine wall may **separate** at the site of a previous scar. If the fetal membranes stay intact and the fetus stays in the uterus, a **dehiscence** has occurred. When the uterine wall **ruptures** and part or the entire fetus extrudes into the peritoneal cavity, death can quickly occur in the fetus and mother without rapid cesarean section. Symptoms of both can include sharp, tearing uterine pain, FHR decelerations, vomiting, fainting, vaginal bleeding, tachycardia, hypotension, and shock. Factors associated with uterine rupture include uterine hyperstimulation, previous uterine surgery, use of prostaglandins, multiparity, abdominal traumatic injury, and fundal pressure.

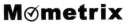

UTERINE INVERSION

Inversion is the turning inside out of the uterus. It can be caused by fundal pressure and traction on the umbilical cord. It can also occur during uterine atony, with large fetuses or short umbilical cords, from adherent placental tissues, and from the use of oxytocin. It can also occur spontaneously without obvious cause. Sometimes only the fundus inverts (partial inversion) and other times the fundus protrudes through the cervical opening (complete inversion).

Inversion may be **visualized** or **occult**. There is sudden severe pelvic pain, hemorrhage, and hypotension. There will be a firm mass below the cervix felt by bimanual exam. The uterus must be immediately replaced manually prior to delivery of the placenta. Tocolytics or general anesthesia may be required to do this. IV fluids and blood are given to replace blood loss as needed. Antibiotics and a nasogastric tube may also be needed.

PROLAPSED UMBILICAL CORD

A prolapse of the umbilical cord occurs when the umbilical cord precedes the fetus in the birth canal and becomes entrapped by the descending fetus. An **occult cord prolapse** occurs when the umbilical cord is beside or just ahead of the fetal head. About half of prolapses occur in the second stage of labor and relate to premature delivery, multiple gestation, polyhydramnios, breech delivery, and an excessively long umbilical cord. Some cases are precipitated by obstetric interventions, such as amniotomy, external eversion, and application of scalp electrode for monitoring. As contractions occur and the head descends, this applies pressure to the umbilical cord, occluding blood flow and causing hypoxia and bradycardia. The decrease in blood flow through the umbilical vessels can cause impaired gas exchange, and if pressure on the cord is not relieved, the fetus can suffer severe neurological damage or death. **Management** includes elevating the presenting part off the cord, having the mother elevate her knees to the chest, and preparing for C-section.

VELAMENTOUS CORD INSERTION

Velamentous cord insertion is an abnormality in which the cord inserts into the membranes rather than the middle of the placenta, traveling through the chorion and amnion to reach the placental margin, leaving exposed vessels unprotected by Wharton's jelly. This can cause shearing of the blood vessels during delivery, leading to hemorrhage. Additionally, the exposed vessels are vulnerable to compression, which can result in fetal anoxia. Velamentous cord insertion is most common with placenta previa and multiple gestations. While incidence is only about 1% for singletons, the incidence increases to almost 9% with twins, so the nurse must be alert for indications. Velamentous cord insertion is associated with about 25% of spontaneous abortions. Velamentous cord insertion may result in vasa previa if the velamentous vessels are lower than the presenting part because they may rupture, causing the fetus to exsanguinate, especially during onset of labor or amniotomy. Indications of velamentous cord insertion include excessive bleeding and fetal distress. Treatment includes careful monitoring and cesarean.

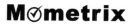

Impact of Methods of Delivery on the Neonate

VAGINAL DELIVERY

EXPULSIVE PERIOD

During the **expulsive period of delivery**, the mother will need to be coached to achieve effective pushing effort. Two types of pushing are effective: open glottis physiologic pushing and closed glottis (Valsalva) pushing. The mother should be coached on the method most effective for her. During crowning, the mother should be instructed to "pant like a puppy." The integrity of the perineum needs to be taken into consideration. Most mothers would like to avoid an episiotomy if at all possible; however, there are several factors that may make an episiotomy necessary:

- Fetal malposition
- Anticipation of the delivery of a large baby
- Possibility of shoulder dystocia, where the anterior shoulder cannot pass below the symphysis pubis
- Poor elasticity of the perineal tissue
- Difficulty in maintaining adequate control of the patient's expulsive efforts

DELIVERY OF THE PLACENTA

The **placenta** will generally deliver 5-30 minutes after delivery of the fetus. The mechanism of **placental separation** starts with the change in the size of the uterus and then proceeds with the formation of a hematoma between the placenta and uterine wall, the separation of the placenta, the descent of the placenta through the lower uterine segment and vagina, and then expulsion. Signs and symptoms of placental separation include a sudden increase in vaginal bleeding, lengthening of the umbilical cord, and the rising of the uterus in the abdomen. Management of placental delivery includes obtaining cord blood samples after the cord is clamped, inspecting the cord for the number of vessels, and avoiding uterine massage and cord traction until the placenta is separated. Pushing by the mother may assist in expulsion of the placenta. If membranes follow the placenta, hold the placenta and carefully roll it over and over until the membranes separate and are delivered. This helps prevent retained membranes.

PERINEAL LACERATIONS

The four types of perineal lacerations are described below:

- **First degree**: The perineal skin and the mucous membranes of the vagina are torn.
- **Second degree**: The perineal skin and vaginal mucous membranes are torn as well as the fascia and muscle of the perineum.
- **Third degree**: The perineal skin, vaginal mucous membranes, and fascia and muscle of the perineum are torn and the tear extends into the rectal sphincter.
- **Fourth degree**: The perineal skin, vaginal mucous membranes, and fascia and muscle of the perineum are torn, the tear extends into the rectal sphincter, and the inner lumen of the rectum is exposed.

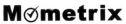

OPERATIVE DELIVERY

FORCEPS-ASSISTED BIRTH

Forceps-assisted birth utilizes a variety of specialized tools to assist with the birth of the fetus by providing traction and a method of rotating the fetal head into proper occiput-anterior position. Most forceps are used with the fetus in the head-down position and the forceps positioned on the sides of the head.

- **Outlet forceps application** can be used when the perineum is bulging, the scalp is visible between contractions, or the sagittal suture is not >45 degrees from midline. The fetal skull must be at station +2 or below.
- **Midforceps application** requires that the head be engaged with the leading edge above +2 station.
- **High forceps** are no longer used.

Indications for forceps-assisted birth include conditions that pose a risk to the mother or fetus and are relieved by birth. Maternal risks of forceps-assisted birth include infection, cervical and birth canal lacerations, extension of episiotomy, anal sphincter injury, and weakening of pelvic floor muscles. Neonatal risks include bruising and edema of face, caput succedaneum, cephalhematoma, transient low Apgar score, retinal hemorrhage, ocular trauma, Erb's palsy, and elevated bilirubin.

VACUUM-ASSISTED BIRTH

Vacuum-assisted birth utilizes a soft suction cup attached to a suction pump that creates negative pressure of 50-60 mmHg. The suction cup is applied to the **occiput** of the fetus, and traction is applied with contractions. Suction use should be limited to 20-30 minutes, with scalp trauma more likely after 10 minutes of use. If the suction cup dislodges more than 3 times, its use should be discontinued. Indications include prolonged second stage of labor or nonreassuring heart pattern. Vacuum-assisted birth may also be used if the mother is too fatigued to push. Neonatal risks include scalp lacerations, subdural hematoma, cephalohematoma, intracranial hemorrhage, subconjunctival hemorrhage, Erb's palsy, sixth and ninth cranial nerve trauma, retinal hemorrhage, and death. A caput forms on the neonate's head, but this should subside in 2-3 days. Maternal risks include perineal trauma, lacerations, pain, and infection.

CESAREAN SECTION

Cesarean sections are done if there is increased risk of uterine rupture, maternal hemorrhage, dystocia, fetal-pelvic disproportion, breech presentation, active herpes infection, and emergent situations such as fetal distress or impending maternal death. Regional anesthesia (spinal, epidural) is associated with lower mortality than general anesthesia, so it is the preferred anesthetic approach. Additionally, there is less fetal depression, reduced risk of maternal pulmonary aspiration, and an opportunity to provide neuraxial analgesia for postoperative pain relief. Regional anesthesia must provide a T4 sensory level, which causes a high sympathetic blockade. In some cases, general anesthesia may be administered for Cesarean section, although the risks to the mother are intensified, so general anesthesia is usually limited to emergent situations in which the mother or fetus is at risk. Reasons for Cesareans are:

- Fetal distress during the second stage of labor
- Tetanic uterine contractions
- Patient confused, uncontrollable, and unable to cooperate (such as psychiatric patients)
- Inverted uterus
- Retained placenta
- Breech extraction or other position requiring version and extraction

VBAC

There has been decreasing interest in **vaginal birth after Cesarean section (VBAC)** with only 10% attempting it in recent years, but many mothers are able to undergo vaginal delivery after a Cesarean section without complications. Risks include hemorrhage and uterine rupture (1%). Women who attempt vaginal birth have a 60-80% success rate. Below are the guidelines for vaginal delivery after Cesarean.

- A woman with one previous Cesarean section and a low transverse uterine incision should be advised to try vaginal birth. A woman with 2 or more previous Cesarean sections may attempt vaginal birth.
- In all cases, a physician, an anesthesiologist, and adequate staff must be present and available throughout labor to provide a Cesarean section if necessary.

Contraindications to attempting a VBAC are:

- T or classic incision
- History of myomectomy
- Contracted pelvis
- Obstetrical complications precluding vaginal birth
- Inadequate facilities or staff to provide emergency Cesarean section if it is needed

DELAYED CORD CLAMPING

Practice since the 1950s has been to clamp the umbilical cord within about 15 seconds of birth, but recent research indicates benefits to delayed cord clamping to 30-60 seconds with some recommending 2-5 minutes to allow increased blood to flow to the newborn (approximately 80 mL within the first minute and 100 mL in the first three) as well as fetal stem cells and immunoglobulins. Benefits to the term infant include increased hemoglobin and improved iron status for the first few months of life. Benefits to preterm infants include lower rates of intraventricular hemorrhage and necrotizing enterocolitis. Delayed cord clamping is contraindicated in infants that require positive pressure ventilation or if mothers are hemodynamically unstable. While there are some concerns that the infant may develop polycythemia, studies have not supported this; however, there is some increase in jaundice and the need for phototherapy. Delayed cord cutting does not appear to increase risk of maternal hemorrhage.

Gestational Age Assessment

ESTIMATING GESTATIONAL AGE

Accurate determination of gestational age (GA) predicts neonatal morbidity and mortality. Compare GA with the birth weight to determine if the patient is large or small for GA. Respiratory distress syndrome affects 1% of neonates. The prognosis for a premature infant with respiratory distress who is an appropriate weight for GA (e.g., 33 weeks and 2,000 grams), is better than the prognosis for a full term, small for gestational age (SGA) baby (e.g. 40 weeks and 2,000 grams). These infants have identical birth weights, but the SGA baby is more likely to require mechanical ventilation and has a greater chance of mortality.

The obstetrician **calculates prenatal GA** throughout a pregnancy by the:

- Reported date of last menstrual period (LMP)
- Periodic physical examinations of the mother
- Ultrasound examinations of the fetus
- Date the fetal heartbeat is first heard
- Date fetal movements are first felt (quickening)

The **Modified Ballard examination** is the first comprehensive postnatal test of the neonate, and when scored correctly, it gives a very accurate estimate of the GA.

INITIAL METHODS FOR GESTATIONAL AGE ESTIMATION

The initial marker for measuring gestational age is the date of the last menstrual period (LMP). Various calculators are available for this, but they are limited by both the reliability of the mother's report of the dates of her LMP and the typical variability in menstrual periods and ovulatory times. Ultrasound that utilizes various measurements of fetal dimensions is a more accurate method of estimating gestational age. Ultrasound is most accurate during the first trimester, when it has been shown to have a 95% accuracy of ±6 days. As the fetus grows, its size becomes more dependent on the environment, rather than the date of conception, making ultrasound dating during the second and third trimesters less accurate. Clinical examination by the obstetrician is less accurate in determining gestational age than ultrasound.

MODIFIED BALLARD SCORE OVERVIEW

The Modified Ballard Score is used to estimate **maturity and gestational age** in newborn infants. It is most reliable when performed within the first 12 hours of life. The Ballard Score was modified to include evaluation of extremely premature infants with gestational ages as low as 20 weeks (score 10) and as high as 50 weeks (score 44). It scores 6 measurements of **neuromuscular maturity** and 6 signs of **physical maturity** on a scale of -1 to +4 or +5, depending upon the category. The total score indicates the estimated gestational age for the infant.

NEUROMUSCULAR MEASUREMENTS

1. Observation of the **infant's posture** while lying supine indicates the total amount of muscle tone the infant possesses. Increased amounts of flexion of the elbows and knees correlates with increased gestational age.
2. **Square window test** measures the resistance to stretching of extensor muscles in the infant's forearm. Increased ability for the tester to flex the infant's wrist correlates with greater gestational age.

3. **Arm recoil test** measures the tone of the biceps muscle. Increased amount of arm recoil (flexion by the infant after the infant's arms are extended) correlates with greater gestational age.
4. **Popliteal angle measurement** assesses the flexor tone of the knee joint. Increased resistance to flexion at the knee is associated with greater gestational age.
5. **Scarf sign test** measures the tone of shoulder flexor muscles. Increased resistance to movement of the infant's arm across the chest is associated with greater gestational age.
6. **Heel-to-ear test** measures the tone of pelvic girdle muscles. Increased resistance to movement of the infant's foot to its ear is associated with greater gestational age.

PHYSICAL SIGNS OF MATURITY

1. **Skin**: Immature infants have thin, transparent skin. The vernix caseosa begins development at the beginning of the third trimester. Dried, cracked skin occurs as this protective coating disappears after the fortieth week.
2. **Lanugo**: Fine, usually unpigmented hairs begin to appear at 24-25 weeks of gestation and thin as the neonate matures.
3. **Plantar surface of feet:** Very immature infants have no creases on the soles of their feet. Creases develop first on the anterior portion, and more mature infants will have creases over the entire sole.
4. **Breast buds**: These are fatty tissue underneath the areola which increase in size as the fetus matures.
5. **Ears**: Increased cartilage content produces a more rigid pinna; ear recoil increases as the infant matures.
6. Genitalia
   a. **Male**: The testes descend from the abdomen into the scrotum at 30 weeks of gestation, and the scrotum develops rugae as the fetus matures.
   b. **Female**: Initially, the female fetus has a large clitoris and small labia majora. As the fetus matures, the labia majora enlarge, while the clitoris shrinks.

PRETERM INFANT

A preterm infant is one born prior to 37 weeks gestational age. In the United States, preterm birth is the most important factor influencing infant mortality; preterm infants account for 75-80% of all neonatal morbidity and mortality. **Health problems associated with premature birth** include:

- Respiratory distress syndrome because of inadequate surfactant production (hyaline membrane disease)
- Hypothermia because of inadequate subcutaneous fat, small amounts of brown fat, and large skin surface area to mass ratio
- Hypoglycemia secondary to poor nutritional intake, poor nutritional stores, and increased glucose consumption associated with sepsis
- Skin trauma or infection secondary to fragile, immature skin
- Periods of apnea because of an immature respiratory center in the brain
- Intraventricular hemorrhage

The original cause of the preterm birth (such as maternal infection) may also play an integral role in the likely health problem associated with prematurity.

CHARACTERISTICS OF PRETERM INFANTS BORN AT 24-25 WEEKS

Characteristics of preterm infants born at 24-25 weeks include the following:

- **Skin**: very thin with visible veins; absent or minimal vernix caseosa as it is just beginning to be secreted at 2 weeks
- **Lanugo**: sparse
- **Feet**: smooth plantar surfaces or faint marks on the anterior surfaces
- **Areolae**: newly developing, breast bud not yet present
- **Eyes**: open
- **Ears**: no or very limited recoil
- **Posture**: immature, indicated by limited flexion of the limbs while the infant is in a supine position
- **Square window sign**: shows decreased flexion at the wrist of approximately 60-90°
- **Range of motion**: increased ROM (lone tone) when performing the popliteal angle, scarf sign, and heel to ear examinations
- **Arm recoil**: limited or no recoil

NEUROMUSCULAR CHARACTERISTICS OF FULL-TERM INFANTS

Neuromuscular characteristics of full-term infants include the following:

- **Supine resting posture**: hips, knees, and arms all flexed past 90°, indicating mature muscular tone
- **Square window**: wrist flexes to 0°, reflecting very little resistance to the extensor muscles of the wrist
- **Arm recoil**: arms recoil past 90°; contact between the infant's fist and face demonstrates mature tone in the biceps muscles
- **Popliteal angle**: <90° knee flexion
- **Scarf sign**: the arms cannot be drawn past the ipsilateral axillary line because of the mature tone of the posterior shoulder girdle flexor muscles
- **Heel to ear**: resistance is felt in the knee and hip when the heel is at the femoral crease because of the tone of the posterior pelvic girdle flexor muscles

CHARACTERISTICS OF POSTTERM INFANTS

Posterm infants are those born >42 weeks of gestation. Many are normal in size and appearance, but some continue to grow *in utero* and weigh >4000 g. Some may exhibit post-maturity syndrome (about 5%), which puts the infant at increased risk. **Characteristics** include:

- **Appearance**: alert (this may indicate intrauterine hypoxia)
- **Skin**: loose, dry, cracking, parchment-like, and lacking lanugo or vernix; may have meconium staining, yellow to green (indicating recent meconium release)
- **Fingernails**: long (sometimes with meconium staining)
- **Scalp hair**: long and thick
- **Body**: long and thin (fat layers absent)
- **Hypoglycemia** from nutritional deprivation
- **Hypothermia** due to decreased brown fat and liver glycogen
- **Meconium aspiration** (risk increases with oligohydramnios), increasing risk of impaired gas exchange
- **Polycythemia** as response to hypoxia, increasing risk of impaired tissue perfusion
- **Seizures** resulting from hypoxia

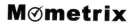

- **Cold stress** (lack of fat stores)
- **Congenital anomalies**

BIRTH WEIGHT AND GESTATIONAL AGE ACRONYMS

These terms do not take into account the estimated gestational age of the infant:

- **ELBW (Extremely Low Birth Weight)**: birth weight of less than 1,000 g (2.2 lb)
- **VLBW (Very Low Birth Weight)**: birth weight of less than 1,500 grams (3.3 lb)

The following terms take into account the estimated gestational age of the infant in comparison to the birth weight:

- **SGA (small for gestational age)**: below the tenth percentile for gestational age
- **AGA (appropriate for gestational age)**: between the tenth and ninetieth percentiles for gestational age
- **LGA (large for gestational age)**: above the ninetieth percentile for gestational age

SGA

Small for gestational age (SGA) infants are those whose weight places them below the 10th percentile for their gestational age. SGA is also called dysmaturity and intrauterine growth restriction. SGA babies commonly aspirate meconium and have a low APGAR score, asphyxia, hypoglycemia, and polycythemia. Common **causes of SGA** include:

- Multiple gestation (twins, triplets, quadruplets)
- Constitutional SGA because both parents are small
- Many genetic defects, such as trisomy 18 (Edwards syndrome), Down syndrome, and Turner syndrome
- Placental malfunction or misplacement (inadequate fetal nutrition from reduced blood flow, sepsis, placenta previa, or abruptio placentae)
- Maternal disease (pre-eclampsia; high blood pressure; malnutrition; advanced diabetes mellitus; chronic kidney, heart, or respiratory disease; and anemia)
- Infections such as cytomegalovirus, toxoplasmosis, and rubella
- Maternal tobacco, illegal drug, or alcohol use during pregnancy
- Birth defects

LGA

Large for gestational age (LGA) infants are those whose weight places them above the 90th percentile for their gestational age. The main pathologic cause for LGA is maternal diabetes (either gestational diabetes or diabetes mellitus). Infants exposed to elevated levels of glucose produce elevated amounts of insulin, which has an anabolic effect on the developing fetus, causing macrosomia (large body). Poor control of diabetes during pregnancy generally results in a larger infant with these **common health problems**:

- Delivery complications (shoulder dystocia, clavicle fracture, prolonged vaginal exit requiring use of forceps or Cesarian section, and perinatal asphyxia)
- Abnormal blood test results (hypoglycemia developing within 1-2 hours of birth, hyperbilirubinemia, hypocalcemia, hypomagnesemia, hyperviscosity [thickened blood] secondary to polycythemia [elevated hemoglobin])
- Jaundice
- Feeding intolerance
- Lethargy
- Respiratory distress
- Birth defects

INTRAUTERINE GROWTH RESTRICTION

When a fetus does not fulfill his or her growth potential for any reason, the diagnosis is **intrauterine growth restriction (IUGR)**. Prenatal ultrasound is used to diagnose IUGR, which is associated with oligohydramnios (decreased amniotic fluid) and preeclampsia (pregnancy-induced hypertension and proteinuria). IUGR is classified as symmetric or asymmetric, based on the size of the newborn's head:

- **Symmetric IUGR**
  - Both head and body are small (growth-restricted).
  - The restriction occurs early in pregnancy.
  - Common causes are chromosomal abnormalities and infections.

- **Asymmetric IUGR**
  - The head is large in proportion to the body; the head is spared.
  - The head is normal in size for gestational age, while the body is growth-restricted.
  - Restriction occurs late in pregnancy.
  - Common causes include placental insufficiency and preeclampsia.

Physical Assessment

PHYSICAL ASSESSMENT

The neonate should undergo three different types of physical assessment:

- **Immediate**: The first examination is done in the delivery room to determine the need for resuscitation or other intervention. This includes the APGAR assessment.
- **1-4 hours after birth**: The second examination includes gestational age assessment, which must be completed within 24 hours for accuracy, and brief physical assessment to determine if there are any problems that might place the infant at risk. This includes assessment of respiratory and cardiac status, cord color, skin color, and movement. The Modified Ballard scoring system is often used.
- **≥24 hours after birth (or prior to discharge)**: The final examination should include a complete physical and behavioral assessment that includes all systems and evaluation of reflexes. All weights and measurements are taken and reviewed. This exam requires observation, palpation, and auscultation. In some cases, instead of a separate examination at 1-4 hours, only this complete physical examination is completed.

RAPID ASSESSMENT

The infant should be given a rapid assessment within seconds of birth to determine if the infant is at term, if the amniotic fluid is clear, if there is muscle tone, and if there are respirations or crying. If any of these conditions are not met, then the child should be placed under radiant heat and further resuscitation done. The basic **steps to resuscitation** include:

- Warming the infant after drying
- Positioning the infant and clearing the airway if necessary
- Stimulating and repositioning the infant

The child should be evaluated throughout the initial procedures:

- **Respirations**: Rate and character of respirations should be noted as well as observation of chest wall movement.
- **Heart rate**: Should be >100 bpm, assessed with stethoscope or at the base of the umbilical cord.

APGAR DELIVERY ROOM ASSESSMENT

Dr. Virginia Apgar developed the **APGAR** test in 1952. APGAR stands for **A**ppearance, **P**ulse, **G**rimace, **A**ctivity, and **R**espiration. The APGAR is the first test given to a newborn. It is used as a quick evaluation of a newborn's physical condition to determine if any emergency medical care is needed and is administered 1 minute and 5 minutes after birth. The test is administered more than once, as the baby's condition may change rapidly. It may be administered for a third time 10 minutes after birth if needed. The baby is rated on the five subscales and the scores are added together. A total score of ≥7 is a sign of good health.

SCORING CHART

Sign	0	1	2
Appearance (Skin Color)	Cyanotic or pallor over entire body	Normal, except for the extremities	Entire body normal
Pulse (Heart Rate)	Absent	<100 bpm	>100 bpm
Grimace (Reflex Irritability)	Unresponsive	Grimace	Infant sneezes, coughs, and recoils
Activity (Muscle Tone)	Absent	Flexed limbs	Infant moves freely
Respiration (Breathing Rate and Effort)	Absent	Bradypnea, dyspnea	Good breathing and crying

> **Review Video: Newborn APGAR Score**
> Visit mometrix.com/academy and enter code: 253451

APPEARANCE, WEIGHT, MEASUREMENTS, AND VITAL SIGNS

The neonate's general appearance, measurements, and VS should be evaluated:

- **Head**: disproportionately large for body
- **Body**: long
- **Extremities**: short and in flexed position (Feet are usually dorsiflexed after breech birth.)
- **Hands**: clenched
- **Neck**: short and chin resting on chest
- **Abdomen**: prominent
- **Hips**: narrow
- **Chest**: rounded
- **Weight**: 2500-4000 g (average about 3400); physiologic weight loss is 5-10% for full term and up to 15% for preterm
- **Length**: 45-55 cm (average 50 cm)
- **Head circumference**: 32-38 cm (usually 2 cm greater than chest circumference)
- **Chest circumference**: 30-36 cm
- **Temperature**: Temperature drops rapidly (skin temperature falls 0.3 °C/minute) after birth with exposure to ambient room temperature but stabilizes within 8-12 hours. Temperature is usually measured by axillary method (for 3 minutes) and ranges from 36.3-37.0 °C.
- **Blood pressure**: 56-77/33-50 mmHg
- **Pulse**: 120-160 bpm awake; 100 bpm asleep; 180 bpm crying
- **Respiration**: 30-60 per minute

CARDIAC RATES

Normal cardiac rates can vary widely from one neonate to another, so it's important to understand the normal range in order to determine if the infant has an abnormal pulse. Rates will also vary depending upon whether the infant is awake, sleeping, or active. Pulse rate should be taken with a stethoscope, because the pulse may be difficult to palpate or count accurately manually. The neonatal **point of maximal intensity (PMI)** is located at the intersection between the 4th intercostal space and the midclavicular line (versus the adult PMI located at the 5th intercostal). Additionally, this allows for assessment of heart murmurs.

Newborn infant:

- At rest: 100-180
- Asleep: 80-160
- Active/sick: ≤220

1-12 weeks:

- At rest: 100-220
- Asleep: 80-200
- Active/sick: ≤220

Monitoring of heart rate is particularly important as alterations of heart rate occur with periods of apnea. A period of apnea is usually followed by decreased heart rate, as well as decreased oxygen saturation. Respiratory rates should be monitored as well as heart rate. **Color** should be noted. Pink coloring indicates good perfusion. Generalized mottling or central cyanosis should be investigated further.

BLOOD PRESSURE

Normal blood pressure values for **term infant**:

- Systolic: 56-77 mmHg
- Diastolic: 33-50 mmHg
- MAP: 42-60 mmHg
- Hypertension: Systolic >90 and diastolic >60.

In a **preterm infant**, normal systolic and diastolic values will vary depending on the gestational age and size of the infant. A preterm infant should have a mean arterial pressure that is a number matching the gestational age in weeks of that infant. For example, an infant born at 28 weeks gestation should have an MAP of 28 mmHg. Hypertension in this instance would be systolic >80 and diastolic >50.

Proper **fit of the blood pressure cuff** is imperative to obtain an accurate reading. One must measure the width of the infant's arm in the area that the cuff will be applied. The cuff should be approximately 25% wider than this measurement. A cuff too small results in a BP reading too high and a cuff too large results in a BP reading too low.

HEART SOUNDS
S1

S1 is the heart sound heard as the mitral and tricuspid valves close at the beginning of the contraction of the ventricle (systole). S1 is easiest to hear if the stethoscope is placed at the fourth intercostal space while the infant is supine and calm. If the S1 heard is louder than normal, that means **cardiac output** and **blood flow** are higher than normal. The conditions that can cause this are:

- Patent ductus arteriosus
- Ventricular septal defect
- Tetralogy of Fallot

If the S1 heard is softer or quieter than normal, this is an indication of **lowered cardiac output**, which could be caused by these problems:

- Congestive heart failure
- Myocarditis

S2

S2 is the sound heard when the pulmonic valve and the aortic valve close at the end of the contraction of the ventricles (systole). S2 is easiest to hear at the upper left border of the sternum. S2 is normally split, as the aortic valve closes slightly ahead of the pulmonic valve. In the presence of a cardiac defect, the S2 split becomes wider (the difference in time between the closing of the aortic and pulmonic valve becomes greater). Conditions that cause a **widened S2 split** include:

- Atrial septal defect
- Tetralogy of Fallot
- Pulmonary stenosis
- Ebstein anomaly

Conditions that cause **no split** in the S2 (the two valves close at the same time or one is not closing) include:

- Pulmonary or aortic atresia
- Aortic or pulmonary stenosis
- Persistent pulmonary hypertension

PERIPHERAL PULSES

Peripheral pulses, usually palpated at the brachial or femoral arteries, are graded according to strength. Peripheral pulses may be difficult to palpate in a neonate and should not be relied upon for cardiac assessment. Pulses should always be verified by auscultation:

- 0 = absent
- 1+ = weak
- 2+ = weak to average
- 3+ = strong
- 4+ = bounding

Weak pulses are noted in conditions that cause a decrease in cardiac output. Some of these conditions include:

- Any defect resulting in obstructed blood flow leaving the left ventricle
- Failure of the heart muscle itself
- Shock

Bounding pulses (4+) are noted when there is too much blood coming from the aorta. Some of the conditions that would cause this are:

- Patent ductus arteriosus
- Aortic insufficiency
- Shunts

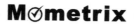

RESPIRATORY RATE OF NEONATE AND BREATH SOUNDS FOUND ON AUSCULTATION

The average **respiratory rate** for newborns is about 35 to 40 (ranging from 30 to 60) times per minute. Tachypnea (>60/min) may occur within the first hour after birth and during the second period of reactivity, but it should not be prolonged. While mild substernal retractions may occur during the first hour, they should not persist, and movement of the chest should be symmetric (asymmetry may indicate pneumothorax). Nasal flaring may also occur during the first hour, but continued flaring may indicate inadequate oxygenation. After birth, the **lungs should be auscultated anteriorly and posteriorly** with almost all lung fields clear. However, during the first hour or two after birth, some fluid may remain in the lungs, so fine rales may be noted. If the newborn was delivered by Cesarean, more fluid may remain in the lungs, so the rales may sound coarse. If the breath sounds are absent (apneic periods of more than 20 seconds) or diminished, breathing is labored, seesaw respirations are evident, or expiratory grunting occurs, these are indications of respiratory distress.

CHEST AND RESPIRATORY ASSESSMENT

The neonate's chest and respiratory status should be evaluated by observation and auscultation. The chest should be symmetric and the ribs flexible. The xiphoid process may protrude slightly. Breasts are sometimes engorged, and the nipples may secrete small amounts of white fluid. Accessory nipples may be noted. Pulmonary function assessment should include anterior and posterior auscultation. Abdominal movement should synchronize with respirations. Periodic breathing is common, but apneic periods should be <20 seconds or they can result in cyanosis or bradycardia. The **Silverman-Anderson Index** is used to evaluate respiratory status. A score of 0 indicates normal findings, and higher scores indicate respiratory distress.

Characteristic	0	1	2
Chest/Abdomen	Rise together with inspiration	Rising abdomen with sinking or lagging upper chest	See-saw movement
Intercostals	No retraction	Minimal retraction	Pronounced retraction
Xiphoid Process	No retraction	Minimal retraction	Pronounced retraction
Nasal Flaring	None	Minimal flaring	Pronounced flaring
Grunt (Expiratory)	None	Grunt heard with auscultation	Audible grunt

GASTROINTESTINAL ASSESSMENT

As the neonate breathes, air enters the **GI system**—first the stomach and then the intestines—within 2-12 hours and enters the colon within 24 hours. Bowel sounds are usually present within 30-60 minutes of birth. The stomach has a capacity of about 50-60 mL and empties intermittently, usually beginning a few minutes after feeding begins and continuing for 2-4 hours after; however, because of immaturity of the cardiac sphincter, the neonate may regurgitate the first few feedings. If regurgitation becomes continuous, further evaluation is indicated. Infants produce little saliva until the salivary glands mature in about 3 months. Term neonates usually pass **meconium** within 8-24 hours, although they may not do so for 48 hours. First meconium is thick, dark, and tarry. **Transitional stools** for the next few days are usually brown to green, after which the child should pass normal stools. Stools of breastfed babies are usually yellow-gold and mushy, and those of formula-fed babies are pale yellow and pasty.

Abdominal and Rectal Assessment

The **abdomen** should be soft, symmetric, and rounded. A distended abdomen with engorged vessels may indicate GI abnormalities. Bowel sounds (present about an hour after birth) should be auscultated prior to palpation. The liver is usually palpable 1-2 cm below the right costal margin, and the tip of the spleen may be palpable in preterm infants only in the left lateral upper quadrant. It should not extend >1 cm below the costal margin. The umbilical cord should be white or blue-white, with two umbilical arteries and one umbilical vein observed and no discharge or bleeding. The presence of only one umbilical artery is associated with GI/GU congenital anomalies. Green/yellow discoloration may indicate meconium staining. The abdomen should be examined carefully for hernias while the infant is at rest and crying.

The **rectal area** should be examined to determine if the anus is present and patent. Meconium is usually passed within 24 hours of birth. Soft swelling in the femoral area may indicate hernia or undescended testicle.

Genitourinary Assessment

Genitourinary assessment requires evaluation of **urinary output**. Many neonates void immediately after birth, although the small amount of urine may be overlooked. About 92% void within 24 hours and 99% by 48 hours. Neonates with **edema** may have higher urinary output as edema recedes. In the first 2 days, most infants void 2-6 times daily, with an output averaging about 15 mL/kg/day. After this, the infant should urinate 5-25 times per day, with volume increasing to 25 mL/kg/day. Urine may appear cloudy because of mucus, and initial voidings have high **specific gravity**, but specific gravity returns to normal levels when the child feeds. Pink stains, referred to as "brick dust spots" often show on the diapers, but these **urate deposits** are of no concern. Female infants may exhibit **pseudomenstruation**—slight bleeding—as maternal hormones are withdrawn.

Male Genitalia Assessment

Male genitalia should be carefully examined to determine if they are clearly male or ambiguous:

- **Penis**: The normal penis is usually about 2.5-3.5 cm long and 1 cm wide with the urinary meatus at the distal end in the glans. Displacement of the urethra is found with epispadias/hypospadias. Micropenis may indicate congenital anomaly. The urethral opening should not be inflamed. The foreskin should adhere to the glans and is tight (if uncircumcised). Small white cysts are sometimes evident on the prepuce.
- **Scrotum**: Skin may be loose/hanging or tight/small with normal slightly darkened skin color and extensive rugae. A large scrotum should be examined by transillumination for hydrocele. If the skin is red and shiny, this may indicate orchitis. Discoloration (bruising) may be present with breech presentation.
- **Testes**: Should be descended and 1.5-2.0 cm in diameter, but may not be in scrotum and may be retractile (moving into the upper scrotum or inguinal canal on stimulation).

Female Genitalia Assessment

Female genitalia should be assessed to determine if there are indications of gender ambiguity, as enlarged clitoris and micropenis may be similar in appearance:

- **Mons**: The labia majora should be symmetric and should cover the clitoris and labia minora in full-term and post-term infants although the labia minora and clitoris are exposed with preterm infants. The urinary meatus should be positioned below the clitoris. Bruising of the labia majora may be evident after vaginal birth.
- **Clitoris**: The clitoris is enlarged in the neonate, and bruising and edema may occur with breech birth. Hypertrophy may indicate hermaphroditism.
- **Vagina**: The vaginal opening should be evident (0.5 cm). Hymenal tag may be observed in the vagina. White or pink-tinged vaginal discharge is common for 2-4 weeks after birth. An imperforate hymen may be indicated by suprapubic mass or mass between labia majora.

Skin Assessment

Skin colors vary with race, but all should be pink-tinged to some degree, as skin pigmentation is slight after birth. Skin characteristics include:

- **Birthmarks**: Dark-skinned infants may have **Mongolian spots** on the buttocks and dorsal area. **Nevus flammeus** (port-wine stain) is a demarcated unraised red-purple lesion caused by capillaries below the epidermis. **Nevus vasculosus** (strawberry mark) is a capillary hemangioma and is a raised, demarcated dark red lesion.
- **Acrocyanosis**: Slight cyanosis of the hands and feet during the 2-6 hours after birth, especially if chilled. Color returns rapidly when skin blanched.
- **Mottling**: Common for hours to weeks after birth and may relate to long periods of apnea/chilling.
- **Harlequin sign**: Deep color on one side of body only for 1-20 minutes; usually transient.
- **Erythema toxicum**: Perifollicular lesions (1-3 mm) white or yellow with pustule appears suddenly over body (except palms and soles); usually transient, cause unknown.
- **Milia**: Small raised white spots on face from exposed sebaceous glands; transient.

Skin Appearance of Neonate

Newborns' skin appearance depends on the development and thickening of their dermis, epidermis, and vernix caseosa. When skin develops during week 15 of gestation, it is initially thin and translucent. By week 20, vernix caseosa production begins. Vernix is a thick, waxy substance secreted by the sebaceous glands and mixed with sloughed-off skin cells, often described as "cheesy." The stratum corneum (protective top layer of the epidermis) develops from weeks 20-24. The epidermis continues to develop and thicken, and is able to form a water barrier by week 32. Near term, the vernix washes away and the skin becomes more wrinkled without its protection:

Gestational Age	Skin Appearance
24-26 Weeks	Translucent, red, many visible blood vessels, and scant vernix
35-40 Weeks	Deep cracks, no visible blood vessels, and thick vernix
42-44 Weeks	Dry, peeling skin, no vernix, and loss of subcutaneous fat

MUSCULOSKELETAL ASSESSMENT

The **musculoskeletal system** should be assessed for muscle tone. Maintenance of fetal position or limp tone may indicate hypoxia, CNS abnormalities, or hypoglycemia. Joint movement should be spontaneous with good muscle tone. Spasticity or floppiness indicates cerebral palsy or other disorders. Jitteriness may indicate hypoglycemia or hypocalcemia.

Extremities should be short, flexed, and able to move symmetrically through range of motion, but without full extension. Arms/legs should be equal in length with feet and hands of normal size (5 digits each). Feet should be flat. Hips should abduct to >60°. Cyanosis or clubbing of nails indicates cardiac anomalies, and yellow-green discoloration indicates meconium staining.

The **back and spine** are examined with the infant in a prone position. The spine should be straight, without a sacral or lumbar curve, which develops only after the child begins to sit. Obvious anomalies, such as spina bifida, and indications of a pilonidal dimple, skin lesions, or tufts of hair that may indicate abnormalities should be noted. C-shaped spine may indicate spina bifida occulta, and lumbar lordosis may indicate myelomeningocele.

ASSESSMENT OF MUSCULAR TONE

Determining the quality of **muscle tone** in a neonate is an important part of neuromuscular assessment. The child is placed supine with the head in neutral position and the LRN nurse moves body parts (arms, legs, head) to determine if the muscle tone is flaccid, jittery, or hypertonic. Neonates are slightly hypertonic so that some resistance should be felt to movement, such as when moving a leg or straightening an arm. Tone should be symmetric. The extremities are usually flexed and legs abducted to the abdomen. This assessment allows the LRN nurse to differentiate common fine tremors or jitteriness found in neonates from seizure activity or nervous system disorders that cause muscular twitching. Normal fine tremors are usually halted by holding or flexing the extremity while seizure activity or twitching does not resolve in this way.

ASSESSMENT OF NEONATAL REFLEXES

Reflex	Eliciting Reflex	Normal Response	Discussion
Palmar Grasping	Stroke the infant's palm.	The infant responds by grasping the finger.	Grasp reflex is stronger in premature infants and fades away at 2 to 3 months of age. Absence indicates CNS deficit or muscle injury.
Rooting	Stroke the side of the infant's cheek.	The infant turns the head in the direction of the touch, and opens mouth to feed.	Rooting reflex helps the infant find and latch onto the mother's breast.
Sucking	Touch the infant's mouth.	The infant sucks.	Premature infants may have an absent or weak suck reflex, as it usually develops around week 32 of gestation. Weak or absent reflex indicates CNS deficit or depression.
Moro (Startle)	Make a loud sound or give the infant a gentle jolt.	The infant extends arms, legs, and neck, then pulls back arms and legs. May also cry.	Moro reflex disappears at 5 to 6 months of age. Asymmetric response indicates peripheral nerve injury, or fracture of long bones, clavicle, or skull.
Blinking	Flash light at eyes.	Eyelids close.	Absence or delay may indicate cerebral palsy, hydrocephalus, and developmental delay.
Tonic Neck (Fencing)	With infant supine, turn head to one side.	Extremities flex on opposite side and extend on same side.	May be incomplete immediately after birth and should diminish by 4 months. Persistence >4 months may indicate neurological abnormalities.
Babinski (Plantar)	Stroke the lateral aspect of the sole from heel to ball of foot.	Hyper-extension of all toes.	Persists until ≤2 years, after which the toes flex.
Trunk Incurvation (Galant)	With infant prone, stroke down one side of the spine (1 inch from spine).	Pelvis turns to stimulated side.	Absence indicates CNS depression or lesion of spinal cord. Should disappear by 4 months.
Tongue Extrusion	Touch tip of tongue.	Neonate pushes tongue out of mouth.	Continuous or repetitive extrusion indicates CNS abnormalities or seizure activity.

> **Review Video: Tonic Neck Response**
> Visit mometrix.com/academy and enter code: 421866

STEPPING REFLEX

If a newborn is held upright with the feet touching a horizontal surface, the contact should make the infant lift one foot and then the other, giving the appearance of walking. This reflex promotes the development of muscles and usually disappears by 4 months. If this reflex is missing, then may be an indication that the infant has a motor nerve defect or other neurological abnormality.

ANAL WINK

The anocutaneous reflex is the reflexive contraction of the anus in response to gentle stroking or stimulation of the skin around the rectum. It occurs in both females and males. Pulling the penis elicits the response in males as well; at one time, this response was believed indicative of sexual abuse, but that has been disproved. Failure of this response indicates that there in an interruption in the reflex arc in the sensory or motor nerves.

ASSESSING MOTOR DEVELOPMENT
PULL-TO-SIT

This test, also known as the head lag test, is conducted with the infant lying in supine position. The infant's arms are grasped with the elbows slightly flexed and the infant pulled into sitting position. The head should be observed carefully as it may lag behind the trunk but should not be completely flexed backward. When the infant reaches the sitting position, the infant should be able to at least briefly bring the head into upright position. If the head consistently lags, this may be an indication of cerebral injury and/or neurobehavioral abnormalities.

TRUNCAL TONE

This test is used to assess hypotonia/floppy infant syndrome. The infant is suspended face down by the abdomen and draped over the examiner's hand. A normal response is for the infant to straighten the back, flex the limbs, and straighten the head while an abnormal response is for the infant to hang in place with the head down and the extremities extended. An abnormal response may indicate CNS disorders or neuromuscular disorders. The most common cause of hypotonia is hypoxic-ischemic encephalopathy.

EYES, NOSE, NECK, AND THROAT ASSESSMENTS

The appearance and movement of the **face** should be symmetric in the neonate and a number of different characteristics examined:

- **Eyes**: Usually blue to blue/gray with white to bluish-white sclera. Small conjunctival hemorrhages and transient strabismus or squint may be evident. Pupils should be equal and reactive. Red retinal reflex should be present. Tears are usually absent during crying. Eye blink test causes lids to close.
- **Nose**: Infants usually breathe through their nose and should be able to breathe easily if mouth is closed. If not, the child should be examined for choanal atresia. Sense of smell is determined if the infant turns toward milk source or away from strong smells, such as alcohol.
- **Neck**: The infant should be able to hold head up slightly while prone, but the head lags when lifted from the supine position because of weak muscles. Neck rigidity may indicate injury to sternocleidomastoid injury.
- **Throat**: The palate should be highly arched, mucous membranes moist, and uvula midline (if bifid, this can indicate submucosal cleft). The infant should exhibit the sucking, rooting, gag, and extrusion reflexes.

MOUTH ASSESSMENT

The mouth should be carefully examined with a gloved finger pressing against the tongue to open the mouth:

- **Lips**: Should be pink, normal-shaped, and symmetric. Thin upper lip with smooth philtrum and short palpebral fissures may indicate fetal alcohol syndrome.
- **Sucking**: Sucking (symmetrical) should occur if lips are touched. Asymmetric movement of the mouth may indicate injury to facial nerve.
- **Gums**: Examined for precocious teeth and Epstein's pearls (keratin-containing cysts).
- **Tongue**: Examined for ridge of frenulum tissue on underside (tongue-tied), although this is not clipped and evidence of protrusion or hypertrophy, which can indicate various disorders, such as Down syndrome and hypothyroidism. Bluish swelling of the frenulum may indicate mucus/salivary gland retention cyst.
- **Mucus membranes**: Examined for color and moisture as cyanosis may indicate respiratory distress and dryness or dehydration. Excessive salivation and drooling may indicate esophageal atresia. White patches on mucus membranes/tongue indicate infection with *Candida albicans*.

STRUCTURES OF THE EAR

The **tympanic membrane** is the eardrum, a thin, semitransparent membrane that separates the external auditory canal from the middle ear. Sound waves cause the membrane to vibrate, transmitting sounds to structures in the middle ear. Three **auditory ossicles** help to transmit the vibrations from the ear drum to structures in the inner ear. These three bones are named the malleus (hammer), incus (anvil), and stapes (stirrup) and are connected to each other by synovial joints. The **cochlea** (snail shell) is located in the inner ear and translates vibrations received from the auditory ossicles into signals that are transmitted to the brain via the vestibulocochlear nerve (cranial nerve VIII).

The following are **structures of the external ear**:

- **Pinna**: All the structures that make up the external ear
- **Helix**: The outermost, curved portion of the ear, which is posterior/superior and has a folded edge
- **Antihelix**: 'C' shaped cartilage that runs on the inside of the helix, separated from the helix by a scooped-out section, called the scapha
- **Tragus**: Small projection just anterior to the external auditory ear canal
- **Antitragus**: Lower cartilaginous portion of the concha, just superior to the fleshy lobe of the ear
- **Concha**: Bowl that surrounds the external auditory canal
- **Lobe**: Fleshy lower portion of the ear that is the traditional site of ear piercing

EAR ASSESSMENT

The ears should be carefully examined for a number of different characteristics:

- **Position**: The insertion point of the top of the ear should be parallel to the inner and outer canthus of the eye. Low-set ears may relate to a number of disorders, such as trisomy 13 and trisomy 18, intellectual disability, and various other disorders.
- **Shape/size**: Ears should be proportionate to head size and symmetric.
- **Pliability**: Ears should be soft and pliable. Cartilage is lacking in premature infants, and the pinna is soft. Cartilage should be firm by 38 to 40 weeks with 2/3 of pinna curving inward.
- **Hearing**: Hearing may be initially assessed by observing response to sudden loud sound. Evoked otoacoustic emissions (EOAE) and auditory brainstem response (ABR) are used for universal hearing screening.
- **Tympanic membrane**: Usually not examined with otoscope because of occlusion with vernix and blood after birth, but should appear gray-white and vascular.

HEAD ASSESSMENT

FONTANELS

The newborn has 8 skull bones and 14 facial bones. Their adjoining edges are bone sutures. Soft spots where the skull flexes along sutures to exit the vagina are **fontanels**. The newborn has 6 fontanels:

- Diamond-shaped anterior fontanel (AF): 2.1 cm
- Triangular posterior fontanel (PF)
- Sphenoid fontanels (2)
- Mastoid fontanels (2)

The AF is the largest and most informative during clinical examination. Fontanels **bulge** when the newborn cries, vomits, lies down, or has hydrocephalus, intracranial tumor, hemorrhage, or meningitis. Fontanels should return to normal when the NNP holds the baby head up and the infant is calm. **Depressed fontanels** indicate the newborn is dehydrated. Conditions associated with an abnormally large AF include hypothyroidism, Down syndrome, achondroplasia, rickets, and increased intracranial pressure. Infants with Down syndrome may have an extra fontanel between the AF and posterior fontanel.

CRANIOTABES

Craniotabes is an area of softened skull found in 30% of newborns. It is softer and more pliable than surrounding tissue and gives way when pressure is applied, as though one is pushing on a ping-pong ball. It is more commonly in premature infants, but can also be found in full-term infants. Usually, craniotabes occurs in the posterior occipital or posterior parietal bones or along the suture lines. Craniotabes is considered to be a normal finding that requires no treatment because it usually resolves by one month of age. Craniotabes may persist longer when it is positioned along a suture line. No work-up is required, but the infant should be carefully examined for indications of disease-related causes of craniotabes, including other conditions that affect bone growth or hardness, such as rickets, syphilis, marasmus, or osteogenesis imperfecta.

CAPUT SUCCEDANEUM AND CEPHALOHEMATOMA

Caput succedaneum and cephalohematoma are both examples of head molding resulting from head trauma during birthing. They can be observed during the newborn period and appear similar upon physical examination because the neonate's head is swollen:

- **Caput succedaneum** is more common. It is a collection of fluid beneath the skin, but superficial to the periosteum. It often occurs when the head presses against the dilating cervix during the birth process. Vacuum-assisted deliveries also contribute to caput succedaneum. The swelling crosses suture lines. Complications are rare. Swelling usually resolves over several days.
- **Cephalohematoma** occurs when blood vessels between the skull and the periosteum rupture, causing a subperiosteal collection of blood. The swelling appears several hours after birth. It does not cross suture lines. Complications such as anemia or hypovolemia may occur if the amount of bleeding is large. The blood will eventually be resorbed and may cause jaundice secondary to the breakdown of red blood cells.

Clinical Laboratory Tests

CAPILLARY BLOOD SAMPLING

Neonatal capillary blood sampling is a common procedure used to acquire small samples of blood for testing of glucose and drug levels, blood gases, electrolytes, urea, blood counts, and other screening tests. If done incorrectly, it can cause pain, trauma, and nerve damage. The lancet should be ≥2.4 mm deep. The baby should be supine. The nurse grasps the foot with one hand holding the ankle with the thumb and index finger and supporting the leg with the other fingers. The infant's heel (bottom, lateral aspect only to avoid nerves in the middle of the foot) should be cleansed thoroughly with water (not alcohol) and air-dried. The skin of the heel should be held tense until after the puncture, and then it is relaxed and the heel lightly compressed to express a drop of blood, which is collected in a capillary tube. Relaxing the pressure and then compressing again will "milk" additional drops. Pressure is applied to the puncture site until bleeding stops and then a dressing is applied.

MICROBIOLOGICAL TESTING

Neonates with exposure to microbiological agents before, during, or after birth may require **microbiological testing:**

- Blood cultures are done to isolate causative agents in order to begin appropriate antibiotic treatment.
- In some cases, microbiological testing of expressed human milk may be indicated.
- Microscopic examination of urine and urine culture may be done to identify urinary pathogens.
- Stool cultures may be done to identify GI pathogens.
- Tracheal secretions may be cultured to identify pathogens causing pneumonia, especially in infants who are ventilated. The findings should be reviewed along with chest radiographs to ensure that positive findings don't just represent tracheal colonization alone.
- Gram stain and scraping of conjunctiva may be done to identify gonococcal conjunctivitis.
- Skin culture may be indicated for the infant with a skin infection.

CLINICAL LABORATORY URINE TESTS

Urine testing includes:

- **pH** should range from 4.5 to 9.0. An alkaline (high) pH can be caused by urinary tract infections, diarrhea, or kidney infection. An acidic (low) pH may reflect lung disease, hyperglycemia, or diarrhea with dehydration.
- **Specific gravity** ranges from 1.001 to 1.040 (usually about 1.015).

About 2% of full-term infants have asymptomatic bacteriuria, but this increases to about 10% for preterm infants. However, urinalysis alone is not an effective test to determine if an infant has a urinary tract infection because the neonate's urine usually contains leukocytes ($\geq 25/mm^3$ in males and $\geq 50/mm^3$ in females), so urine cultures of infants younger than 3 days often show poor results, even in the presence of infection. Thus, blood cultures (and in some cases cultures of CSF) are preferred if infection is suspected, as neonates are more likely to develop kidney infections and sepsis from cystitis than older infants. The most common infective agent is *Escherichia coli* although *Candida* and *Staphylococcus* are common with prolonged hospitalization.

SERUM CREATININE LEVELS AND RENAL FUNCTION

Serum creatinine is a marker of renal function. Creatinine is a byproduct of creatine phosphate metabolism in muscle. **Serum creatinine levels** reflect the balance between the production of creatinine and its clearance by the kidneys. Creatinine is filtered by the kidneys and generally not reabsorbed by the tubules, so it is a good indicator of the glomerular filtration rate (GFR). Elevated serum creatinine at birth may reflect elevated maternal levels, especially if the mother has toxemia. The serum creatinine level normally drops in the first few weeks of life. Premature infants often have a higher serum creatinine level and take longer to reach a normal level, because the GFR is lower in premature infants and immature kidneys allow creatinine to be reabsorbed across leaky tubules. Certain disease states (such as respiratory distress syndrome with mechanical ventilation) are associated with decreased GFR.

CLINICAL LABORATORY TESTS FOR ABGS

Arterial blood gases (ABGs) are monitored to assess the effectiveness of oxygenation, ventilation, and acid-base status and to determine oxygen flow rates. Partial pressure of a gas is that exerted by each gas in a mixture of gases, proportional to its concentration, based on total atmospheric pressure of 760 mmHg at sea level. Normal values for children include:

- Acidity/alkalinity (pH): 7.26-7.44
- Partial pressure of carbon dioxide ($PaCO_2$): 35-45 mmHg
- Partial pressure of oxygen (PaO_2): >80 mmHg
- Bicarbonate concentration (HCO_3^-): 22-28 mEq/L
- Oxygen saturation (SaO_2): >92%

The relationship between these elements, particularly the $PaCO_2$ and the PaO_2, indicates respiratory status. For example, $PaCO_2$ >55 and the PaO_2 <60 in an infant previously in good health indicates respiratory failure. There are many issues to consider. Ventilator management may require a higher $PaCO_2$ to prevent barotrauma and a lower PaO_2 to reduce oxygen toxicity. Premature infants may need lower PaO_2 to prevent retinopathy of prematurity.

INVASIVE BLOOD GAS MONITORING

Invasive blood gas monitoring options include the following:

- **Arterial blood gas (ABG)** is the most informative measurement of blood gas status. If an infant has an umbilical artery catheter, it is easily obtained by aspirating 1-2 mL of blood.
- **Venous blood gas (VBG)** is easier to obtain if an arterial catheter is not in place. In order to compare the values in the VBG with an ABG, make the following calculations:
  o Add 0.05 to the pH of the VBG.
  o Subtract 5-10 mmHg from the $PaCO_2$ of the VBG.
- **Capillary Blood Gas (CBG)** can be obtained with a heel stick, without a venous or arterial line, but the values obtained in a CBG are the least accurate and are rarely useful. The oxygen status of the neonate (reflected in the PaO_2) can be estimated by clinical evaluation of the neonate and a noninvasive pulse oximeter reading.

> **Review Video: Newborn Cord Blood Gases**
> Visit mometrix.com/academy and enter code: 188117

CLINICAL LABORATORY TESTS FOR RED BLOOD CELLS

Red blood cells (RBCs or erythrocytes) are biconcave disks that contain hemoglobin, which carries oxygen throughout the body. The heme portion of the cell contains iron, which binds to the oxygen. RBCs live about 120 days in adults but this is reduced 20-25% in neonates and 50% in preterm infants. The RBCs are destroyed and their hemoglobin is recycled or excreted. **Normal values of red blood cell** count vary by age:

- Neonate: 4.1-6.1 million per mm^3
- 2-6 months: 3.8-5.6 million per mm^3

The most common disorders of RBCs are those that interfere with production, leading to various types of **anemia**:

- Blood loss
- Hemolysis
- Bone marrow failure

The **morphology** of RBCs may vary depending upon the type of anemia:

- Size: normocytes, microcytes, macrocytes
- Shape: spherocytes (round), poikilocytes (irregular), drepanocytes (sickled)
- Color (reflecting the concentration of hemoglobin): normochromic, hypochromic

CLINICAL LABORATORY TESTS FOR HGB, HCT, MCV, RETICULOCYTE COUNT, AND PLATELETS

Additional laboratory tests specific to red blood cells include the following:

- **Hemoglobin:** carries oxygen and is decreased in anemia and increased in polycythemia
  - Neonate: 14.5-22.5 g/dL
  - 2 months: 9.0-14.0 g/dL

- **Hematocrit:** indicates the proportion of RBCs in a liter of blood (usually about 3 times the hemoglobin number)
  - Neonate: 48-69%
  - 3 days: 44-75%
  - 2 months: 28-42%

- **Mean corpuscular volume (MCV):** indicates the size of RBCs and can differentiate types of anemia (For adults, <80 is microcytic and >100 is macrocytic, but this varies with age.)
  - Neonate: 95-121 μm^3
  - 0.5-2 years: 70-86 μm^3

- **Reticulocyte count:** measures marrow production and should rise with anemia
  - 0.5-1.5% of total RBCs

- **Platelets:** essential for clotting
  - 150,000-400,000
  - may increase to >1 million with iron deficiency anemia or decrease to <100,000 during acute infection

CLINICAL LABORATORY TESTS FOR WBCs

Leukocytes are white blood cells (WBCs). Normal total values vary according to age. The differential is the percentage of each type of WBC out of the total. The differential will shift with infection or allergies, but should return to normal values:

Item	Neonate	1 Day	2 Weeks	1 Month
WBCs (1000s/mm³)	9.0-30.0	9.4-34.0	5.0-20.0	5.0-19.5.
Myelocytes	0%	0%	0%	0%
Neutrophils (Bands)	9.1%	9.2%	5.5%	4.5%
Neutrophils (Segs)	52%	52%	34%	30%
Lymphocytes	31%	31%	48%	56%
Monocytes	5.8%	5.8%	8.8%	6.5%
Eosinophils	2.2%	2.0%	3.1%	2.8%
Basophils	0.6%	0.5%	0.4%	0.5%

CLINICAL LABORATORY TESTS FOR PITUITARY HORMONES

The **anterior pituitary gland (adenohypophysis)** produces hormones that are critical for growth and development:

- **Growth hormone** (GH) promotes growth of bones and muscles and promotes protein synthesis and metabolism of fat but decreases carbohydrate metabolism. Normal values:
  - Cord blood: 8-40 µg/L
  - 1 day: 5-50 µg/L
  - 1 week: 5-25 µg/L

- **Thyroid stimulating hormone** (TSH) stimulates secretion of thyroid hormones. Normal values:
  - 0-3 days: <20 mIU/L

- **Adrenocorticotropic hormone** (ACTH) stimulates the adrenal glands to produce glucocorticoids, androgens, and mineralocorticoids. Abnormalities can result in Cushing's disease or Addison's disease. Normal values:
  - Cord blood: 11-25 pmol/L
  - Neonate: 2-41 pmol/L

The **posterior pituitary gland (neurohypophysis)** stores hormones produced by the hypothalamus, critical to renal function. **Antidiuretic hormone (ADH)** controls the reabsorption of fluids in the kidney tubules. Changes in serum osmolality stimulate or depress ADH secretion, so values vary:

- Serum osmolality 270-280 mOsm/kg: ADH 0-1.4 pmol/L
- Serum osmolality 280-285 mOsm/kg: ADH 0.5-2.3 pmol/L
- Serum osmolality 285-290 mOsm/kg: ADH 0.9-4.6 pmol/L

CLINICAL LABORATORY TESTS FOR THYROID HORMONES

The **thyroid gland** produces hormones critical for metabolism and growth. They are amino acids that contain iodine and are stored in the thyroid until needed by the body. The thyroid gland takes iodide from the blood and utilizes it to produce hormones. Thyroid hormone production is controlled by the thyroid-stimulating hormone (TSH) produced by the pituitary gland and the thyrotropin-releasing hormone (TRH) produced by the hypothalamus. Together, the thyroid hormones increase metabolic rate and protein and bone turnover. They are necessary for the growth and development of the fetus and infant. Thyroid hormones include:

- **Thyroxine** (T_4) is a weak hormone that maintains the body's metabolism in a steady state.
  - Neonate: 10-36 pmol/L
- **Triiodothyronine** (T_3) is about 5 times stronger than thyroxine and can respond quickly to metabolic needs.
  - All ages: 4.0-7.4 pmol/L
- **Thyrocalcitonin** is secreted in response to serum calcium levels and reduces the serum level of calcium and phosphate by increasing deposits in bones, aiding ossification and bone development.
  - Male: <19 ng/L
  - Female: <14 ng/L

CLINICAL LABORATORY TESTS FOR INFANTS WITH HIV POSITIVE MOTHERS

The immunological status of infants with **HIV-positive mothers** is assessed in a series of tests performed over the first two years in order to institute treatment and decrease likelihood of transmission to 2% or less.

ELISA and rapid tests are used to identify those neonates who are HIV-positive at birth. Confirmatory testing is done with the neonate's blood (not cord blood due to possibility of maternal contamination), usually using DNA PCR, which is about 99% sensitive by 1 month, but does NOT detect very recent infection (for instance, infection acquired during the birth). RNA PCR may be used for some subtypes of HIV infection.

In the United States, testing is based on identifying mothers with HIV. If the mother's status is not known, then some states require mandatory testing of the infant, but laws vary. Based on positive findings, treatment is begun within 24 hours without waiting for confirmatory test results. Subsequent testing is done at 2, 4, 12, and 18 months.

General Management

Resuscitation and Stabilization

MINIMUM NEONATAL RESUSCITATION EQUIPMENT

The minimal equipment that should be present for neonatal resuscitation includes the following:

- **Temperature**: Thermometer, warmed drying towels, warmed swaddling blankets, radiant warmer, phototherapy equipment.
- **Respiration**: Oxygen tank and hood, flow meter, humidifier, heater, tubing, nasal prongs. Bag and mask set-up (assorted sizes). Laryngoscope with size 0 and 1 blades. Endotracheal tubes, sizes 2.5-4. Bulb syringe, suction catheters (sizes 6, 8, and 10 Fr.), suction canister. Cardiorespiratory monitor, oxygen analyzer.
- **Fluids**: IV needles and tubing, infusion pump, umbilical catheters (sizes 2.5 and 5 Fr.). Blood pressure monitor, pulse oximeter. Isotonic saline, D10W, sodium bicarbonate. If transfusions are done here, blood drainage system, volume expander, and blood warmer.
- **Drugs**: Epinephrine, Naloxone.
- **Procedures**: Various sterile surgical packs, dressings, chest tubes, scalpels, hemostat. Arterial blood gas equipment and portable x-ray machine.

ABCs OF NEONATAL RESUSCITATION

The ABCs of resuscitation are a device to help remember in what order to do the steps of the resuscitation process. In this device, the letters stand for the following:

- **Airway**: An airway should be established as the very first thing to tend to. If there is no airway, air cannot be moved during resuscitation attempts. This step includes clearing the mouth and nose of secretions and properly positioning the infant in the "sniff" position.
- **Breathing**: This step involves initiating breathing after the airway has been established. This can be done with stimulation, supplemental oxygen, or through artificial ventilation. Oxygen should be initiated at 21% (up to 30% in preterm neonates) and titrated as needed.
- **Circulation**: Once an airway is open and breathing has been established, then circulation is considered. Chest compressions or the administration of volume expanders may be indicated. Epinephrine is only indicated if the heart rate remains <60 despite warming, ventilation, and chest compressions.

ESTABLISHING AIRWAY AND STIMULATING RESPIRATIONS

To **establish an airway**, the infant is placed supine with the head slightly extended in the "sniffing" position. A small neck roll may be placed under the shoulders to maintain this position in a very small premature infant. Once the proper position is established, the mouth and nose are suctioned (mouth first, to prevent reflex aspiration of secretions when the nose is suctioned) with a bulb syringe or catheter if necessary. The infant's head can be turned momentarily to the side to allow secretions to pool in the cheek where they can be more easily suctioned and removed to establish the airway. **Stimulating** the newborn is often all that is needed to initiate spontaneous respirations. This tactile stimulation can be accomplished by gently rubbing the infant's back or trunk. Another technique used to provide stimulation is flicking or rubbing the soles of the feet. Slapping neonates as stimulation is no longer practiced and should NOT be used.

ADMINISTRATION OF FREE-FLOW OXYGEN

If an infant remains cyanotic in the chest area (central cyanosis) after the initial steps of resuscitation have taken place, administering **free-flow oxygen** is the next step to take. Free-flow oxygen is administered to the neonate by the use of either a mask hooked up to an oxygen source or by the use of the oxygen tubing itself. If the tubing alone is used, the nurse can hold the tube with a cupped hand to help direct and concentrate the oxygen at the infant's airway. Free flow oxygen should be administered at a rate of 5 L/minute, initiated at 21% (up to 30% in preterm neonates). If the infant starts to turn pink, the oxygen can be carefully and slowly removed while continuing to closely monitor the infant for returning cyanosis. If the infant remains centrally cyanotic after the administration of free-flow oxygen, bag and mask ventilation must be considered as the next step.

BAG AND MASK VENTILATION

Ventilation using a bag and mask is indicated when one or more of the following occurs and has not responded to other resuscitation attempts:

- Apnea that does not respond to tactile stimulation such as rubbing the chest or back or flicking the soles of the feet
- Gasping respirations
- Heart rate of <100 bpm, determined by auscultation at the apex of the heart or palpation of the base of the umbilical cord
- Central cyanosis that persists after administering free-flow oxygen (Acrocyanosis alone is NOT an indication for the need for further oxygenation or ventilation.)

The flowmeter is set at 5-10 L/min, and opening breath pressures of 30-40 cmH$_2$O are used for full term infants and 20-25 cmH$_2$O for preterm. Ventilation is done at 40-60 breaths/min with pressure of 15-20 cmH$_2$O for normal lungs and 20-50 cmH$_2$O for immature or compromised lungs.

FLOW-INFLATING BAG AND MASK VENTILATION

Bag and mask ventilation is indicated for persistent apnea or gasping respirations, bradycardia (<100 bpm), and persistent cyanosis unrelieved by free-flowing oxygen.

Flow-inflating bag and mask (connected to oxygen flow, which inflates bag) equipment includes:

- Oxygen inlet
- Flow control valve
- Pressure manometer attachment
- Patient outlet for mask attachment

Advantages: Flow-inflating bag and mask ventilation has the ability to deliver anywhere from 21% (room air) to 100% oxygen; any pressure desired can be set. This type of bag and mask also has the ability to maintain positive end-expiratory pressure (PEEP) and CPAP.

Disadvantages: Because this bag must be connected to a gas (oxygen) source to inflate, it can only be used where a gas supply exists. It requires some experience to deliver the desired quantity of air with each breath. The high pressures possible with this type of equipment make overinflation of the lungs possible, resulting in pneumothorax. A complete seal is necessary to deliver a tidal volume.

SELF-INFLATING BAG AND MASK VENTILATION

Self-inflating bag and mask (does not require gas source) equipment includes:

- Air inlet
- Oxygen inlet
- Patient outlet for mask attachment
- Valve assembly
- Oxygen reservoir
- Pop-off valve
- Pressure manometer attachment

Advantages: Self-inflating bag and mask ventilation is simple to use and does not require much practice or experience to operate. It can be operated anywhere, even if no oxygen source is near, and can easily deliver a tidal volume.

Disadvantages: These bags usually have a pop-off valve that will open at a pressure set by the manufacturer to prevent over inflation of the lungs. This valve popping off can prevent the ability to deliver enough pressure to ventilate very noncompliant lungs. Another disadvantage is that if 90% or higher oxygen delivery is desired, this equipment must have a reservoir attached to deliver this concentration. The inability to deliver PEEP is also a disadvantage to the self-inflating bag and mask.

GASTRIC SUCTIONING FOLLOWING NEONATAL RESUSCITATION

When an infant is resuscitated using a bag and mask, air is inadvertently pumped into the stomach as it is being pumped into the lungs, so **gastric suctioning** is necessary. Once respirations have been stabilized, either spontaneously or with mechanical ventilation, the stomach should be aspirated to remove any air pumped into it. If the air is left in the abdomen, it remains distended, causing an upward pressure on the lungs; this compromises lung capacity and breathing effort. Use this procedure:

1. Select an orogastric catheter or size 8 Fr. feeding tube.
2. Measure the distance from the nose to the earlobe, then to the xiphoid.
3. Mark the tube at this distance.
4. Advance the tube to the mark.
5. Attach a 20 mL syringe to the tube.
6. Aspirate the contents of the stomach.
7. Leave the tube in place, open to air, and taped to the infant's cheek to keep the stomach decompressed.

CHEST COMPRESSIONS

If **chest compressions** are indicated for resuscitation, these steps should be followed.

1. Position the neonate in the "sniffing" position with the neck slightly extended.
2. Make sure there is firm support for the infant's back.
3. Using a two-finger technique, proceed with the compressions on the lower third of the sternum with a depth of one third of the anterior-posterior diameter of the chest. The compression rate is 90 compressions per minute and 30 breaths per minute, equaling 120 "events" per minute. Essentially, one cycle is 3 compressions and 1 breath every 2 seconds.
4. When performing the compressions, the hands should be placed in a circle around the chest to provide support to the infant's back. The ratio of compressions to breaths should be 3:1.

5. Check the heart rate again after 30 seconds of compressions—about 45 compressions total.
6. If the heart rate is less than 60 beats per minute, continue with another round of compressions, but if the rate is 60 beats per minute or higher, stop compressions.

During chest compressions, oxygen should be delivered at a concentration of 100%.

INDICATIONS FOR STOPPING OR NOT PROVIDING RESUSCITATION TO NEWBORN

The decision to **discontinue or not perform resuscitative efforts** in the newborn (DNR) is very difficult to make. Whenever possible, the decision to withhold or stop resuscitative efforts in the newborn should be made by the attending physician with parental input, especially in situations with variable degrees of morbidity and mortality. Infants born under these conditions associated with certain death should not be resuscitated:

- Extreme prematurity (less than 23 weeks gestation)
- Extremely low birth weight (less than 400 grams)
- Congenital anomalies that are incompatible with life (anencephaly, trisomy 13 or 18)

Discontinue resuscitation of the infant who has not responded to appropriate resuscitation for 10 minutes and shows no signs of life (no heart rate or respiratory effort).

RESUSCITATION MEDICATIONS

EPINEPHRINE

Epinephrine is a naturally-occurring hormone produced by the adrenal glands. Epinephrine is used to resuscitate both adults and children. It is a sympathomimetic that supports the circulatory system by:

- Increasing heart rate
- Increasing contraction strength
- Vasoconstricting vessels in the skin, mucosa, and circulation of the gastrointestinal tract, causing a rise in blood pressure

If positive pressure ventilation and chest compressions have not caused the neonate's heart rate to rise above 60 beats per minute during resuscitation, then epinephrine is indicated. The recommended IV dose is 0.01-0.03 mg/kg. The usual concentration of epinephrine is 1:10,000 or 0.1 mg/mL. Endotracheal administration is not widely recommended, but may be used if no IV access is available. Higher doses are required for endotracheal administration (0.05-0.1 mg/kg).

VOLUME EXPANDERS

Volume expanders used in neonatal resuscitation include:

- Normal saline
- Ringer's Lactate
- O- blood, or blood that has been crossmatched with the mother

Prepare 40 mL in a syringe or IV. Give 10 mL/kg over 5-10 minutes. Repeat if necessary. Rapid infusion of a large volume causes intraventricular hemorrhage. (5% albumin in saline is no longer the solution of choice.) Consider volume expanders in instances where neonatal blood loss is suspected and/or the neonate is showing signs of shock that is not responding to other resuscitative efforts. Blood loss occurs due to trauma of the placenta or umbilical cord, or with neonatal hemolysis. Shock is inadequate perfusion in tissues and organs. Signs and symptoms of shock are pallor, cold extremities, neurological depression, and weak pulse.

Naloxone Hydrochloride

Naloxone hydrochloride, an opiate antagonist, is not used in the routine resuscitation of an infant but is used in one very specific situation following birth. Naloxone is considered the antidote for narcotics administered to the mother of the infant within 4 hours of birth if the infant shows signs of serious respiratory depression from secondary absorption. If the mother of the infant has narcotics in her system as a result of an addiction to narcotics rather than as treatment for labor pain, however, naloxone cannot be given to this infant. If naloxone is given to an infant born to a narcotic-addicted mother, the drug will cause a severe abstinence reaction in the newborn that can result in seizure.

Neonatal Transport

An infant that is severely compromised at birth or <32 weeks gestation often requires **transport** to specialized neonatal care units, usually because of respiratory distress, preterm birth, congenital anomalies, and suspected cardiac abnormalities. The infant should be resuscitated and stabilized prior to transport. Communication with the regional center should be immediate and detailed. The **STABLE program** (**s**ugar, **t**emperature, **a**rtificial breathing, **b**lood pressure, **l**ab work, and **e**motional support) can guide efforts to stabilize the infant. The transport team must take copies of all records and lab reports. Transport teams may include NICU nurses, NNPs, physicians, and respiratory therapists. Adequate supplies (similar to those needed for resuscitation) must be available as well as oxygen, air-blended mixtures, monitors, and transport incubators. The incubator must control temperature while allowing access. Insulating material may be needed for very cold environments.

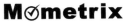

Fluid and Electrolytes and Glucose Homeostasis

RENAL SYSTEM AND FLUID MAINTENANCE

Maintenance of adequate fluid volume can be difficult in neonates. The pediatric renal system matures over the first 3 years of life. The nephrons in the young infant's kidneys are immature and the glomerular filtration rate is low because of impaired ability to filter urine until about 6-12 months of age. Also, the ability to concentrate or dilute urine may not reach adult levels until ages 2-3 years. Premature infants may have additional renal abnormalities, such as decreased creatinine clearance or impaired sodium retention. Infants are less tolerant of both dehydration and fluid overload. The 4-2-1 rule is used to determine maintenance fluid requirements. Sum the following:

- 4 mL/kg/hr for the first 10 kg weight
- 2 mL/kg/hr for the next 10 kg weight
- 1 mL/kg/hr for any remaining weight

Often a programmable infusion pump or buret with microdrip is used to manage fluids because the balance must be maintained within a narrow range.

BODY FLUID/FLUID BALANCE

Body fluid is primarily **intracellular fluid (ICF)** or **extracellular fluid (ECF)**. Infants and children have proportionately more extracellular fluid (ECF) than adults. At birth, more than half of the child's weight is ECF, but by 3 years of age, the balance is more like adults:

- ECF: 20-30% (interstitial fluid, plasma, transcellular fluid)
- ICF: 40-50% (fluid within the cells)

The fluid compartments are separated by semipermeable membranes that allow fluid and solutes (electrolytes and other substances) to move by osmosis. Fluid also moves through diffusion, filtration, and active transport. In fluid volume deficit, fluid is out of balance and ECF is depleted; an overload occurs with increased concentration of sodium and retention of fluid. Signs of **fluid deficit** include:

- Thirsty, restless to lethargic
- Increasing pulse rate, tachycardia
- Fontanels depressed (infants)
- Decreased urinary output
- Normal BP progressing to hypotension
- Dry mucous membranes
- 3-10% decrease in body weight

TOTAL BODY WATER

Total body water (TBW) content is the percentage of the body composed of water. An extremely premature infant (24-26 weeks of gestation) has a TBW content of 90%. The TBW content drops to 75-80% at full term (40 weeks), compared to 60-65% in adults. Because preterm infants have such a high percentage of TBW, any fluid loss can cause severe problems. Physiological diuresis is fluid loss from the extracellular space, and this is the initial type of fluid loss in neonates. Because intracellular space is relatively small in neonates, there is less fluid available to shift into the extracellular space, so the effects of extracellular fluid loss are much more pronounced on infants than adults. Diuresis continues during the first week after birth, so full term infants lose 5-10% of their weight, and premature infants lose 10-15% of their weight. Diuresis diminishes but slowly continues over the first 1-2 years of life. The typical toddler has a TBW content of 60%.

SENSIBLE AND INSENSIBLE WATER LOSS

Sensible water losses occur via urination, stool, and gastric drainage, and can be accurately measured. **Insensible water losses** (IWL) occur as water evaporates from the skin (2/3) or the respiratory tract (1/3). IWL cannot be directly measured. Premature neonates have thin skin that allows for increased amounts of evaporative water loss. As the skin matures and the stratum corneum develops (around 31 weeks of gestation) less water is lost through the skin. A full-term neonate will have an IWL of 12 mL/kg/day at 50% humidity. Factors that increase IWL include prematurity, radiant warmers, phototherapy, fever, low humidity, and tachypnea. Infants who are mechanically ventilated should receive humidified oxygen to negate the IWL through their lungs. The nurse must take into account IWL when providing fluids to neonates.

FLUID DEFICIT

Fluid deficit must also be carefully estimated and managed. For the neonate, **fluid deficit** should be replaced over 3 hours, with half the first hour and a quarter in each of the remaining 2 hours. Fluid deficit is calculated by first finding the **maintenance fluid requirement** using the 4-2-1 rule (4 mL/kg/hr for the first 10 kg of weight of the neonate, then 2 mL/kg/hr for the next 10 kg, and 1 mL/kg/hr for any remaining kg). Preoperative deficits usually are treated with lactated Ringer's or normal saline (which may cause hyperchloremic acidosis). Glucose-containing fluids may contribute to hyperglycemia.

Fluid replacement must account for both blood loss and third-space loss. Blood loss may be replaced with lactated Ringer's (3 mL for each mL of blood loss) or 5% albumin colloid (1 mL for each mL of blood loss) to maintain hematocrit at a predetermined adequate minimal level:

- Infants and neonates: >30% (may be as high as 40-50%)
- Older children: 20-26%

Blood is replaced with packed red blood cells when the allowable blood loss threshold is exceeded. **Allowable blood loss** is calculated by the following formula based on the infant's average hematocrit:

$$\text{Average hematocrit} = \frac{\text{Initial hematocrit} + \text{Final hematocrit}}{2}$$

$$\text{Allowable blood loss} = \frac{\text{Est. blood volume} \times (\text{Initial hematocric} - \text{Final hematocrit})}{\text{Average hematocrit}}$$

Blood loss should be monitored carefully to determine when it exceeds the allowable blood loss. **Volume of packed red blood cell replacement (PRBC)** is based on the weight, current hematocrit, and desired hematocrit of the patient. If a massive transfusion is required (blood loss exceeds 50% of total blood volume in 3 hours), then the transfusion of platelets and FFP is also indicated.

Third space loss after surgery can only be estimated based on the degree of trauma:

- Minor: 3-4 mL/kg/hr
- Moderate: 5-6 mL/kg/hr
- Severe: 7-10 mL/kg/hr

Lactated Ringer's is most commonly used to replace third space loss.

PRETERM NEONATAL FLUID BALANCE
PRETERM NEONATAL URINARY OUTPUT

The pre-term neonate has 3 **phases of urine output**:

1. **Oliguric phase:** Output is lower than intake during the first 12-24 hours after birth. The premature infant's urine output may be less than 1 mL/kg/hr in the oliguric phase.
2. **Diuretic phase:** Output is greater than intake 24-72 hours after birth. The premature infant's urine output may be greater than 5 mL/kg/hr in the diuretic phase, so the infant's weight decreases.
3. **Adaptive phase:** Output is appropriate after 72 hours, as the kidneys adjust to the rate of input. The urine output more closely reflects the real fluid status of the infant.

The appropriate response to decreased fluid intake is to decrease urine output and produce concentrated urine (elevate the specific gravity). The appropriate response to excessive fluids is to increase urine output and produce dilute urine (lower the specific gravity).

FLUID REQUIREMENTS OF PREMATURE NEWBORNS

The nurse must correctly manage fluid for the premature infant, because the infant's immature kidneys have a very limited ability to concentrate or dilute urine. Premature infants are less able to compensate for dehydration or fluid overload than infants who are several months old. **Total fluid requirements** for a newborn are equal to maintenance requirements (sensible plus insensible fluid losses), in addition to the amount required for growth. Typically, the total requirement ranges from 100-150 mL/kg/day of fluid, but many conditions exist that either increase or decrease fluid requirements. Closely monitor these indicators of hydration status: daily weight change, urine output, and urine osmolality. Conditions that increase fluid requirements include:

- Prematurity
- Elevated body and environmental temperatures
- Phototherapy
- Decreased environmental humidity
- Gastroschisis or omphalocele secondary to increased evaporation from exposed tissue

NEONATAL ELECTROLYTE BALANCE

SODIUM, HYPONATREMIA, AND HYPERNATREMIA

Sodium (Na) regulates fluid volume, osmolality, acid-base balance, and activity in the muscles, nerves and myocardium. It is the primary cation (positive ion) in ECF, necessary to maintain ECF levels needed for tissue perfusion:

- Normal neonatal value: 133-146 mEq/L
- Hyponatremia: <133 mEq/L (critical value <120)
- Hypernatremia: >146 mEq/L (critical value >160)

Hyponatremia develops with excessive water gain or excessive sodium loss. Late symptoms include apnea, irritability, twitching, and seizures when serum sodium drops below 120 mEq/L, but infants are often asymptomatic. In the first days after birth, hyponatremia is usually secondary to excessive water gain (dilutional hyponatremia), reflected in a weight gain or absence of expected weight loss. Conditions causing dilutional hyponatremia include syndrome of inappropriate antidiuretic hormone (SIADH), renal dysfunction with decreased urine output, and overhydration. **Treatment** involves identifying and treating underlying cause, restricting fluid, and replacing sodium if necessary.

Hypernatremia is caused by dehydration, excess use of sodium-containing solutions, and diabetes insipidus. Late symptoms include seizures. The **underlying cause** must be identified and treated.

HYPOCALCEMIA

The ionized form of **serum calcium** is the only biologically available form in the body.

- Cord: 8.2-11.2 mg/dL
- 0-10 days: 7.6-10.4 mg/dL
- 11 days to 1 yr: 9.0-11.0 mg/dL
- Critical value for hypocalcemia: <7 mg/dL

Signs of **hypocalcemia** include jitteriness, irritability, stridor, tetany, high-pitched cry, seizures, and decreased myocardial contractility, with decreased cardiac output. An electrocardiogram may show a prolonged QT interval and a flattened T-wave. Early-onset hypocalcemia usually presents in the first 3 days of life and is associated with prematurity, birth asphyxia, and infants of diabetic mothers. Late-onset hypocalcemia presents after the first week of life and is associated with DiGeorge syndrome, hyperphosphatemia, vitamin D deficiency, magnesium deficiency, diuretic therapy, and hypoparathyroidism. Hypocalcemia is treated with a slow infusion of calcium gluconate. Rapid infusion may cause bradycardia. Tissue infiltration with calcium causes necrosis, so the administration site must be monitored.

HYPERCALCEMIA

Hypercalcemia (>12 mg/dL) is rare, occurring less often than hypocalcemia. Signs of hypercalcemia include vomiting, constipation, hypertension, hypotonia, lethargy, and seizures. Possible causes of hypercalcemia include congenital hyperparathyroidism, maternal hypoparathyroidism, hypervitaminosis D, hyperthyroidism, hypophosphatasia, subcutaneous fat necrosis, Williams syndrome, and adrenal insufficiency. Idiopathic hypercalcemia is diagnosed when no other cause can be found. Iatrogenic hypercalcemia occurs because of excess administration of calcium or vitamin D or phosphate deprivation. Treatment depends on the exact cause but may include:

- Correction of the underlying cause
- Furosemide (Lasix) after adequate hydration to increase calcium excretion
- Glucocorticoids to inhibit intestinal absorption of calcium
- Use of low calcium and low vitamin D formulas

MAGNESIUM, HYPERMAGNESEMIA, AND HYPOMAGNESEMIA

Magnesium is the second most abundant intercellular cation:

- Normal neonatal value: 1.5-2.2 mg/dL
- Critical values for neonates: <1.2 mg/dL and >3 mg/dL

Hypermagnesemia most commonly results from maternal administration of magnesium prior to delivery. Maternal serum chemistries are reflected in newborn blood values. Magnesium is used in the pregnant woman as a tocolytic agent to stop pre-term labor and also for treatment of pre-eclampsia. Signs of hypermagnesemia in an infant include hypotonia, hyporeflexia, constipation, low blood pressure, apnea, and marked flushing secondary to vasodilatation. Elevated magnesium blocks neurosynaptic transmission by interfering with the release of acetylcholine. Treatment is usually supportive, as the elevated serum magnesium will be cleared by the infant's kidneys. In severe cases, the infant may require respiratory and/or blood pressure support.

Hypomagnesemia in neonates occurs with preterm birth, respiratory distress syndrome, and neonatal hepatitis. **Symptoms** include:

- Neuromuscular excitability/tetany
- Seizure and coma
- Tachycardia with ventricular arrhythmias
- Respiratory depression

Treatment includes diagnosing the underlying cause and administering magnesium replacement.

SERUM POTASSIUM CHANGES AFTER BIRTH

Electrolyte levels in the newborn reflect those of the mother at birth. Shortly after birth, within the first 24-72 hours, **serum potassium** concentrations are expected to rise without exogenous potassium delivery and with normal renal function, resulting from a shift of potassium from the intracellular space to the extracellular space. **Potassium shift** is more extreme in premature infants and can result in life-threatening hyperkalemia. Over the next several days, the potassium level will fall to normal in an infant with normally functioning kidneys. Preterm infants' serum electrolytes, including potassium, should be carefully monitored in the first 48 hours of life and until values have stabilized.

- Normal neonatal values: 3.7-5.9 mEq/L
- Hyperkalemia: >6 mEq/L (critical value: >6.5 mEq/L)
- Hypokalemia: <3.5 mEq/L (critical value: <2.5 mEq/L)

HYPERKALEMIA

Hyperkalemia is a serum potassium level greater than 6 mEq/L in a non-hemolyzed blood sample. Squeezing the infant's heel too hard during blood collection can cause the sample to hemolyze and give an artificially elevated laboratory value. Causes of hyperkalemia in the newborn fall into 3 categories:

- Excessive potassium supplementation
- Transcellular shift, where potassium concentrated inside cells moves outside cells, due to low pH, cellular damage, intraventricular hemorrhage, or trauma
- Decreased potassium secretion by the kidneys, due to congenital adrenal hyperplasia with elevated secretion of aldosterone or renal failure

Cardiac manifestations of hyperkalemia include potentially fatal arrhythmias like bradycardia, tachycardia, supraventricular fibrillation, and ventricular fibrillation. EKG shows peaked T waves (earliest sign), and a widened QRS complex.

Hyperkalemia must be treated promptly because it may develop into a lethal cardiac arrhythmia, especially if the blood potassium value is >7 mEq/L and the infant's electrocardiogram shows abnormalities. Follow these steps to lower potassium levels:

- Discontinue all potassium administration.
- Elevate the blood pH by inducing hyperventilation.
- Give sodium bicarbonate to shift extracellular potassium back inside cells.
- Administer insulin and/or inhaled albuterol to enhance the shift of extracellular potassium back inside cells. *Monitor glucose levels closely.*
- Increase excretion of potassium by giving furosemide (Lasix) or sodium polystyrene sulfonate (Kayexalate).
- Give calcium gluconate concurrently to help stabilize the myocardium and lessen the chance of the infant developing an arrhythmia.
- In extreme cases, consider dialysis or exchange transfusion.

HYPOKALEMIA

Hypokalemia is a serum potassium level <3.5 mEq/L. Common causes of hypokalemia are chronic diuretic use and excessive nasogastric drainage. Alkalosis accentuates hypokalemia by triggering the sequestration of potassium from the extracellular fluid to inside the cell. Electrocardiograph manifestations of hypokalemia include a flattened T wave (earliest manifestation), ST segment depression, and appearance of U waves (second recovery wave following the T wave). These changes are identical to those seen with hypomagnesemia. Hypokalemia is usually not of concern until the level drops below 3.0 mEq/L. Signs of hypokalemia include cardiac arrhythmias, ileus, and lethargy. Treatment is with Slow-K and can be intravenous or oral. Rapid administration of potassium is associated with possible life-threatening cardiac dysfunction.

PARENTERAL INFUSION

Many inpatient infants require intravenous fluids, and there are a number of different types of access for **parenteral infusions**:

- **Umbilical cord catheterization (arterial, venous)**: This is limited to a few days only.
- **PICC line:** This allows for long-term use without repeated IV insertions. It is particularly useful for ELBW babies although they pose the danger of thrombosis, infection, and infiltration. Percutaneous insertion sites include the saphenous, antecubital, axillary, basilic, cephalic, and external jugular veins.
- **Peripheral venous access**: This is used for short-term access. Extremely small catheters and introducers (Quick-cath) may extend use to 5-7 days. There is increased risk of infiltration and skin necrosis, especially in the foot.

The catheter or needle should be secured, but must allow visualization, and the site should be checked at least every hour during administration of fluids.

INFUSION TECHNIQUES AND EQUIPMENT
UMBILICAL ARTERY CATHETERIZATION

Umbilical catheters may be arterial or venous, depending on primary need. Arterial catheterization indications include ABG monitoring, continuous arterial BP monitoring, and infusion of parenteral fluids.

Umbilical artery catheter placement: A sterile field must be maintained, so the infant's arms and legs are restrained to prevent contamination. The infant's temperature must be monitored and maintained at 36-37 °C (by placing on a radiant heater or in a heated incubator). The child is placed in supine position and the umbilical cord and surrounding skin cleansed with povidone iodine and then alcohol or sterile water. For infants <1250 g, a 3.5 Fr. catheter is used, and for those >1250 g, a 5 Fr. catheter. After sterile draping, iris forceps are used to dilate one of the arteries and the catheter inserted. If resistance is felt at the umbilical cord tie, it may need to be loosened. The inserted length correlates to the infant's length (using chart), traveling inferiorly and then superiorly (leg loop). Blood should be aspirated and extremities observed for circulatory compromise. Radiograph verifies correct placement.

UMBILICAL VEIN CATHETERIZATION

Umbilical catheters may be inserted into the umbilical vein. This is easy to identify as there is only one, it is larger than the arteries, and it is usually open and does not require dilation. Indications for using the umbilical vein include exchange transfusions, CVP monitoring, and emergency administration of fluids.

Umbilical vein catheter placement: Catheter size is 3.5 Fr. for ELBW infants or 5 Fr. (most common). Length of placement is estimated by measuring the length from the umbilicus to the sternal notch and multiplying this number by 0.6. The procedure for insertion is similar to that for the umbilical artery, but insertion is usually easier. The catheter should be in the inferior vena cava, above the diaphragm but below the right atrium. Placement should be verified by echocardiography, as radiograph may not provide adequate visualization.

PICC LINES

Percutaneously inserted central catheters (PICC) are used for extended intravenous access or those with limited access and as a transition from umbilical catheters. Insertion sites include the scalp, axilla, and brachial cephalic saphenous veins. The catheter insertion length is measured:

- **Hand/arm:** insertion site to axilla and to 1 cm above nipple line
- **Scalp:** insertion site to 1 cm above nipple line
- **Leg:** insertion site to 1 cm above umbilicus

Topical (EMLA) or local anesthetic is used and the infant's temperature maintained at 36-37 °C. Limbs are restrained to prevent contamination of sterile field. If the catheter is inserted in the hand or arm, the infant's head is turned toward insertion site to partially occlude the jugular vein and reduce risk of catheter entering the jugular. After insertion above the waist, the catheter should be in the superior vena cava above the right atrium. PICC lines in lower extremities should lie in the inferior vena cava below the right atrium. AP and lateral radiographs, ultrasound, or echocardiogram verify correct placement.

BROVIAC CATHETERS

Broviac catheters are large-bore silastic indwelling catheters that may be surgically (cutdown) or needle inserted if percutaneous insertion is not possible. The most common sites for insertion are the internal or external jugular vein and the common facial vein. **Broviac catheters** are most commonly used if long-term access (months, years) is required, such as for parenteral nutrition or medications. A Broviac catheter is tunneled subcutaneously and exits through the anterior chest. Placement is confirmed with radiograph. The Broviac catheter is cuffed at the exit point to decrease infection, but the catheter still poses a high risk of infection, especially with frequent administration of parenteral nutrition. Complications include pneumothorax, hemothorax, air embolism, misplacement or occlusion of catheter. The catheter must be secured as it is easily dislodged, so length and positioning should be carefully documented and the catheter checked frequently. The catheter is flushed with heparin to maintain patency and prevent thrombus formation.

Nutrition and Feeding

DIGESTION AND ABSORPTION

Digestion is the processes by which food is converted into chemicals that are used by the body. These processes are immature at birth and most don't function until 3-6 months. Digestion begins in the mouth as milk is mixed with saliva, but salivary amylase, which begins the digestion of starch, has little effect on milk because milk passes into the esophagus and stomach quickly. Protein digestion begins in the stomach where hydrochloric acid acts on curds formed by the enzyme renin. The curds slow the progress of the milk to allow digestion. Pancreatic and liver enzymes further digest protein and fat in the small intestine. Infants cannot adequately absorb fat until 4-5 months or complex carbohydrates until 4-6 months. Simple carbohydrates break down into glucose and monosaccharides and fat into fatty acids and glycerol. Trypsin levels are sufficient to convert proteins into polypeptides and amino acids. **Absorption**, the transfer of digestive end products (electrolytes, vitamins, fluids, nutrients) into the circulation, takes place primarily in the small intestine and is facilitated by villi.

NUTRITIONAL NEEDS

CALORIC REQUIREMENTS OF NEONATES

The caloric needs of a neonate (pre-term or term) depend on postnatal age, activity, current weight, growth rate, thermal environment, and route of nutritional intake. Cold stress increases caloric requirements. Infants who receive parenteral nutrition need fewer calories, as they do not have any fecal loss, and the nutrients are not absorbed by the gastrointestinal tract. These are the general requirements for adequate growth:

- **Full-term infant**: 100-120 cal/kg/day
- **Premature infants**: 110-160 cal/kg/day
- Infants who are recovering from **surgery** or have a **chronic illness**, such as bronchopulmonary dysplasia (BPD): ≤180 cal/kg/day

Most human breast milk and unfortified formulas supply 20 calories per ounce. To ingest 120 cal/kg/day, an infant needs to ingest 6 ounces/kg/day of unfortified formula or human breast milk. Special formulas designed for premature infants and fortifiers that can be added to human breast milk provide higher calorie contents per ounce (22-24 calories per ounce).

PROTEIN REQUIREMENTS

Neonates require adequate **protein** to sustain growth, with intake requirements depending on gestational age. A positive nitrogen balance exists when the intake of protein meets or exceeds the infant's requirements. A negative protein balance occurs when protein is provided in inadequate amounts, leading to catabolism (muscle breakdown). Generally, the USDA recommends newborns through 6 months of age receive 9.1 g/day of protein. Premature neonates have higher protein requirements relative to body weight than do full term infants:

- **Full term**: 2.0-2.5 g/kg/day
- **Preterm**: 3.5-4.0 g/kg/day

Preterm infants should be started on parenteral nutrition supplemented with protein as soon as possible to avoid negative protein balances. Special formulas designed for premature infants are available with elevated protein contents. Human breast milk fortifiers are also available to enhance the protein levels and caloric content of human breast milk for premature infants although the content of human breast milk adjusts automatically for the needs of preterm infants.

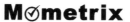

CARBOHYDRATE AND FAT REQUIREMENTS

Nutritional requirements of carbohydrates and fats vary according to whether a neonate is full-term or preterm and the type of feeding (human breast milk, enteral, parenteral).

Lactose is the primary **carbohydrate** in human breast milk. A full-term neonate requires 60 g of carbohydrate daily for the first 6 months of life according to the USDA, and a preterm neonate requires 12-14 g/kg/day. Preterm infants may require supplemental glucose via infusion, starting at 6 mg/kg/min, and increased daily by 1 mg/kg/min, up to 12-13 mg/kg/min until blood glucose levels are stabilized and can be maintained by the neonate. Lactose is metabolized into galactose and glucose, the main energy source for the brain. Human breast milk is approximately 40% carbohydrates. Inadequate intake may result in hypoglycemia, while excess intake may result in weight gain and hyperglycemia.

Fats provide the primary energy source for neonates and should comprise at least 30% of calories but no more than 54%. Fat intake needs are 31 g/day for full-term neonates, according to the USDA, and 5-7 g/kg/day for preterm neonates. Because preterm neonates are more susceptible to essential fatty acid deficiency, they should be closely monitored, and administered IV 20% emulsion lipids (0.5-1.0 g/kg/day) if necessary, until stabilized. Fats provide energy for the body and contribute to the development of the CNS and tissue growth. Excess fat may contribute to weight gain, impaired cholesterol metabolism, and later cardiac morbidity. Deficiency may result in impaired development and dermatitis (from lack of adequate fatty acids).

VITAMINS

Nutritional requirements of vitamins are generally met with human breast milk or formula in the healthy neonate. Daily vitamin requirements vary according to the neonate's condition and whether preterm or term. **E**=Enteral, **P**=Parenteral.

Vitamin	Preterm/Term	Notes
A	**E:**700-1500/1250 IU **P:** 700-1500/2300 IU	**Deficiency:** Vision impairment/blindness, impaired growth, depressed immune system **Excess:** Poor feeding, weight loss, fever, diarrhea
C	**E:** 20-60/30-50 mg **P:** 35-50/80 mg	**Deficiency:** Impaired brain development, weakness, bleeding **Excess:** Diarrhea, skin irritation, GI upset
D	**E:** 400/300 IU **P:** 120-260/400 IU	**Deficiency:** Impaired skeletal growth, calcium malabsorption **Excess:** Hypercalcemia, dehydration, cardiac and renal impairment, bone loss, hearing impairment
E	**E:** 6-12/5-10 IU **P:** 2-4/7 IU	**Deficiency:** Peripheral neuropathy, retinopathy, IVH, spinocerebellar impairment, hemolytic anemia **Excess:** GI upset, bleeding
K	**E:** 0.05/0.2 mg **P:** 0.06-0.1/0.05 mg	**Deficiency:** Bleeding **Excess:** Hemolysis, hyperbilirubinemia
Vitamin B1 (Thiamine)	**E:** 0.2-0.7/0.3 mg **P:** 0.8-0.8/1.2 mg	**Deficiency:** Cardiovascular and neurological damage **Excess:** rash, tachycardia, irritability
Vitamin B2 (Riboflavin)	**E:** 0.3-0.8/0.4 mg **P:** 0.4-0.9/1.4 mg	**Deficiency:** Thyroid hormone insufficiency, stomatitis, hepatic and neurological impairment, anemia **Excess:** Vomiting, hypotension
Vitamin B3 (Niacin)	**E:** 5-12/5 mg **P:** 5-12/7 mg	**Deficiency:** GI upset, diarrhea, cognitive impairment **Excess:** Flushing, hives, hepatic impairment

Vitamin	Preterm/Term	Notes
Vitamin B6 (Pyridoxine)	E: 0.3-0.7/0.3 mg P: 0.3-0.7/1.0 mg	**Deficiency**: Impaired development of neurological system, seizures **Excess**: Peripheral nerve damage, respiratory distress, hypotonia, lethargy, GI upset
Vitamin B12 (Cobalamin)	E: 0.3-0.7/0.3 mg P: 0.3-0.7/1.0 mg	**Deficiency**: Vomiting, diarrhea, hypotonia, lethargy, anemia, megaloblastic anemia **Excess**: Skin irritation, diarrhea, tachycardia, poor sleeping

MINERALS

Daily mineral requirements vary according to the neonate's condition and whether preterm or term. **E**=Enteral, **P**=Parenteral.

Minerals	Preterm/Term	Notes
Biotin	E: 6-20/10 mcg P: 6-13/20 mcg	Deficiency: Hypotonia, seizures, skin disorders, hearing loss, conjunctivitis, lethargy Excess: Hyperglycemia
Calcium	E: 210-250/130 mg/kg P: 60-90/60-80 mg/kg	Deficiency: Jitteriness, irritability, stridor, tetany, high-pitched cry, seizures, and cardiac dysfunction Excess: Vomiting; constipation, hypertension, hypotonia, lethargy, seizures
Chloride	E: 2-3/2-3 mEq/kg P: 2-3/2-3 mEq/kg	Deficiency: Weakness, lethargy, irritability, impaired absorption of iron and vitamin B_{12} Excess: Metabolic acidosis
Chromium	E: 2-4/2 mcg/kg P: 0.2/0.2 mcg/kg	Deficiency: peripheral neuropathy, impaired glucose tolerance, muscle weakness, loss of weight Excess: Skin irritation
Copper	E: 100-150/75 mcg/kg P: 20/20 mcg/kg	Deficiency: Hypochromic anemia, bone demineralization, neutropenia Excess: Gastroenteritis, hepatic injury
Folate (Folic acid)	E: 50/25-50 mcg P: 40-90/140 mcg	Deficiency: Lethargy, pallor, tachycardia, low weight, general weakness Excess: GI upset, poor sleeping
Iodine	E: 4/7 mcg/kg P: 1.0/1.0 mcg/kg	Deficiency: Intellectual disabilities, hypothyroidism, thyroid enlargement Excess: Abdominal pain, fever, hypothyroidism, skin irritation
Iron	E: 1-2/1-2 mg/kg P: 0.09-0.2/0.1-0.2 mcg/kg	Deficiency: Anemia, lethargy, impaired development Excess: GI upset, tachycardia, hyperpnea, hypotension, seizures, coma, liver failure
Magnesium	E: 8-15/7 mg/kg P: 4-7/5-7 mg/kg	Deficiency: Tetany, seizure, coma, tachycardia, ventricular arrhythmias, respiratory depression Excess: Hypotonia, hyporeflexia, constipation, hypotension, apnea, vasodilatation/flushing
Manganese	E: 10-20/85 mcg/kg P: 1.0-1.0 mcg/kg	Deficiency: Weakness, hearing impairment Excess: Impaired iron absorption
Molybdenum	E: 2-3/2 mcg/kg P: 0.25/0.25 mcg/kg	Deficiency: Inability to metabolize sulfites, seizures Excess: growth restriction, diarrhea

Minerals	Preterm/Term	Notes
Phosphorus	E: 112-125/45 mEq/kg P:40-70/40-45 mEq/kg	Deficiency: Impaired bone metabolism, muscle weakness, tremors, seizures, impaired immune response Excess: GI upset, tachycardia, hyperreflexia, tetany
Potassium	E: 2-3/2-3 mEq/kg P: 2-3/2-3 mEq/kg	Deficiency: Cardiac arrhythmias, ileus, and lethargy Excess: Cardiac arrhythmias (bradycardia, tachycardia, VF)
Selenium	E: 1.3-3/1.6 mcg/kg P: 1.5-2/2.0 mcg/kg	Deficiency: Impaired immune response Excess: Diarrhea, lethargy, respiratory depression
Sodium	E: 2-4/2-3 mEq/kg P: 2-3.5/2-3 mEq/kg	Deficiency: Apnea, irritability, twitching, weight gain, and seizures Excess: weight loss, irritability, lethargy, fever, seizures (late)
Zinc	E: 800-1000/830 mcg P: 400/250 mcg	Deficiency: Impaired growth, impaired immune response, dermatitis Excess: Vomiting and diarrhea, neurological damage

HUMAN BREAST MILK

Human breast milk is the food of choice for newborn infants. **Colostrum**, produced during the first few days after birth, is scant, thick, yellowish, and high in protein and antibody content. Colostrum stimulates the passage of meconium. **Transitional milk** (days 3-14) is thinner and white, with a composition closer to that of mature milk. By the second week, most mothers produce 23-27 ounces of bluish-white **mature human breast milk**. Most neonates nurse every 1-3 hours for 20-40 minutes. Benefits of human breast milk are as follows:

- Human breast milk provides appropriate amounts of carbohydrate, protein, fat, vitamins, minerals, enzymes, and trace elements.
- It contains maternal antibodies that help bolster the infant's immature immune system.
- Breastfed babies have reduced risks of eczema, asthma, obesity, and elevated cholesterol later in life.
- Breastfeeding enhances the bond between the mother and the infant by physical contact and promotes recognition of communication signals.
- The maternal cost is an extra 500 calories a day and extra water.
- It eliminates the possibility of kidney damage caused by incorrectly mixed formula.

COMPOSITION

Human breast milk has immunologic benefits that formulas lack, resulting in decreased morbidity in breastfed infants. Human breast milk contains these important substances:

- **Antibodies**: Secretory IgA to provide protection from respiratory, enteric, and viral pathogens
- **Primary nutrients:** Protein with whey-to-casein ratio of 60:40 (including IgM, IgG, lactoferrin, lysozyme, casein [40%], and fibronectin), carbohydrate (about 40% of total calories), and fat (free fatty acids)

The following are **secondary nutrients:**

- Nucleotides
- Vitamins A, C, D, E; vitamin D content ≤25 IU/L; supplement if ≤2 months of age
- Enzymes: anti-inflammatory and antibacterial properties, including lipase, which breaks down fat
- Growth factors
- Hormones: prolactin, cortisol, thyroxine, insulin, and erythropoietin
- Cells: beta-lymphocytes, macrophages (90%), neutrophil, T-lymphocytes, cytokines, interleukin 1b, 6, 8, 10, 12 (both inflammatory and anti-inflammatory properties)

FEEDING

FEEDING CUES

The infant gives a number of feeding cues to show hunger. Mothers should be taught to recognize these cues, as it's more difficult for a frantically hungry baby to latch on. These are some indications that the infant is hungry:

- Licking the lips
- Sucking motions of the mouth
- Rooting or bobbing of the head
- Keeping hands in fists
- Bringing hands near mouth or face
- Turning the head toward and trying to suck on a finger stroking the baby's cheek or lower lip
- Crying (usually the last indication)

Infants who are consistently not receiving adequate nutrition usually appear sleepy and listless. They often stop gaining weight or lose weight. Skin turgor may be poor. Urinary output and stools decrease. The infant may appear disinterested in nursing. On the other hand, an infant who is satisfied usually stops sucking and may turn the head away from the breast or resist nursing. The infant will appear relaxed and may doze. Some infants take short breaks while nursing and then resume.

Early Feeding Cues

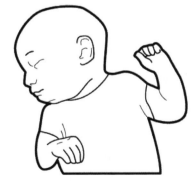 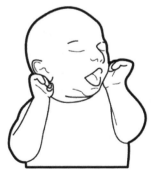 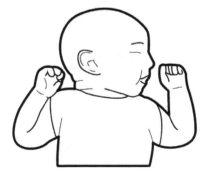

Mid-Active Feeding Cues

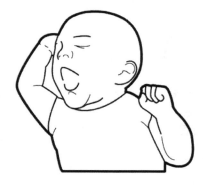 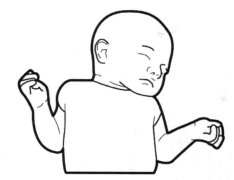 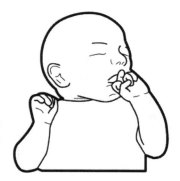

Late Feeding Cues

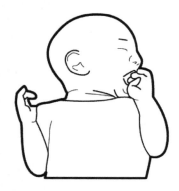 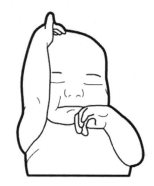 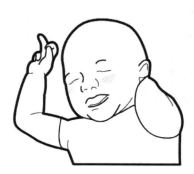

BREASTFEEDING FREQUENCY AND DURATION

Most infants initially nurse every 1-3 hours, but during **growth spurts** (2-3 weeks, 6 weeks, 3 months, and 6 months), the infant may nurse every half to one hour for 2-3 days, stimulating the breasts to increase production. Nursing usually takes 20-45 minutes, with 15-20 minutes on each side. Nursing should begin on the last breast used. Infants may nurse more frequently in the late afternoon and evening. Infants should be fed every 3 hours until they regain their birth weight, even if the infant must be awakened. Infants vary in **demand schedules**. Some eat 5-10 times over a 3-hour period and then sleep for about 4 hours. The schedule is less important than assuring that the child nurses **8-12 times** every 24 hours and appears satisfied. By 8-12 weeks, infants begin sleeping longer at night. Some may sleep through the night at 4 months, while others continue to nurse at night.

LATCHING ON AND LET-DOWN

Once the infant is in position, the mother should grasp the breast using a C-hold or U-hold (to make the breast firmer) and lean toward the baby, guiding the nipple toward the infant's mouth. Brushing the nipple against the infant's mouth usually causes the infant to open the mouth and lunge toward the breast. Then, the mother guides the nipple into the infant's mouth while pulling the infant toward the breast. The infant's lower lip should be low on the areola so the baby **latches** on to both the areola and the nipple.

Proper Latch

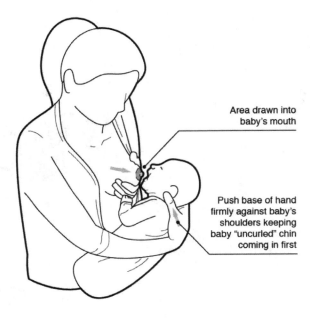

Area drawn into
baby's mouth

Push base of hand
firmly against baby's
shoulders keeping
baby "uncurled" chin
coming in first

C-Hold

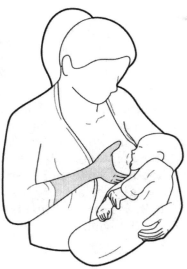

U-Hold

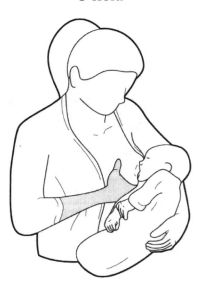

Suckling stimulates nerves in the areola and nipple, increasing production of prolactin and oxytocin, which in turn stimulate contraction of cells about the areola, causing milk to be ejected in a **"let-down"** (milk-ejection) reflex, which is sometimes associated with a tingling sensation, usually within a few minutes of nursing. It may take up to 2 weeks before letdown is efficient.

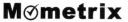
PROBLEMS ASSOCIATED WITH LATCH-ON

Most problems associated with latch-on result from poor maternal technique and are easily resolved with demonstration and support:

- **Infant latches on to the end of the nipple,** resulting in pain and limited milk flow: The mother should learn to brush the nipple against the infant's lips until the baby opens the mouth completely before inserting the nipple.
- **Infant's mouth on just the nipple and not the areola**: The mother should use a C-hold or U-hold to guide the nipple into the infant's mouth, making sure that most of the areola (1.0-1.5 inches) is covered by the infant's mouth.
- **Inverted nipples**, making latching on difficult: If the nipple is so flat that the infant cannot easily latch on, using a silicone nipple shield for the first few minutes may help to elongate the nipple, at which point the shield should be removed because the shield doesn't allow adequate breast stimulation, and the infant must work harder to suckle.

NIPPLE SHIELDS

Silicone nipple shields, which fit over the mother's nipple and areola, are sometimes used if a mother's nipples are inverted or flat, but they should not be used with cracked nipples if the mother can tolerate feeding. The breast does not receive adequate stimulation if the infant feeds with the shield in place, so milk production decreases and the baby may not be able to get adequate nutrition. Also, because the silicone nipple feels different from the breast, the infant may be reluctant to wean from the shield. If it is absolutely necessary to use a nipple shield for a flat or inverted nipple, it should be used only for the first few minutes, as even a flat nipple will usually elongate during that time. Then the rest of the feeding can be done without the shield.

SUCK-SWALLOW SEQUENCE

A neonate usually **sucks** and then **swallows** when the mouth becomes full. Each suck usually fills the mouth, a **suck to swallow ratio** of 1:1. Infants do not breathe while swallowing, so a 1:1 ratio means the child must breathe quickly, resulting in a rapid suck-hold breath and swallow-breathe sequence. During a swallow, the soft palate rises to block access to the nasal passages, the larynx rises, and the epiglottis covers the airway to prevent aspiration. If milk flow is inadequate, the child may need to suck twice for each swallow (2:1). If the flow is too fast, the child may need to swallow twice or more for each suck (1:2) and some milk may run down the pharynx and into the airway, resulting in aspiration. Or, the child may need to swallow so rapidly there is no time to breathe, and apnea may occur. A newborn usually sucks twice a second for about a minute and then about once per second as the milk flow increases.

EXPRESSING AND STORING HUMAN BREAST MILK

A mother can **express and store milk** for her infant if the infant is unable to nurse or if she must be separated from the infant. The most efficient method is to use a **bilateral electric breast pump**. The **pulsatile electric pump** provides adequate stimulation in the early postpartum period to establish and maintain the mother's milk supply, usually emptying the breasts within 15-20 minutes. If the child is not nursing, the pump should be used at least 8 times in each 24-hour period. Other methods of expressing milk include manual expression and use of a hand pump. Electric pumps usually have collection systems, so the milk flows into a bottle that can be used for feeding. Human breast milk can be stored for later use using the following guidelines:

- **Room temperature**: 4 hours
- **Refrigerated**: ≤4 days (best used within 48 hours)
- **Frozen**: 3-4 months in a separate-door freezer-refrigerator, and 6 months in a deep freezer at 0 °F

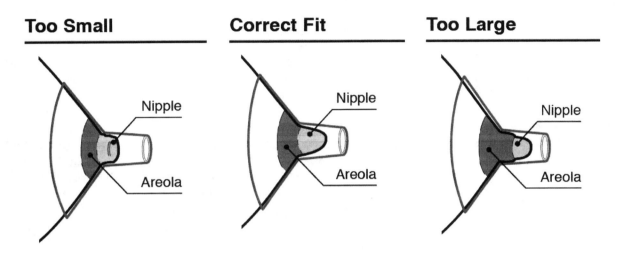

SUPPLEMENTAL NURSING SYSTEM

Supplemental nursing systems allow the mother to provide supplemental nutrients or medication to the infant while breastfeeding. A typical system has a container for the liquid supplement and a tubing system with a tubing clamp to adjust flow. The tubing is taped to the breast and the end extends about 2-3 mm past the end of the nipple on the top, so the baby encloses both the nipple and the tubing in the mouth when nursing. The tubing should be under the baby's upper lip. Once the baby begins to nurse, the clamp is released so the supplement begins to flow. The bottom of the container is usually positioned level with the breast or slightly lower, so the child must suckle in order to gain the supplement. If the container is higher than the breast, the solution may flow too freely and may choke the child.

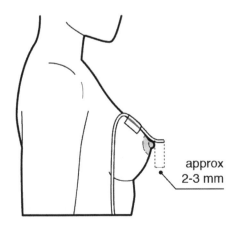

DONOR MILK

While the mother's milk is most highly recommended for her newborn's nutrition, some mothers are not able to express sufficient milk for newborn growth and development. Low birth weight infants may also need more human breast milk than available. In these instances, the first recommendation for supplemental nutrition is donor milk, followed by formula. **Donor milk** has an association with lower rates of gut disorders (such as necrotizing enterocolitis) and other infections. Donor milk is generally collected by hospitals and nonprofit milk banks that receive human breast milk donations from mothers that overproduce milk. These mothers have been approved by their physician, by the infant's physician, and through a screening process to ensure the milk is safe to donate.

INFANT FORMULAS

A wide variety of infant formulas are available, but there are 3 primary types:

- **Cow-milk-based formulas** (Enfamil, Similac, Good Start): These are appropriate for most infants. These are enriched with various components, including vitamins, minerals, iron, tyrosine, phenylalanine, and carnitine.
- **Soy-based formulas** (Isomil, Soyalac, ProSobee, Nursoy): These are appropriate for infants with primary lactose deficiency or galactosemia and those allergic to cow-milk-based formulas.
- **Therapeutic formulas** (Nutramigen, Pregestimil): Many preparations are available to meet special needs.

Formula may be purchased in ready-to-feed bottles or cans that require no preparation, liquid concentrate, or powder. Concentrate and powder require the addition of water, so a clean water supply and the ability to measure correctly are necessary to avoid inadequate or unsafe nutrition. Babies who are bottle-fed with formula usually feed less frequently than those who are breastfed. Neonates usually take 2-3 ounces of formula every 3-4 hours. Neonates require approximately 2.5 ounces of formula for each pound (0.5 kg) of weight within each 24-hour period.

NUTRITIONAL VALUE OF FULL TERM FORMULA AND PRETERM FORMULAS

The nutritional value of full term formula and preterm formulas is discussed below:

- **Carbohydrates**: One gram of carbohydrates provides 3.4 calories. Carbohydrates provide approximately 1/3 of the caloric content in infant formulas. Lactose is the predominant carbohydrate. Premature infants may be deficient in the enzyme lactase (enzyme that breaks down lactose), so premature infant formulas utilize lesser amounts of lactose, combined with glucose polymers.
- **Lipids**: One gram of fat provides 9 calories. Lipids supply approximately 2/3 of the caloric content in infant formulas. Common sources of lipids include palm, soybean, coconut, and safflower oils. Premature infant formulas have a higher percentage of fat supplied as medium-chain triglycerides (MCT). MCTs can be absorbed without pancreatic lipase or bile salts that are deficient in premature infants.
- **Proteins**: One gram of protein provides 4 calories. Proteins provide less than 5% of the caloric content in infant formulas. Proteins provide amino acids that are used as building blocks for muscle and other tissues. Preterm formulas have higher protein content than term formula to help meet the increased growth requirements of preterm infants.

SPECIAL PRETERM FORMULAS

Preterm formulas are designed with the special requirements of the premature infant in mind. These infants often have an increased caloric requirement to meet growth expectations. **Preterm formulas** differ from full-term formulas because they provide:

- 24 cal/oz as opposed to the 20 cal/oz found in human breast milk and in formulas for full-term infants.
- Increased levels of protein, vitamins, and minerals, particularly increased amounts of vitamin D, calcium, and phosphorus to prevent osteopenia of prematurity.
- Less lactose than term formulas, so they are less likely to cause diarrhea.

Human breast milk can be **fortified** with the addition of human breast milk fortifiers to achieve the same results. Infants are typically switched to a transitional or cow milk-based formula prior to discharge.

FAT-SOLUBLE VITAMINS IN FORMULAS

Vitamins found in formulas are organic nutrients required in small amounts to maintain growth and normal metabolism. **Fat-soluble vitamins** include:

- **Vitamin A:** Important for growth and development of tissues as well as proper functioning of the immune system. Vitamin A supplementation in extremely low birth weight infants has been shown to reduce the incidence of bronchopulmonary dysplasia.
- **Vitamin D:** Required for adequate calcium and phosphorus absorption. Vitamin D deficiency leads to rickets (soft bones, bowed legs).
- **Vitamin E:** An antioxidant that is limited in preterm infants, making them susceptible to developing hemolytic anemia without proper supplementation.
- **Vitamin K:** Important in the clotting process. Infants receive an injection of Vitamin K shortly after birth to prevent hemorrhagic disease of the newborn.

Excessive fat-soluble vitamins A and D are toxic because they accumulate in adipose tissue and the liver. Water-soluble vitamins include thiamine (B_1), riboflavin (B_2), niacin (B_3), pantothenate (B_5), pyridoxine (B_6), cobalamin (B_{12}), C, biotin, and folic acid. Excessive water-soluble vitamins are excreted in the urine.

ENTERAL FEEDING

Enteral (tube) feeding provides nutrition to infants with a functioning gastrointestinal tract but the inability to take an adequate amount of milk/formula orally. Ideally, human milk is provided for enteral feedings because it provides antimicrobial factors (IgA, leukocytes, complement, lactoferrin, lysozyme) lacking in formula. However, preterm infants don't grow at adequate rates on human milk alone, so human milk is usually supplemented with formula that contains additional carbohydrates, protein, fatty acids, vitamins, and minerals. Enteral feeding is indicated in infants requiring endotracheal intubation, or weak infants with an inability to suck, swallow, gag, or coordinate these activities (<34-36 weeks). Feedings may be continuous or intermittent (over 30 to 60 minutes). Feedings should be given slowly and tube position checked frequently to prevent aspiration. If feedings must be prolonged, oral aversion and gastroesophageal reflux may occur, so gastrostomy tube placement may be done. Oral feedings must be introduced slowly once per day, then once per 8 hours, every third feeding, every other feeding, and finally every meal.

PROCEDURE

A feeding tube for enteral feeding should be measured (tip of ear to midpoint between xiphoid process and umbilicus) and marked before insertion. The infant should be swaddled and supine. Oral tubes are used for infants <1 kg and those with NCPAP, on a ventilator, or with a high need for oxygen. Nasal tubes are used for infants >1kg or those taking oral feedings or with a strong gag reflex. Short-term tubes (polyvinyl chloride) are changed every 24-72 hours and long-term tubes (polyurethane) every month. Prior to feeding, stomach contents are aspirated for assessment but then re-instilled to prevent electrolyte loss unless blood, bile, stool, or thick mucus is in aspirate. Feeding should be by gravity flow 5-8 inches above infant, usually over 30 minutes for intermittent feeding, and the tube should be cleared with 1-2 mL water at end. For continuous feeding, the placement of the tube and residual milk/formula should be checked every 2 hours. Usually, a 4-hour amount of milk/formula feeding is hung at one time.

GAVAGE FEEDING

Gavage feeding per a nasogastric or orogastric tube is indicated for neonates who are preterm, critically ill, or unable to adequately swallow to obtain sufficient nutrition. Calories and nutrition provided are based on gestation, development, and laboratory findings (such as electrolytes). Typical caloric feedings:

- Preterm, 24-34 weeks: 15-20 g/kg/day.
- Preterm, 33-36 weeks: 14-15 g/kg/day.
- Full-term, 37-40 weeks: 7-9 g/kg/day.
- Full-term 0-3 months of age: 30 g/day.

Non-nutritive sucking should be provided during gavage feeding with the mother/caregiver holding the neonate with skin-to-skin (kangaroo care) contact during feeding if possible. The neonate has increased risk of gastroesophageal reflux if fed in the supine position, so prone or left lateral position with head elevated to 30 degrees during feeding is preferred. Additionally, one hour after feeding, position the neonate in the right lateral position for one hour followed by the left lateral position to facilitate gastric emptying.

BOLUS VS. CONTINUOUS FEEDINGS

Bolus gavage feedings are generally administered over a 15-30-minute period while continuous feedings are administered over a number of hours. There is not yet consensus as to which method is better and study results are often conflicting on the effects of each type, such as which method is most likely to increase apneic periods. Bolus feedings are generally more common but continuous feedings are becoming more popular and require less direct nursing time. Intermittent feedings are usually done with gravity flow and require constant attendance during feeding, but continuous feedings are usually provided with an automatic pump.

Bolus feedings:

- Simulates normal feeding patterns
- May cause metabolic instability
- Increases risk of gastroesophageal reflux
- May overwhelm immature GI system
- May improve splanchnic oxygenation

Continuous feedings:

- Improves feeding tolerance
- Promotes metabolic stability
- Decreases risk of gastroesophageal reflux
- May result in increased weight gain
- May increase risk of bacterial contamination
- May result in fat separation and decreased fat intake

TROPHIC FEEDINGS

Trophic feedings (also called minimal enteric nutrition) are very small enteral feeds given soon after birth to extremely premature infants not expected to tolerate enteral feeds for several weeks. Studies have shown that trophic feeds prevent atrophy of the gut and enhance gastrointestinal maturation and small intestine motility. They may also protect the preterm infants from developing necrotizing enterocolitis (NEC). Trophic feeds can be started within 24-48 hours of birth in stable infants. The fluids of choice are colostrum, human milk, or preterm infant formula. Trophic feedings are non-nutritive (not designed to add significant calories or nutrition to the infant). Typical volumes are 1-2 mL/kg per feeding, with a total volume not to exceed 15 mL/kg/day.

TOTAL PARENTERAL NUTRITION

A preterm or compromised infant may not tolerate enteral feedings for several weeks, so the infant's nutritional needs are met with IV **total parenteral nutrition** (TPN). The goals of TPN are to:

- Provide normal metabolism
- Support growth without significant morbidity
- Prevent essential fatty acid deficiency
- Balance nitrogen
- Prevent muscle wasting (catabolism)

TPN is started after birth. Dextrose provides the majority of calories, but to avoid elevated blood glucose levels, dextrose is administered at 6mg/kg/min and increased to 10-12 mg/kg/min over several days. The infant's serum glucose is monitored regularly for hyperglycemia. Protein content is slowly increased over several days to 3-3.5 g/kg/day. Lipids, required for calories and the absorption of fat-soluble vitamins like A, D, and E, are started at 0.5 g/kg/day and increased to 3-3.5 g/kg/day. Other components of TPN include sodium, potassium, calcium, phosphorus, magnesium, trace elements, and vitamins. TPN may be administered through a peripheral IV line for <one week and a central line for longer periods.

INTRAVENOUS LIPIDS

Intravenous lipids are an important component of total parenteral nutrition (TPN) because they provide essential fatty acids, a concentrated calorie source (9 calories per gram of fat), and improve delivery of fat-soluble vitamins to infants who cannot tolerate enteral feeds. General guidelines for the administration of IV lipids are to start with 0.5/g/kg on the third day of life and advance slowly to a final administration rate of 3-3.5/g/kg/day by 7-10 days. Delivery of IV lipids should be continuous over 18-24 hours each day. Serum lipid levels should be monitored for hyperlipidemia. Potential **complications** include:

- Risk of kernicterus in infants with elevated unconjugated bilirubin (Free fatty acids displace bilirubin from albumin binding sites. Infusion of lipids should be at the lower level in infants with elevated unconjugated bilirubin.)
- Exacerbation of chronic lung disease
- Exacerbation of persistent pulmonary hypertension

TPN COMPLICATIONS

Complications of total parenteral nutrition (TPN) result from the presence of the intravenous access (usually a central line) and the development of cholestasis. Both of these events are more common in infants receiving TPN for longer than 2-3 weeks. The longer an infant receives TPN, the more likely complications will occur. Consequences of prolonged venous access include sepsis, thrombophlebitis, and extravasation of fluid into soft tissue with possible tissue necrosis. Premature infants have an immature hepatobiliary system. One hypothesis for the development of cholestasis is that a lack of fat in the duodenum leads to biliary stasis. Infants requiring TPN are often very ill, may have episodes of shock, or require surgical interventions, all of which contribute to the development of TPN-associated cholestasis. Jaundiced infants show an elevated direct bilirubin in blood serum. Treatment usually involves the discontinuation of TPN, along with the slow introduction of enteral feeds (if possible).

SUPPLEMENTARY OR COMPLEMENTARY FEEDING

Supplementary or complementary feeding with breastfed babies is usually discouraged because it may weaken the suckling reflex or cause the child to lose interest in breastfeeding, especially if a bottle is offered before breastfeeding is well established. To breastfeed, the child must latch on differently to the breast than to a bottle nipple, with the mouth opened more widely for the breast. Additionally, the tongue moves front to back when nursing (expressing milk) and up and down (squeezing the nipple) when feeding from a bottle. Changing from one to the other can be confusing for the infant, and some cannot adjust. Once the infant nurses well, usually after about 4 weeks, mothers who want to pump for supplementary feedings may try to slowly introduce the bottle. Neonates do not need water and should not be given juice or sugar water.

DIETARY SUPPLEMENTS

Dietary supplements include:

- **Human milk fortifiers**: HMFs are added to human milk to improve nutritional values. Contains nutrients (protein, carbohydrates, fats), vitamins, and minerals. Some fortifiers are derived from cow's milk and others from human milk. Human milk fortifiers are generally used for preterm and VLBW (very low birth weight) neonates.
- **Glucose polymers**: Glucose polymers are derived from starches (such as rice and tapioca) and are alternatives to glucose used as nutritional supplements to increase carbohydrate intake. Glucose polymers and lactose are commonly found in formulas intended for preterm neonates.
- **Medium chain triglycerides**: This nutritional supplement is provided to preterm neonates in order to increase fat absorption to promote growth.
- **Probiotics**: Live bacteria and yeast supplements are added to feedings of preterm neonates to reduce the risk of necrotizing enterocolitis.

IRON SUPPLEMENTATION

The premature infant is especially susceptible to iron deficiency because of the lack of maternal iron transfer during the third trimester and the multiple blood samplings that occur with the extensive monitoring of the premature infant. To minimize the risk of iron deficiency anemia, premature infants fed human milk should be started on **iron supplementation** once they receive full enteral feeds. Studies have shown that premature infants fed a premature formula have better iron stores when that formula is supplemented with 15 mg/L of iron compared to those receiving formula with only 3 mg/L of iron. All formula-fed term infants should receive iron-fortified formulas. Breastfed term infants should be given iron supplementation when they are several months old.

CARNITINE SUPPLEMENTATION FOR PREMATURE INFANTS

Carnitine is a quaternary amino acid that is synthesized from methionine and lysine in the liver and kidney. Carnitine aids in the metabolism of long chain fatty acids by helping to transport them across the mitochondrial membrane. Carnitine is present in human milk and formulas in sufficient amounts. Infants who are born premature have low tissue stores of carnitine, as much of it is transferred to the fetus during the third trimester. Symptoms of carnitine deficiency include increased episodes of apnea, decreased muscle tone, and poor growth. Infants who are not being enterally fed and are receiving TPN may benefit from supplementation with carnitine because it makes them better able to metabolize fats.

COMPLICATIONS OF BREASTFEEDING

ENGORGEMENT

Production of milk sometimes outstrips demand in the first 2-3 days as the mother is starting to nurse, and the breasts become **engorged** (enlarged, taut, and painful). The mother should be reassured that this is normal and can be relieved, as new mothers may feel they should stop nursing or be afraid they are doing something wrong. Nursing frequently (every 2-3 hours) and gently massaging the breast toward the nipple during nursing should reduce engorgement. If the areola is hard, some milk should be manually expressed to soften the areola before the infant latches on. Breast pumps and heat (except in a shower) may increase engorgement. Cold compresses, acetaminophen, or ibuprofen may provide relief. Engorgement usually recedes within 24-48 hours.

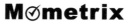

INSUFFICIENT MILK

Only about 1.5% of women are physiologically unable to produce **sufficient milk** for an infant. In almost all cases, the mother is simply not nursing correctly or frequently enough to stimulate milk production.

BLOCKED MILK DUCT

A palpable, localized lump or an area of hard, swollen erythematous tissue usually indicates a **blocked duct**. Causes include nursing the baby in the same position or wearing a constricting or poorly-fitting bra. Painful, blocked ducts generally open within 24-48 hours, with symptoms receding, as opposed to mastitis which tends to worsen. Massaging the affected area while breastfeeding, manually expressing the breast during a warm shower, applying heat to the area, and using a breast pump to completely empty the breast after feeding may alleviate the blockage. Additionally, while breastfeeding on the affected side, the infant should be positioned so the chin points toward the blocked area, usually using the football position. If blockage is not alleviated, blocked milk ducts may progress to mastitis.

MASTITIS

Indications that the breast has become infected (**mastitis**) with bacteria include induration, swelling, erythema, increasing fever, and acute pain. Without prompt treatment, painful abscesses may form. The infected area may be localized, sometimes appearing similar to blocked milk duct, or generalized, encompassing the whole breast. The mother may have chills and flu-like symptoms before obvious inflammation of the breast. Usually, the mother becomes infected from the infant, most commonly with *Staphylococcus aureus,* so breastfeeding does not endanger the neonate. Treatment includes antibiotics, usually penicillin G, dicloxacillin, or erythromycin, and nursing, pumping, or expressing on the affected side to prevent abscess formation. Applying heat or massaging the breasts in a warm shower may increase circulation. Pain relief includes alternating warm and cold compresses, and acetaminophen or ibuprofen.

CRACKED NIPPLES

Nipples often become sore when the mother begins breastfeeding, but this typically lessens in a few days. However, **cracked nipples** may lead to infection. These are some of the causes:

- The baby latching on improperly to just the nipple and not the areola
- Use of drying lotions or soaps
- Use of a breast pump with too much suction
- Monilial infection from thrush in the baby's mouth

Sometimes changing the baby's **position** or rotating positions during nursing may reduce discomfort. Nursing should begin on the least sore nipple, as the infant nurses more strongly at first. The breasts should be cleansed only with water and a small amount of human milk applied to the nipple after nursing, unless the baby has thrush. One hundred percent USP modified **lanolin** (Lansinoh or PureLan) applied to the nipples may promote healing. It does not need to be removed for breastfeeding. Acetaminophen or ibuprofen may be taken 30 minutes before nursing. Nipple shields should be avoided if possible, as they interfere with latching on.

Oxygenation, Ventilation, and Acid-Base Homeostasis

OXYHEMOGLOBIN DISSOCIATION CURVE

The oxyhemoglobin dissociation curve is a graph that plots the percentage of hemoglobin saturated with oxygen (Y-axis) and different partial pressures of oxygen (PaO_2 levels) (X-axis.) The neonate has about 70-90% fetal hemoglobin, which carries less oxygen but has a higher affinity for oxygen and greater oxygen saturation than adult hemoglobin, so the curve is different. A curve shift to the right represents conditions where hemoglobin has less affinity for oxygen (greater amounts of oxygen are released). A shift to the left has the opposite implications. Low pH shifts the curve to the right, enabling increased off-loading of hemoglobin to tissues. Elevated oxygen shifts the curve to the left, causing increased affinity of hemoglobin for oxygen in the lungs. Small changes in fetal PaO_2 result in greater loading or unloading of oxygen compared to adult hemoglobin. Because of the increased affinity for oxygen, lower tissue oxygen levels are needed to trigger the unload of oxygen. Thus, the infant will have a lower PaO_2 and oxygen saturation before cyanosis is evident.

MONITORING

NON-INVASIVE MONITORING OF INFANT ON OXYGEN

Non-invasive monitoring of the neonate receiving oxygen includes:

- **Heart rate monitor**: Should show beats per minute as well as a visual depiction of the heart rhythm.
- **Respiratory monitor**: Should show respiratory rate as well as a visual wave showing the pattern of breathing. Alarms should be turned on for apnea and tachypnea.
- **Blood pressure monitor**: Peripheral cuff type monitoring, this does not need to be continuous but needs to be done at regular intervals determined by the physician or practitioner.
- **Pulse oximetry**: Should be a continuous monitoring with alarms set for ordered lower limits.
- **Oxygen analyzer**: Shows the oxygen level being delivered to the neonate.

NEONATAL PULSE OXIMETRY

Pulse oximetry is a means of monitoring the saturation level of the **hemoglobin** in the blood. For example, a reading of 98% indicates that 98% of the hemoglobin available is bound to oxygen or saturated with oxygen. A machine uses infrared light to read the hemoglobin. Several things can affect the accuracy of this reading.

- The **perfusion status** of the neonate. If the infant is suffering from a condition that results in poor perfusion (hypovolemia, hypotension, etc.), the pulse oximetry reading will be inaccurate, as the machine will have difficulty reading the blood.
- **Phototherapy** used for jaundice will also cause inaccurate readings because, like the tool used in pulse oximetry, it is a light.
- Use of **dopamine**, a potent vasoconstricting drug, which causes problems reading the blood for oxygen levels if the veins are constricted, affecting blood flow.

Pulse oximetry is now a recommended screening tool for congenital heart defects. While not diagnostic, it provides information that can either rule out congenital heart defects or trigger further investigation.

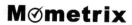

NON-INVASIVE TRANSCUTANEOUS O_2/CO_2 MONITORING

Non-invasive transcutaneous O_2/CO_2 monitoring includes **skin oxygen tension (TCPO$_2$)** and **carbon dioxide tension (TCPCO$_2$)**. One or two leads are placed on the infant's skin over any part of the body that allows good contact. O_2 and CO_2 diffuse through the skin and monitors provide a digital display. If right-to-left shunting is suspected, then leads are usually placed on right shoulder and lower abdomen or leg (above and below the ductus arteriosus). The electrodes are calibrated (usually every 4 hours to ensure accuracy), and then heat (43-44 °C) the underlying skin, but they must be left in place for 15 minutes after calibration to ensure adequate heating of the skin. The electrodes can cause erythema (first-degree burns), so they should be repositioned every 2-4 hours. The electrodes should not be placed beneath the infant because the pressure against it can impede circulation.

CARDIOPULMONARY MONITORING

Cardiopulmonary monitoring includes **electrocardiogram (ECG)** and **respiratory sensors**. Usually, 3 chest ECG leads that record the electrical activity of the heart and sense respiratory movement are placed, and the patterns are recorded on a visual screen. Many computerized monitors have memory capability so that data can be analyzed out of real time. They can also be set to record certain events, such as periods of apnea. Alarm thresholds are set so that an alarm indicates dangerous changes. Apnea alarms should be both visual and auditory. False alarms may occur and should be thoroughly evaluated for a cause, such as loose leads or movement. Home monitors include records of compliance so that a review of data shows the time the monitor was actually in use. Home monitors are used for infants at risk for SIDS. Because of interference problems that might provide inaccurate readings, monitors should never be used as a sole evaluation of cardiopulmonary status. Observation and examination must be used to verify the infant's condition.

END-TIDAL CO_2 MONITORS

End-tidal CO_2 monitors are used to confirm correct placement of endotracheal tubes during intubation and to ensure adequate oxygenation. Both sidestream analysis with a double lumen endotracheal tube (ETT) and mainstream analysis within the ventilator circuit are used. Clinical assessment alone is not adequate.

Capnography is attached to the ETT and provides a waveform graph, showing the varying concentrations of CO_2 in real time throughout each ventilation (with increased CO_2 on expiration) and can indicate changes in respiratory status. A typical waveform rises with expiration (indicating CO_2 level), plateaus, and then falls with inspiration (and intake of oxygen). Changes in the height or shape of the waveform can indicate respiratory compromise. Pressure of end-tidal CO_2 (PETCO$_2$) is useful for neonates with normal lung function or in premature infants with mild-moderate lung disease, but results may be inaccurate if there is a large alveolar-arterial gradient.

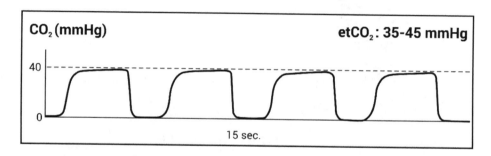

NEONATAL OXYGEN ADMINISTRATION

Principles of neonatal oxygen administration:

- Oxygen administration should be titrated to the need of the particular infant. The determining factor to titrate to should be PaO_2 levels as measured from arterial blood. Oxygen concentration should be titrated to keep the arterial PaO_2 level between 50 and 80 mmHg.
- Supplemental oxygen concentration should be initiated at 21% (30% in preterm infants) and then titrated up to prevent injuries from excessive oxygenation.
- Oxygen should never be given without some method of monitoring the level of oxygen in the infant's blood at all times, such as with pulse oximetry or arterial blood gas studies.
- Oxygen given to a neonate should always be humidified at 30-40%. Oxygen administered without humidification dries the nasal passages, increasing respiratory distress.
- Oxygen should also be warmed to 31-34 °C. Failing to warm the oxygen can cause cold stress for the infant.
- Any adjustments to the concentration of oxygen must be done slowly because an abrupt change can cause sudden vasoconstriction.

OXYGEN HOOD

Oxygen can be delivered through a clear **oxygen hood** (usually made of plastic) fitted over the infant's head. This type of delivery is appropriate for an infant who has a mild form of RDS and can maintain normal carbon dioxide levels in his blood, only needing supplemental oxygen. A blender that mixes the oxygen with water, thus humidifying it, is usually used with a hood. When the hood is being used for oxygen delivery, it is important that it fit the infant correctly. A hood too large will allow oxygen to escape and lower the concentration the infant is receiving, a hood too small will irritate the infant's skin at contact points. If the infant is to be held for feedings or otherwise removed from the hood, a secondary delivery tool should be available.

NASAL CANNULA DELIVERY OF OXYGEN

A nasal cannula is used for the delivery of a neonate who has a long term need for oxygen and is starting to develop motor skills needing the mobility that a cannula allows. The cannula should be the correct size for the infant. The application of a cannula involves putting some kind of skin protection on the infant's cheeks, such as a piece of OpSite or some other kind of barrier. The tubing is then taped to this barrier to avoid skin irritation. The nares should be frequently assessed for patency. Infants are obligatory nose breathers (they must breathe through their nose) and if mucous or formula plugs the holes in the cannula, they will not be getting the concentration of oxygen they need. Suction the nares as often as needed to keep them clear.

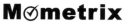

NON-INVASIVE POSITIVE PRESSURE VENTILATORS

Non-invasive positive pressure ventilators provide air through a tight-fitting nasal or facemask, usually pressure cycled, avoiding the need for intubation and reducing the danger of hospital-acquired infection and mortality rates. It can be used for acute respiratory failure and pulmonary edema. There are 2 types of non-invasive positive pressure ventilators:

- **CPAP** (Continuous positive airway pressure) provides a steady stream of pressurized air throughout both inspiration and expiration. CPAP improves breathing by decreasing preload and afterload for patients with congestive heart failure. It reduces the effort required for breathing and improves compliance of the lung.
- **Bi-PAP** (Bi-level positive airway pressure) provides a steady stream of pressurized air as CPAP, but it senses inspiratory effort and increases pressure during inspiration only. Bi-PAP pressures for inspiration and expiration can be set independently. Machines can be programmed with a backup rate to ensure a set number of respirations per minute.

MECHANICAL VENTILATION

ENDOTRACHEAL INTUBATION

The difficult airway of neonates makes choosing an age-appropriate **endotracheal tube** (ETT) very important. Generally, a 2.5 mm ETT is recommended for preterm neonates and a 3 mm ETT is recommended for term infants under the age of 1 year. Length-based tape (such as the Broselow Tape) can also be utilized for ETT size estimation in emergency situations. While uncuffed ETTs have been the traditional recommendation for newborns requiring intubation, cuffed ETTs that are low pressure and high volume have recently proven safe for neonates. Regardless, additional ETTs that are a size larger and a size smaller should be immediately available in the case of difficulty intubating.

An acceptable ETT leak is 15-20 cmH$_2$O pressure. The ETT may be inserted nasally or orally. Premedication (morphine or fentanyl and midazolam) is used to relieve stress on the neonate. Atropine may be given to block vagal response. ETT placement should immediately be verified by auscultation and radiograph, ultrasound, or disposable end-tidal carbon dioxide detectors. Esophageal intubation is indicated if no air exchange is detected bilaterally or if there is air sound over left upper abdomen. The tube may be too high if air sounds are diminished and too low if the right lung is better ventilated than the left.

POSITIVE PRESSURE VENTILATORS

Positive pressure ventilators assist respiration by applying pressure directly to the airway, inflating the lungs, forcing expansion of the alveoli, and facilitating gas exchange. Generally, endotracheal intubation or tracheostomy is necessary to maintain positive pressure ventilation. There are 3 basic kinds of positive pressure ventilators:

- **Pressure cycled**: This type of ventilation is usually used for short-term treatment in adolescents or adults. The IPPB machine is the most common type. This delivers a flow of air to a preset pressure and then cycles off. Airway resistance or changes in compliance can affect volume of air and may compromise ventilation.
- **Time cycled**: This type of ventilation regulates the volume of air the infant receives by controlling the length of inspiration and the flow rate. This type of ventilator is used almost exclusively for neonates and infants.
- **Volume cycled**: This type of ventilation provides a preset flow of pressurized air during inspiration and then cycles off and allows passive expiration, providing a fairly consistent volume of air.

HIGH FREQUENCY JET VENTILATION

High frequency jet ventilation (HFJV) (Life Pulse) directs a high velocity stream of air into the lungs in a long spiraling spike that forces carbon dioxide against the walls, penetrating dead space and providing gas exchange by using small tidal volumes of 1-3 mL/kg, much smaller than with conventional mechanical ventilation. Because the jet stream technology is effective for short distances, the valve and pressure transducer must be placed by the infant's head. Inhalation is controlled while expiration is passive, but the rate of respiration is up to 11 per second ("panting" respirations). HFJV may be used in conjunction with low-pressure conventional ventilation to increase flow to alveoli. HFJV reduces barotrauma because of the low tidal volume and low pressure. HFJV is used for numerous conditions, including evolving chronic lung disease, pulmonary interstitial emphysema, bronchopulmonary dysplasia, and hypoxemic respiratory failure. It reduces mean airway pressure (MAP) and the oxygenation index. Treatment with HFJV may reduce the need for ECMO.

HIGH FREQUENCY OSCILLATORY VENTILATION

High frequency oscillatory ventilation provides pressurized ventilation with tidal volumes approximately equal to dead space at about 150 breaths per minutes (bpm). Pressure is usually higher with HFOV than HFJV in order to maintain expansion of the alveoli and to keep the airway open during gas exchange. Oxygenation is regulated separately. HFOV has both an active inspiration and expiration, so the respiratory cycle is completely controlled. HFOV reduces pulmonary vascular resistance and improves ventilation-perfusion matching and oxygenation without injuring the lung, reducing the risk of barotrauma. HFOV is used for respiratory distress syndrome, persistent pulmonary hypertension of the newborn (PPHN) associated with meconium aspiration syndrome (MAS). Other indications are air leak syndromes, pulmonary interstitial emphysema, and congenital diaphragmatic hernia. Infants in respiratory distress may be placed on HFOV immediately after birth instead of on conventional ventilation to avoid pulmonary damage.

VENTILATOR MANAGEMENT

There are many types of ventilators now in use, and the specific directions for use of each type must be followed carefully, but there are general principles that apply to all **ventilator management.** The following should be monitored:

- **Type of ventilation**: volume-cycled, pressure-cycled, negative-pressure, HFJV, HFOV, CPAP, Bi-PAP.
- **Control mode**: controlled ventilation, assisted ventilation, synchronized intermittent mandatory [allows spontaneous breaths between ventilator controlled inhalation/exhalation], positive-end expiratory pressure (PEEP) [positive pressure at end of expiration], CPAP, Bi-PAP.
- **Tidal volume** (T_v) range should be set in relation to respiratory rate.
- **Inspiratory-expiratory ratio** (I:E) usually ranges from 1:2 to 1:5, but may be outside of that range.
- **Respiratory rate** will depend upon T_v and $PaCO_2$ target.
- **Fraction of inspired oxygen** (FiO_2) [percentage of oxygen in the inspired air], usually ranging from 21-100%, usually maintained <40% to avoid toxicity.
- **Sensitivity** determines the effort needed to trigger inspiration.
- **Pressure** controls the pressure exerted in delivering T_v.
- **Rate of flow** controls the L/min speed of T_v.

VILI

Ventilation-induced lung injury (VILI) is damage caused by mechanical ventilation. It is common in acute distress syndrome (ARDS) but can affect any ventilation patient. VILI comprises 4 interrelated elements:

- **Barotrauma**: damage to the lung caused by excessive pressure
- **Volutrauma**: alveolar damage related to high tidal volume ventilation
- **Atelectotrauma**: injury caused by repetitive forced opening and closing of alveoli
- **Biotrauma**: inflammatory response

In VILI, essentially the increased pressure and tidal volume over-distends the alveoli, which rupture, and air moves into the interstitial tissue resulting in pulmonary interstitial emphysema. With continued ventilation, the air in the interstitium moves into the subcutaneous tissue and may result in pneumopericardium and pneumomediastinum, or rupture the pleural sac. This can cause tension pneumothorax and mediastinal shift, leading to respiratory failure and cardiac arrest. VILI has caused a change in ventilation procedures with lower tidal volumes and pressures used as well as newer forms of ventilation, HFJV and HFOV, preferred to mechanical ventilation for many patients.

TRACHEOSTOMY

A tracheostomy in the neonate is done in emergent situations, such as upper airway obstruction or abnormalities, and elective situations, such as for prolonged ventilation or subglottic stenosis related to endotracheal intubation. The tracheostomy tube should extend to 1 cm superior to the carina. Because of small size (2.5-3.0 cm inner diameter), neonatal tracheostomy tubes have no inner cannula and are usually not cuffed. Humidity must be provided by attaching the tracheostomy to a warmed humidified air source or use of heat-moisture exchangers. Suctioning to maintain patency is done every 4 hours with the suction catheter extending slightly below (3-5 mm) the tracheostomy tube, and the suctioning length should be prominently posted. There is no consensus on the use of saline instillation during suctioning. Tubes should be changed regularly, usually at least once weekly. Skin about the stoma should be inspected twice daily and drainage cleansed with saline or hydrogen peroxide/saline (if crusting). In some cases, a thin gauze or hydrocolloid dressing may be placed under the flanges.

RISK FACTORS WITH ADMINISTRATION OF OXYGEN/VENTILATION

There are risk factors associated with administration of oxygen/ventilation:

- High oxygen concentration can result in **retinopathy of prematurity (ROP) and blindness**.
- The mechanical ventilation used to treat a neonate's respiratory disease exerts pressure on the vascular system feeding the lungs; this includes pressure on the pulmonary artery, which comes out of the heart. If this pressure on the pulmonary artery is great enough, **cardiac output can be lessened**. Lowering the positive pressure settings on the ventilator can alleviate some of this pressure, thus improving cardiac output. Cardiac output can also be supplemented by giving the infant an infusion of extra fluid. This helps to raise cardiac output by enough to compensate for the increased pressure from the ventilator pressures that the heart must overcome to keep the body well oxygenated.
- Oxygenation during resuscitation has been recommended to start at 21% (up to 30% in a preterm newborn) to prevent injuries that can occur from hyperoxygenation. During CPR, oxygen should be administered at 100%.

CHEST TUBE INSERTION/REMOVAL FOR PNEUMOTHORAX

Chest tubes are inserted in the neonate to treat pneumothorax causing cardiac or respiratory compromise or pleural effusion. **Transillumination** may be used to identify the area of pneumothorax but a **chest x-ray** is more accurate. An 8-12 Fr. chest tube is placed anteriorly for collections of air and posteriorly/laterally for fluid. The infant is supine with the arm at 90° on the insertion side. The insertion sites are

- **Anterior**: midclavicular line, second or third intercostal space
- **Posterior/lateral**: anterior axillary line, fourth, fifth, or sixth intercostal space

Lidocaine is instilled and an incision made over the rib below the target intercostal space. The tissue is spread and the pleura punctured above the rib with a hemostat, expelling air. The chest tube is inserted 2-3 cm for preterm infants and 3-4 cm for full-term infants. The purse-string suture is tightened and the chest tube attached to 2 or 3 bottles or a self-contained Pleur-evac underwater seal system. An x-ray is taken to confirm placement. The chest tube is removed quickly and pressure dressing applied if there is no bubbling for 24 hours and the radiograph is clear.

PLEUR-EVAC SYSTEM

A chest tube is attached to a three-chamber system called a **Pleur-Evac.** As the name indicates, there are three separate chambers in this collection system:

- The first chamber is the **collection chamber**. This chamber is where the air and/or fluid that is being drained from the pleural space collects as a result of a pulmonary leak. Bubbling in this chamber is the result of air being pumped out of the pleural space and is expected.
- The second chamber is the **water seal chamber**; this chamber is where the water in an amount prescribed by the physician is placed to create the vacuum necessary to pull the fluid and/or air out of the pleural space. The amount of water placed in this chamber affects the amount of pressure and should be carefully monitored to make sure it remains at the ordered level. Bubbling in this chamber indicates a leak and must be investigated.
- The third chamber is the **suction chamber**, which is responsible for the suction that creates the pressure removing the air from the pleural space.

NEEDLE ASPIRATION FOR PNEUMOTHORAX

Neonates receiving bag and mask ventilation or mechanical ventilation risk developing a **pneumothorax**. Signs of pneumothorax include rapid deterioration, poor oxygenation, tachypnea, increased work breathing, impaired circulation, unequal air entry into lungs, displaced apical heartbeat, and increased transillumination on the affected side. If the neonate's clinical status allows it, a chest x-ray will confirm the diagnosis. Air is removed by **needle aspiration.**

The **equipment** for needle aspiration:

- Oral sucrose
- 1% lidocaine
- Fentanyl
- 21-gauge butterfly needle
- 10 mL syringe
- 3-way stopcock attached to the syringe
- 70% isopropyl alcohol swab
- Sterile gloves

The **procedure** for needle aspiration is as follows:

1. Give oral sucrose.
2. Place infant in supine position.
3. Swab second and third intercostal spaces in midclavicular line with alcohol.
4. Infiltrate site with 1% lidocaine 0.5-1.0 mL.
5. Drape insertion site.
6. Give 250 mcg fentanyl over 2-3 minutes IV.
7. Insert needle directly into second or third intercostal space in mid-clavicular line until air is aspirated into the syringe.
8. Expel air through stopcock.

Thermoregulation and Integumentary

NEUTRAL THERMAL ENVIRONMENT

A neutral thermal environment (NTE) is a place in which the infant's body temperature is maintained within a normal range without alterations in metabolic rate or increased oxygen consumption (i.e., environmental temperature in which oxygen consumption and glucose consumption are lowest). Infants who are in an NTE are not utilizing energy to maintain their body temperature in the normal range. Just because an infant has a normal body temperature does not mean he/she is in an NTE. The infant may still be utilizing mechanisms, such as non-shivering thermogenesis, to maintain body temperatures, as evidenced by increased oxygen consumption and poor weight gain over time. Charts are commercially available that outline the appropriate NTE for infants based on current weight and birth weight.

HEAT TRANSFER MECHANISMS

There are four heat transfer mechanisms to consider when caring for a neonate, especially a premature one:

- **Conduction**: The transfer of heat between solid objects of different temperatures in contact with each other. Heat is transferred from the body of the infant to a cold surface it may come into contact with, such as a scale. Care should be taken to make sure the scales are warmed before use. Conduction can also be used to warm the infant by placing a warmed blanket next to the skin.
- **Convection**: The transfer of heat through air currents moving around and across an infant's body. Incubators use convection of warm air being pumped into the incubator to keep an infant warm. Heat can be lost this way if a cool draft is allowed near the infant.
- **Radiation**: Heat transferred between two objects not in contact with each other. This is the transfer of heat through emission of infrared rays. Radiant warming beds use this mechanism to warm the infant. Heat loss occurs when an infant is in an incubator and the walls of the incubator are cooler than body temperature. The neonate in an incubator with this situation will lose body heat through radiation from its body to the cooler walls despite the warm air being pumped in.
- **Evaporation**: Loss of heat occurs when moisture evaporates from the surface of the skin. Evaporation is the result of the conversion of liquid into a vapor and is a major concern at birth, as a wet infant can experience a 3-degree drop in body temperature in only about 10 minutes. Thus, it is critical to dry the neonate at birth and to replace wet linens with warm, dry ones.

EVAPORATIVE HEAT LOSS AND HUMIDITY RELATED TO PRETERM INFANTS

Evaporative heat loss occurs when moisture vaporizes from the skin of an infant. In infants born younger than 31 weeks gestation, **evaporative heat loss** is greatly enhanced by the poor keratinization of the infant's skin. Poor keratinization makes skin highly permeable, which promotes both fluid and heat loss. This permeability decreases 7-10 days after birth. The amount of evaporation is dependent on the relative humidity of the environment. The more **humid the environment**, the more that evaporation and its associated heat loss are suppressed. A dry environment promotes evaporative heat and fluid loss through the skin. An incubator with humidity controls should be used for infants who are vulnerable to evaporative heat loss. Infants prone to temperature instability should be kept in a highly humid environment.

COLD STRESS/HYPOTHERMIA
SIGNS OF COLD STRESS

Cold stress/hypothermia in the neonate is a body temperature measurement of less than 36.5 °C rectally with associated symptoms. Preterm neonates are especially vulnerable to cold stress, as they have limited ability to intrinsically create or conserve body heat. They do not shiver, have limited ability to constrict superficial blood vessels and have limited amounts of both subcutaneous and brown fat. **Signs of cold stress** include:

- Body is cool to touch
- Central cyanosis and acrocyanosis
- Mottling of skin
- Poor feeding, weak suck, increased gastric residuals, and abdominal distension
- Bradycardia
- Shallow respirations with tachypnea
- Restlessness and irritability
- Apnea
- Lethargy and decreased activity
- Weak cry
- Hypoglycemia
- Central nervous system depression with hypotonia
- Edema

RISK FACTORS IN PRETERM INFANTS

Preterm infants have not yet developed many of the features that full term infants use to help protect them from heat loss. The characteristics that make premature infants especially **vulnerable to cold stress** include:

- Larger surface area to body mass ratio that allows for quicker transfer of body heat to the environment
- Decreased amounts of subcutaneous fat that provides insulation from heat loss
- Decreased amounts of brown fat used for non-shivering thermogenesis
- Immature skin that is not completely keratinized is more permeable to evaporative water and heat loss
- Inability to flex the body to conserve heat
- Limited control of skin blood flow mechanisms that conserve heat

NON-SHIVERING THERMOGENESIS

Non-shivering thermogenesis (NST) is the major route of rapid increase of body temperature in response to cold stress in the term neonate. NST is the oxidation of brown fat to create heat. Brown adipose tissue contains a high concentration of stored triglycerides, a rich capillary network, and is controlled by the sympathetic nervous system. Brown fat cells have a rich supply of mitochondria that are unique, in that when fat is metabolized ATP is not produced, but instead heat is created. Temperature regulation is controlled by the posterior hypothalamus. When a cold body temperature is detected, the posterior hypothalamus responds by triggering the adrenal glands to release norepinephrine and the pituitary gland to release thyroxine. Both norepinephrine and thyroxine stimulate NST. Brown adipose production begins around 26-28 weeks of gestation and continues until 3-5 weeks after delivery. Premature infants have limited amounts of brown fat and limited ability to create heat via NST.

THERMOREGULATION TO TREAT HYPOTHERMIA

There are a number of steps in the treatment of hypothermia:

1. Determine if the cause of hypothermia is from an abnormal physiological process in the infant or from environmental conditions.
2. Rewarm the infant slowly, as rewarming too rapidly may result in apnea or hypotension.
3. Maintain the ambient temperature at 1.0-1.5 °C higher than the infant's temperature. Oxygen consumption is not elevated when the difference between the skin temperature and the environmental air temperature is less than 1.5 °C.
4. Increase the air temperature by approximately 1 °C every hour until the infant's temperature is in the normal range and stable.
5. Warm IV fluids with a blood-warming device prior to infusion, to enhance warming of the child.
6. Closely monitor the infant's blood glucose levels, vital signs, and urinary output during rewarming.

HYPERTHERMIA

Hyperthermia (rectal temperature greater than 37.0 °C) can be caused by excessive heat from an external source (such as a radiant warmer set too high) or internally from a hypermetabolic state (such as a fever):

External heat source	Hypermetabolic
Core temperature < skin temperature	Core temperature > skin temperature
Skin warm and flushed	Skin cool to touch

Infants who are physiologically competent attempt to cool themselves when hyperthermia is caused by an external heat source by an extended posture, diaphoresis, and flushed, warm skin. Hyperthermia in the neonate can cause increased metabolic demands, vasodilatation, and increased fluid loss. An increased metabolic demand leads to an increased oxygen requirement, hypoxia, cyanosis, and breathing irregularities, such as tachypnea. Increased glucose consumption leads to hypoglycemia and its associated signs (jitteriness, lethargy, vomiting, or seizures). Peripheral vasodilatation helps cool the infant but may cause tachycardia and hypotension. Increased fluid losses contribute to tachycardia and hypotension. Signs of shock may develop with lethargy and decreased urine output. Dehydration may also cause electrolyte abnormalities.

MINIMIZING HEAT LOSS

At delivery, minimize heat loss while evaluating the newborn by following these steps:

- Dry the infant thoroughly (including hair) to minimize evaporative heat loss and remove wet towels.
- Place a cap on the infant's head, as the head is the most significant area of heat loss.
- When the infant is to be weighed, cover the scales with a warm cloth to minimize conductive heat loss.
- Place the infant in a warm environment such as:
  o Skin-to-skin contact with the mother and covered with a warm blanket.
  o Bundled in warm blankets and given to the mother to hold.
  o Underneath a preheated warmer for further evaluation or resuscitation.

Minimizing heat loss is especially important if the newborn is premature or has intrauterine growth restriction, but full-term newborns also suffer if they become chilled.

Kangaroo Care

Dr. Edgar Ray invented kangaroo care in the late 1970's in Bogotá, Colombia, when morbidity and mortality rates rose in his NICU, but he had limited technological resources. **Kangaroo care** consists of placing the infant, after drying and warming, in minimal clothing in an upright position on the mother's bare chest between her breasts. This allows for skin-to-skin contact with the infant's head next to the mother's heart. A precipitous drop was noted in premature infant mortality after this method of care was instigated. The concept is to provide the neonate with closeness similar to that experienced with the mother while in the womb. Kangaroo care is maintained for as long as the neonate allows. Preterm infants attached to ventilators and IV infusions also benefit from kangaroo care. There are physiological and psychological benefits for both the neonate and the mother. Enhanced bonding between the neonate and the mother, shorter hospital stays, low cost, and decreased morbidity and mortality are all documented benefits.

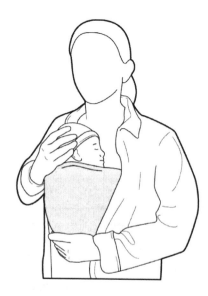

The following are specific **benefits** of kangaroo care for the mother, the neonate, and the institution:

- **Mother's benefits:**
  - Enhanced bonding with the infant
  - Increased production of milk with higher rates of successful breastfeeding
  - Increased confidence in caring for the infant
  - Increased opportunity for teaching and assessing maternal care by nursing staff
- **Neonate's benefits:**
  - Regulation of temperature, heart and respiratory rates
  - Calming effect with decreased stress
  - Decreased episodes of apnea
  - Increased weight gain
  - Enhanced bonding with the mother
  - Fewer nosocomial infections

- **Institutional benefits**:
  o Earlier discharge from hospital
  o Decreased morbidity and mortality (especially in developing countries)
  o Decreased use of financial resources

INCUBATORS

The goal of placing an infant in an incubator is to provide a neutral thermal environment (NTE) that places minimal stress on the infant. Most incubators are rigid, box-like structures like an isolette, in which an infant is kept in a controlled environment to receive medical care. The infant is allowed to grow and mature here before being transitioned to the more "uncontrolled" environment of an open crib. Features that incubators possess that enhance the production of an NTE include a heater, a fan to circulate warmed air, and a humidity control system. They also usually have a way to increase the oxygen content of the environment and ports to allow for nursing care without removing the infant. A servo-control is used in conjunction with a temperature-sensing thermistor that is attached to the infant to help regulate the infant's temperature within a set range. Some incubators may have double walls that lessen radiant heat loss. Infants who are in need of close monitoring are not placed in an incubator but instead are placed under a radiant warmer with minimal covering. This allows the nurse to monitor the infant's skin color and breathing patterns more closely.

RADIANT WARMERS

Radiant warmers are devices that provide overhead heat directly to the infant. Radiant heaters provide an area for direct observation and free access to the infant, which is very useful in the initial evaluation and resuscitation (if necessary) of the newborn or for procedures such as intubation or line placement. Radiant heat devices work best if the room temperature is kept above 25 °C. Two **problems related to radiant warmers** include:

- Promote dehydration if an infant is placed under them for a prolonged amount of time, especially if the infant is premature
- Risk overheating the infant or cause first-degree burns

Temperature sensors must be appropriately placed and the infant's temperature monitored frequently to ensure the infant is not being over or under heated.

SKIN TEMPERATURE PROBES

Skin temperature probes are often used to monitor the temperature of the infant in an isolette or radiant warmer. Incorrect placement of the probe can alter the reading, causing the warming device to deliver too much or too little heat. The temperature probe should not be placed over a bony area of the body or over an area where brown adipose tissue is abundant. Brown adipose tissue is abundant around the neck, the midscapular region of the back, and the mediastinum and organs in the thoracic cavity, kidneys, and adrenal glands. A common probe placement area for an infant who is supine is over the liver. If the probe is not making good skin contact, it will indicate that the infant is cold, and the warmer will deliver increased amounts of heat, possibly causing hyperthermia. If the probe is underneath the infant, it may indicate an artificially warm temperature and decrease heat to the infant, causing hypothermia.

SERVOCONTROL

The servocontrol is a **thermistor probe** used to monitor the temperature of the infant in an incubator or radiant warmer. The servocontrol is essentially the automatic thermostat that adjusts the environmental temperature in response to the infant's body temperature. Typically, the infant's temperature should be maintained at 36.0-36.5 °C. Incorrect placement of the probe can alter the reading, causing the warming device to deliver too much or too little heat. The servocontrol should avoid a bony area of the body or an area where brown adipose tissue is abundant (neck, midscapular region, mediastinum, and organs in the thoracic cavity, kidneys, and adrenal glands). If the infant is supine, the probe is placed on the abdomen at the midpoint between the xiphoid process and the umbilicus. If prone, the probe is placed over either flank. If in a radiant warmer, a special foil shield should protect the probe. As mentioned above, the probe must make proper skin contact, and the nurse should be sure that is not reading artificially warm or artificially cool. An incorrect reading can put the infant at risk for hyperthermia or hypothermia.

SKIN DEVELOPMENT AND CARE

The **neonate's skin** comprises 4% of its body weight and is the largest organ, but it is still developing and doesn't reach maturity until adolescence or later:

- Neonatal skin is about 1 mm thick (2 mm at maturity) and has little subcutaneous fat, so thermoregulation is impaired, making the infant lose heat rapidly. The neonate's temperature must be maintained, but overheating must be avoided. The thinness of the skin increases chemical absorption, so care must be used when applying lotions, chemicals, or topical medications.
- The epidermis and dermis are loosely connected, increasing the danger of separation and blister formation with friction.
- Eccrine glands function and produce sweat but are immature and may not be adequate for temperature control, increasing the danger of overheating. Apocrine glands are small and nonfunctional.
- Melanin levels are low at birth, so skin is light-colored and more susceptible to damage from the sun. As such, infants must be shielded from direct sunlight.

CAFÉ AU LAIT SPOTS

Café au lait spots (CAL) are flat skin lesions with increased melanin content and regular or irregular borders. If the CAL spots are faint, use a Wood lamp to make them easier to see. Fewer than 3 café au lait spots have no clinical significance. However, 6 or more café au lait spots with a diameter larger than 5 mm occur in 95% of patients with **neurofibromatosis type 1 (NF1)**, a disorder of chromosome 17. Lisch nodules on the irises and Crowe's sign (freckles on the axillae and inguinal area) corroborate the diagnosis of NF1. The pediatrician must be alerted that this child should receive future monitoring for the symptoms that occur with NF1, such as bowed legs, rib lesions, scoliosis, neurofibromas, glaucoma, and corneal opacification. Café au lait spots are also associated with tuberous sclerosis, McCune-Albright syndrome, ataxia-telangiectasia, Gaucher disease, basal cell nevus syndrome, and Fanconi anemia. CAL affects 18% of black infants, 3% of Hispanic infants, and 0.3% of white infants.

HEMANGIOMA

Hemangioma is a bright red vascular tumor that occurs in 1-3% of neonates, especially in girls, preterm infants <1500 g, and those whose mothers had chorionic villus sampling. The head and neck are the most common sites. **Hemangiomas** may initially appear as a faint telangiectasia or red macule, but they proliferate rapidly during the first year, after which they go through a slow involution in which they decrease in size, usually complete in 95% by adolescence. Hemangiomas may be superficial, deep, or mixed and may involve skin as well as other organs. Complications, such as airway compromise, vision problem, ulceration, renal abnormalities, imperforate anus, and skeletal anomalies may occur as the hemangioma grows, depending upon adjacent structures. Imaging of hemangiomas is indicated only in infants that display evidence or possibility of underlying structural abnormalities. Treatment may include just monitoring or systemic or localized treatment with corticosteroids to slow proliferation. Oral propranolol is the first-line therapy for infantile hemangiomas in infants age 5 weeks to 5 months. Pulsed dye laser treatment is a common treatment to reduce proliferation.

SUBCUTANEOUS FAT NECROSIS

Subcutaneous fat necrosis is a nodular skin lesion disorder that usually occurs ≤6 weeks of birth in full-term or post-term infants caused by necrosis of subcutaneous fatty tissue. Onset is usually between days 2-21. **Subcutaneous fat necrosis** is commonly associated with hypothermia, trauma to tissue from forceps, neonatal stress (various causes), and hypercalcemia. Single or multiple lesions may develop, ranging in size from about 1 cm in diameter to much larger, with erythema obvious over lesions. Lesions are usually rubbery and often distributed across the buttocks, upper legs, shoulders, upper back, upper extremities, and cheeks. In some cases, fluctuant lesions may open and drain or require aspiration. The lesions usually resolve over time with no treatment. Serum calcium should be monitored and hypercalcemia evaluated for cause and treated as necessary.

ECCHYMOSIS, PETECHIAE, HYPERPIGMENTATION, AND HYPOPIGMENTATION

Ecchymosis (large blue-purple discolored bruising) and **petechiae** (pinpoint <1 mm hemorrhagic areas) may be the result of birth trauma, particularly difficult births, breech births, or forceps-assisted birth and is most noticeable on the presenting part. These types of bruising usually fade within 24-48 hours, but if they persist, they may indicate underlying pathology. **Ecchymosis** and petechiae can indicate clotting disorders and bleeding in the tissue, such as can occur with DIC. They may also be evidence of thrombocytopenia (especially diffuse petechiae) and vitamin K deficiency.

Hypopigmentation may be caused by a number of disorders, including PKU, Addison's disease, vitiligo, albinism, and herpes simplex virus. It may also result from post-inflammatory changes.

Hyperpigmentation, while rare in the newborn, can occur with severe toxoplasmosis infection, Addison's disease, liver disease, porphyria, pellagra, sprue, lentiginosis, and melanism. Untreated syphilitic lesions may cause hypo- or hyperpigmentation after regression.

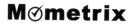
ERYTHEMA TOXICUM

Erythema toxicum is a skin eruption of erythematous papules, vesicles, and sometimes pustules that is essentially benign and occurs in ≥50% of newborns. It is a generalized rash that resembles that of herpes simplex, occurring on the face, limbs, and trunk (everywhere except the palms and soles of the feet). It usually occurs 2-3 days after birth. The lesions are surrounded by a mottled erythematous halo of about 0.5-1.5 cm. Individual lesions often appear and resolve within hours but new lesions occur. Lesions may be limited to a few on the face or may cover the body. Erythema toxicum is often associated with eosinophilia and occurs in the first few weeks of life before the immune system matures, so it is hypothesized that the rash may be an allergic response. The rash usually resolves in about 2 weeks without treatment.

NEONATAL PUSTULAR MELANOSIS

Neonatal pustular melanosis is a benign rash (vesicles and macules) that is present at birth in about 2.2% of white infants and 4.4% of black infants. Usually, in preterm infants, vesicles (2-4 mm) with milky fluid are present at birth and rupture, leaving a halo of white scaly tissue and a pigmented macule at the center. Erythema is not associated with this rash. Full-term infants may exhibit only the macular stage as the vesicles ruptured prior to birth. The pigmented discoloration fades with time but may persist for ≤3 months. The cause of neonatal pustular melanosis is not known. The rash may be localized and sparse or profuse (beneath chin, neck, upper chest, upper back, and buttocks). No treatment is indicated, and there appears to be no long-term sequelae, but the lesions must be differentiated from congenital herpes infection, especially if erythema is evident.

PREAURICULAR SKIN TAG

A preauricular skin tag is a small extension of skin located anterior to the ear. They may be single or multiple in number, and they may be pedunculated (attached by a narrow stalk) or sessile (flat). Occasionally, skin tags are associated with hearing loss and dysmorphic features in some congenital syndromes (e.g., cat eye syndrome). At one time, it was believed that a **preauricular skin tag** was an indication of renal anomalies, but this has not been supported by research. A skin tag with a narrow stalk may be simply ligated, but one with a thicker stalk should be removed by a surgeon, as the stalk may contain cartilage that extends into the subcutaneous tissue. Removal of a cartilaginous skin tag requires anesthesia.

PORT-WINE STAIN

A port-wine stain (capillary angioma) is a birthmark comprised of dilated capillaries below the epidermis. The lesion is usually on the face or neck and is light pink at birth but darkens with age. The lesion alone is benign, but it may be an indication of other disorders, such as Sturge-Weber syndrome (neurological disorder with seizures, paralysis, and glaucoma) or Klippel-Trenaunay-Weber syndrome (disorder with hypertrophy of bones and soft tissue as well as varicose veins and multiple port-wine stains), so the infant should be evaluated and have an eye examination, especially if the lesion is on the eyelids, as this is associated with glaucoma. Over time, the capillary angioma may thicken and form nodules, so early treatment is advisable. The most common treatment is laser therapy, which destroys the capillaries without damaging other tissue, usually done in infancy to prevent psychological trauma and to prevent changes in the skin, such as thickening.

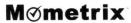

Pharmacology, Pharmacokinetics, and Pharmacodynamics

PRINCIPLES OF DRUG ADMINISTRATION TO NEONATES

DOSAGE AND INTERVAL

The half-life of a drug ($t_{1/2}$) is the time required to reduce serum concentrations by half, and half-life must be considered when determining **dosage and interval** of drugs for neonates. Steady state is usually achieved within 4-5 half-lives. Half-life is a factor of clearance, and small or preterm infants often have reduced clearance because of slow metabolism, resulting in longer half-life. In determining dosage, the infant's weight, gestational age, and post-natal age must be considered.

One major problem with dosing and interval for neonates is that most drugs are not tested on infants, so about 98% are prescribed off-label. There are a number of reference tools available, including software programs, to assist with determining proper dosage and interval for neonatal medications.

NEONATAL TOLERANCE AND WEANING

Tolerance and weaning from drugs are often concerns with the administration of opiates. **Tolerance** occurs after repeated administration results in a lessening of effects, requiring an increase in dosage to achieve the same results. When a neonate is weaned from a medication or a dosage is decreased, only one class of medications should be involved. Thus, if the infant is receiving both an opiate and a benzodiazepine, they should not be weaned from both at the same time. The infant should be evaluated for level of pain prior to weaning and reassessed at least every 4 hours during the weaning process. Usually medications are reduced at a rate of 10% per day or 20% every other day. Infants often tolerate an initial reduction in dose better than subsequent reductions, so careful observation for signs of increased pain or withdrawal must be made. Careful control of the environment—temperature, light, and noise—should be done to reduce infant stress during the **weaning process**.

PRINCIPLES OF NEONATAL ABSORPTION

Principles of neonatal absorption can be discussed specific to various elements of the process of absorption:

- **GI tract**: Medications may have increased or decreased rates of absorption depending on the rate of gastric emptying, the acidity of the GI tract, the availability of pancreatic or other enzymes, the presence of intestinal bacteria, and GI perfusion as well as disease processes, such as vomiting or diarrhea, and medical procedures, such as GI suctioning.
- **Skin/muscle**: Skin maturation occurs between 23 and 33 weeks of gestation and continues to mature in the weeks after birth. The neonate's skin is thinner and more readily absorbs topical preparations because of increased permeability. Muscle is thinner and generally has less perfusion, so absorption may be slow in the premature or seriously ill neonate, but if perfusion increases, the faster absorption of retained medication may result in overdose.
- **Blood drug levels**: Medications are absorbed immediately but distribution to some organs may vary, and therapeutic levels must be monitored carefully as toxic concentrations may occur if medication administered by IV push or over a short period. Dosage and concentration may be inconsistent because clearance is prolonged.
- **Drug incompatibilities**: Occur when two drugs undergo a reaction when combined that results in the deterioration of one or both of the drugs and can result in inadequate therapeutic effect. Parenteral drugs/solutions may appear cloudy or develop precipitates. The greater the number of drugs administered, the greater the risk of incompatibilities.
- **Drug withdrawal** (therapeutic drugs): Withdrawal protocols vary according to the medication. Some medications, such as some heart medications, must be withdrawn slowly in decreasing doses to avoid a negative response while others can be stopped abruptly. Because clearance may be slowed, the effects of the drug may continue after the medication has been discontinued, so this must be considered when changing medications.
- **Drug resistance**: Ineffectiveness of a drug to treat an infection or condition. For example, some forms of *Staphylococcus* are resistant to vancomycin because of antimicrobial resistance.

PROTEIN BINDING IN NEONATAL DRUG THERAPY

Protein binding is an important consideration for neonatal drug therapy because when drugs are bound by proteins in the blood, they are not available to be biologically active. The portion of the drug that is **not** bound to a plasma protein is the active portion. **Protein binding** is significant in premature neonates because they typically have:

- Lower levels of plasma proteins, such as albumin.
- Lower binding capacity.
- Susceptibility to competition from endogenous substances like bilirubin, which also attaches to plasma proteins.

Drugs that are normally highly protein bound in the adult have a higher free percentage (activity) in the neonate. Lower than expected dosages may give clinical results. Examples of drugs that are highly protein bound include phenobarbital and indomethacin. If a drug with a high affinity for plasma proteins is administered, it may displace bilirubin from binding sites, increasing the neonate's risk for kernicterus.

PLACENTAL TRANSFER OF DRUGS

The **placenta** acts as a barrier to protect the fetus, but its main function is to provide oxygen and nutrients for the fetus by linking the maternal and fetal circulation. Virtually all **drugs** cross the barrier to some degree, some by active transport. Some drugs are readily diffused across the placental barrier and can affect the fetus. Drugs that are non-ionized, fat-soluble and have low molecular weight diffuse easily as glucose does. Once a substance crosses the barrier, the lower pH of the fetal blood allows weakly basic drugs, such as local anesthetics and opioids, to cross into fetal circulation where they become ionized and accumulate because they can't pass back into maternal circulation (ion trapping). Giving an intravenous injection during a contraction, when uterine blood flow decreases, reduces the amount of the drug that crosses the placental barrier. A few drugs with large molecules (heparin, insulin) have minimal transfer, and lipid soluble drugs transfer more readily than water-soluble.

ANTICOAGULANTS

Neonates may require **anticoagulant therapy** for thrombosis, sometimes associated with catheters used for critical care or thrombocytosis associated with iron-deficiency anemia. Anticoagulant therapy poses fewer risks than fibrinolytic therapy although excessive bleeding may occur. Anticoagulants include:

- **Unfractionated heparin**:
  o Preterm infants: initial bolus of 50 units/kg and maintenance of 15-35 units/kg/hr to maintain level of 0.3-0.7 units/mL
  o Full-term infants: initial bolus of 100 units/kg and maintenance of 25-50 units/kg/hr to maintain level of 0.3-0.7 unit/mL
- **Low-molecular-weight heparin**: 1.7 mg/kg subcutaneously every 12 hours or as needed to maintain level of 0.5-1.0 units/mL 4 hours after administration
- **Warfarin**: may be used in rare cases, such as genetic deficiencies of protein C or S (purpura fulminans), for long-term therapy

Infants that are heparin resistant may be administered fresh frozen plasma (1 mL/kg every 24-48 hours) or AT concentrate (50-150 units/kg every 24-48 hours) to enhance effect of heparin.

ANTICONVULSANTS

Anticonvulsants are used to treat seizures, which often indicate central nervous system dysfunction. Seizures are more common during the neonatal period than later in infancy/childhood and are associated with low birth weight. Treatment is critical to prevent brain damage, but drugs may cause sedation, rash, and blood dyscrasias:

- **Phenobarbital** (Luminal) is the neonatal drug of choice. Loading dose is 20 mg/kg IV in 10-15 minutes and then 5 mg/kg to maximum 40 mg/kg to control seizures. Maintenance dose is 3-4 mg/kg/24 hours in 2 doses beginning ≥12 hours after loading dose. Infant should be provided oxygen and ventilation as needed.
- **Fosphenytoin** (Cerbxy) is used if phenobarbital is ineffective. It has high water solubility and neutral pH and does not cause tissue injury. It can be administered IV or IM. Loading dose is 15-20 mg PE/kg and maintenance is 4-8 mg PE/kg/day. Blood pressure should be monitored and caution exercised with hyperbilirubinemia.
- **Phenytoin** (Dilantin) is sometimes used instead of fosphenytoin if phenobarbital is ineffective. It is incompatible with other drugs and glucose and can cause hypotension, bradycardia, and dysrhythmias if administered too quickly and cannot be given IM or in central lines. Loading dose is 15-20 mg/kg IV over 30 minutes, and maintenance is 4-8 mg/kg/day. Line must be flushed with NS.
- **Lorazepam** (Ativan) is used if other drugs are ineffective in controlling seizures. Onset is action is very rapid (<5 minutes), so the infant must be monitored carefully for respiratory depression. Medication is administered by slow IV push over a number of minutes at 0.05-0.10 mg/kg.

In some cases, seizures are triggered by hypoglycemia, and treatment includes glucose 10% solution. Pyridoxine (B_6) deficiency may also cause seizures and is treated with IV or IM Vitamin B_6.

ANTIBIOTICS

Antibiotics are frequently prescribed to neonates with suspected infection or sepsis, but dosing must be carefully calculated to account for the larger volume of extracellular fluid and the clearance rate of their renal system. Neonatal exposure to antibiotics also increases the risk of future health problems (due to their influence on the development of the neonate's gastrointestinal system/gut) or antibiotic resistance. Antibiotics may be classified according to their chemical nature, origin, action, or range of effectiveness. **Broad-spectrum antibiotics** are useful against both gram-positive and gram-negative bacteria. **Medium-spectrum antibiotics** are usually effective against gram-positive bacteria, although some may also be effective against gram-negative bacteria. **Narrow-spectrum antibiotics** are effective against a small range of bacteria. Antibiotics kill the bacteria by interfering with their biological functions (bacteriocidal) or by preventing reproduction (bacteriostatic).

ANTIBIOTIC THERAPY FOR NEONATAL SEPSIS

For the treatment of **early-onset sepsis**, the American Academy of Pediatrics recommends a broad-spectrum antibiotic (such as ampicillin) every 12 hours combined with an aminoglycoside (gentamicin) or cephalosporin every 24 hours until the causative bacteria is/are identified and treatment can be more specified. In the case of **late-onset sepsis,** ampicillin (or vancomycin if the neonate has remained hospitalized since birth) is usually combined with gentamicin. In either case, once blood cultures return negatively for infection, antibiotics should be discontinued no more than 48 hours from incubation.

GENTAMICIN

Gentamicin is an inexpensive aminoglycoside antibiotic commonly used to treat neonates with gram-negative bacterial infections, like *Staphylococci*. It works by interfering with bacterial protein synthesis, resulting in a defective bacterial cell membrane. **Gentamicin** is excreted unmetabolized by the kidneys and renal function is directly related to clearance. Clearance is slower in premature neonates secondary to immature kidneys. The peak level (highest concentration in the blood) of gentamicin is measured 30 minutes after infusion is completed, and trough level (lowest concentration of the drug in the blood) is measured 30 minutes prior to the next dose. Potential toxicities from elevated gentamicin levels are ototoxicity (ear damage potentiated by concurrent use of furosemide) and nephrotoxicity (kidney damage), so patients with renal failure may only require dosing once every several days. If the pre-dose level falls below 0.5 mg/L and the post-dose level falls below 4 mg/L, the gentamicin is sub-therapeutic and will not kill the bacterial infection.

NEONATAL ANTI-VIRAL DRUGS

Drug	Dosage	Use
Acyclovir	IV: 60 mg/kg/day for 14-21 days	Indicated for herpes simplex and varicella zoster infections. Complications include rash, TTP, hemolytic uremic syndrome, increased liver enzymes, urea, and creatinine.
Ganciclovir	IV: 6 mg/kg every 12 hr for 6 weeks	Indicated for cytomegalovirus (disseminated, pneumonia). Complications include neutropenia, thrombocytopenia, phlebitis, rash, increased liver function tests, and seizures.
Palivizumab (Synagis)	IV or IM: 15 mg/kg monthly during season or while at risk	Humanized monoclonal antibody indicated to treat or protect against respiratory syncytial virus for neonates with severe respiratory disease, such as bronchopulmonary dysplasia. Complications include fever, poor feeding, bleeding, irritability, wheezing, and allergic reaction.
Respiratory Syncytial Virus Immune Globulin (RSVIG/RespiGam)	IV: 750 mg/kg (15 mL/kg) with slow infusion	Indicated for prophylaxis against respiratory syncytial virus but less potent than palivizumab and requires IV administration and larger volume. Complications include fever, wheezing, GI upset, allergic reaction, muscle rigidity.

ANTI-HYPERTENSIVES AND OTHER CARDIAC DRUGS

Antihypertensives are used to control congestive heart failure and reduce the cardiac workload:

- **Captopril** is an ace inhibitor is used to control hypertension.
- **Propranolol** is a beta-blocker used to control hypertension.
- **Labetalol** (Normodyne, Trandate) is an alpha-1 and beta-adrenergic blocker that slows the heart rate and decreases peripheral vascular resistance and cardiac output.

Miscellaneous cardiac drugs are used for specific purposes:

- **Calcium chloride/Calcium gluconate** is given intravenously after surgery to increase myocardial contractibility.
- **Brevibloc** (Esmolol) is a beta-blocker given intravenously after surgery to control systemic hypertension, arrhythmias, and outflow obstruction.
- **Indomethacin** (Indocin) is a NSAID that is given intravenously to inhibit the production of prostaglandin, thereby speeding the closure of the ductus arteriosus.
- **Prostaglandin** is given intravenously before surgery to maintain the patency of the ductus arteriosus for structural cardiac abnormalities in conditions such as coarctation of the aorta or transposition of the great arteries.

DIURETICS

Diuretics are used in the cardiac patient to increase renal perfusion and filtration, thereby reducing preload. Dosages are weight and age related. Diuretics commonly used include:

- **Bumetanide** (Bumex) is a loop diuretic (acting on the renal ascending loop of Henle) given intravenously after surgery to reduce preload.
- **Ethacrynic acid** (Edecrin) is a loop diuretic given intravenously after surgery to reduce preload.
- **Furosemide** (Lasix) is a loop diuretic and is used for the control of congestive heart failure as well as renal insufficiency. It is used after surgery to decrease preload and to reduce the inflammatory response caused by cardiopulmonary bypass (post-perfusion syndrome).
- **Spironolactone** (Aldactone) is a potassium-sparing synthetic steroid diuretic that increases the secretion of both water and sodium and is used to treat congestive heart failure. It may be given orally or intravenously.

LOOP, THIAZIDE, AND POTASSIUM-SPARING DIURETICS

Diuretics decrease the fluid load in infants with heart failure or lung disorders, such as bronchopulmonary dysplasia. Different **classes of diuretics** have different mechanisms of action and different side effect profiles:

- **Loop diuretics** (e.g., furosemide) are the most potent of the diuretics and work on the ascending limb of the loop of Henle. They disrupt the Na+/K+/2Cl- transporter and also limit K+ reabsorption. Hypokalemia, hyponatremia, and increased calcium excretion are the adverse reactions seen with chronic use.
- **Thiazide diuretics** (e.g., chlorothiazide) work by inhibiting Na+/Cl- transport in the distal convoluted tubule. They are less potent than loop diuretics. Hyponatremia, hypokalemia, and hypomagnesemia are the adverse reactions from chronic use.
- **Potassium-sparing diuretics** (e.g., spironolactone) work by inhibiting the action of aldosterone. Aldosterone promotes K+ secretion and Na+ reabsorption at the distal nephron. These diuretics are the least potent, but do not cause hypokalemia.

Vasodilators and Anti-Arrhythmics

Vasodilators may be used for arterial dilation or venous dilation. These drugs are used to treat pulmonary hypertension or generalized systemic hypertension. Dosages are weight and age related. Vasodilators include:

- **Nitroglycerine** is used intravenously after surgery to improve myocardial perfusion by dilating the coronary arteries. It can be used as a venous dilator and decreases the diastolic pressure of the left ventricle and reduces systemic vascular resistance (SVR).
- **Nitroprusside** is given intravenously before and after surgery for peripheral vascular dilation to decrease afterload and SVR in order to increase cardiac output.

Antiarrhythmics are used to control arrhythmias and slow the heart rate:

- **Amiodarone** is given intravenously after surgery to reduce AV and SA conduction, slowing the heartbeat. It is used to control both ventricular dysrhythmias and junctional ectopic tachycardia.
- **Lidocaine** is given intravenously before and after surgery to control ventricular dysrhythmias.
- **Procainamide** is given intravenously after surgery to control supraventricular tachycardia and is effective for both atrial and ventricular tachycardia.

Vasopressors/Inotropes

Drugs used to increase cardiac output and improve contractibility of the myocardium are the vasopressors/inotropes. Dosage and administration of pediatric medications is weight and age related. Inotropes include:

- **Dobutamine** is given intravenously before and after surgery to improve cardiac output and treat cardiac decompensation.
- **Dopamine** is given intravenously before and after surgery to increase cardiac output, blood pressure, and the excretion of urine.
- **Digoxin** is given intravenously or by mouth and is used to increase the strength of myocardial contractions, resulting in better cardiac output.
- **Epinephrine** is given intravenously before and after surgery to increase blood pressure and cardiac output, but it must be used judiciously because it also increases consumption of oxygen.
- **Milrinone/Amrinone** is given after surgery to increase cardiac output and stroke volume, decrease systemic vascular resistance (SVR), and control congestive heart failure.

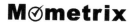

DIGITALIS

Digitalis is a cardiac glycoside that is used to treat congestive heart failure (CHF) and several different cardiac arrhythmias. Digitalis slows and strengthens the heartbeat. It has both a direct action on the myocardium and an indirect action mediated through the autonomic nervous system. The direct effect on the myocardium works by inhibiting the action of the sodium/potassium pump across cardiac cell membranes. The net result is an increase in intracellular sodium and calcium and an increase in extracellular potassium. The intracellular calcium is responsible for the increased strength of contractions of the heart (positive ionotrope). The indirect action of digitalis causes the heart rate to slow (negative chronotrope) by decreasing electrical conduction through the AV node. Digoxin has a narrow therapeutic index, meaning the lethal dose is close to the therapeutic dose. Signs of **digitalis toxicity** in infants include:

- GI signs: anorexia, nausea, vomiting, and diarrhea
- Cardiac arrhythmias: most commonly conduction disturbances, such as first-degree heart block, a supraventricular tachyarrhythmia such as atrial tachycardia, or bradycardia

Assume any alteration in cardiac conduction in an infant taking digoxin is a consequence of digitalis toxicity.

VOLATILE ANESTHETICS

Small infants have a high water content (70-75%) compared to adults (50-60%), and a lower muscle mass. These factors, coupled with slow renal and hepatic clearance, increased rate of metabolism, decreased protein binding, and increased organ perfusion affect the pharmacological action of drugs. Pediatric doses are calculated according to the child's weight in kilograms, but other factors may affect dosage. **Anesthetic agents** must be chosen with care because of the potential for adverse effects:

INHALATIONAL

Infants are more likely to develop hypotension and bradycardia with inhalational anesthetic agents. Inhalation induction is rapid because infants and young children have high alveolar ventilation and decreased FRC compared to older patients with depression of ventilation more common in infants. There is increased risk of overdose. Sevoflurane is usually preferred for induction and isoflurane or halothane for maintenance as desflurane and sevoflurane are associated with delirium on emergence.

NONVOLATILE ANESTHETICS

Infants may need higher proportionate (based on weight) doses of propofol because it is eliminated more quickly than with adults. It should not be used for infants who are critically ill, as it has been correlated to increased mortality rate and severe adverse effects leading to multi-organ failure. Thiopental is also used in higher proportionate doses for infants and children although this is not true for neonates. Neonates are especially sensitive to opioids, and morphine should be avoided or used with caution. Clearance rates for some drugs (sufentanil, alfentanil) may be higher in infants. Ketamine combined with fentanyl may cause more hypotension in neonates and small infants than ketamine combined with midazolam. Midazolam combined with fentanyl can cause severe hypotension. Etomidate is not used for infants but is reserved for children >10.

MUSCLE RELAXANTS

Onset with muscle relaxants is about 50% shorter in infants than adults, and pediatric patients may have variable responses to muscle to non-depolarizing muscle relaxants. Drugs that are metabolized through the liver (pancuronium, vecuronium, and cisatracurium) have prolonged action, so atracurium and cisatracurium, which do not depend on the liver, are more reliable. Succinylcholine can cause severe adverse effects (rhabdomyolysis, malignant hyperthermia, hyperkalemia, arrhythmias), so its use requires premedication with atropine, but succinylcholine is usually avoided in pediatric patients except for rapid sequence induction for children with full stomach and laryngospasm. Rocuronium is frequently used for intubation because of fast onset, but it has up to 90 minutes duration, so mivacurium, atracurium, and cisatracurium may be preferred for shorter procedures. Nerve stimulators should be used to monitor incremental doses, which are usually 25-30% of the original bolus. Blockade by non-depolarizing muscle relaxants can be reversed with neostigmine or edrophonium and glycopyrrolate or atropine.

BRONCHODILATORS AND RESPIRATORY STIMULANTS

Bronchodilators and respiratory stimulants are used to treat respiratory distress in the neonate:

- **Aminophylline and theophylline** both stimulate the sympathetic nervous system and dilate the bronchi. These medications are used for apnea of prematurity in the neonate and bronchospasm in infants with respiratory distress. Apnea of prematurity is treated with loading dose of 6 mg/kg aminophylline with maintenance doses of 2.5-3.5 mg/kg intravenously every 12 hours. Further treatment may be done orally with theophylline. Side effects include tachycardia, seizures, and irritability.
- **Albuterol** is a selective β2-adrenergic agonist bronchodilator that can be administered orally (100-300 µg/kg 3-4 times daily) or inhaled (100-500 µg/kg 4-8 times daily).
- **Caffeine citrate,** a stimulant, is the first line treatment for apnea of prematurity as it is safer than theophylline and can be administered orally. Loading dose is usually 20 mg/mg with one-time daily maintenance dose of 5mg/kg.
- **Epinephrine** is used to treat stridor with effect on β-adrenoreceptors. It is delivered with nebulizer at 50-100 µg/kg as needed.

CAFFEINE FOR NEONATAL APNEA

Apnea of prematurity occurs when the neonate stops breathing for 20 seconds or longer because the respiratory centers are immature. Apnea of prematurity is an exclusionary diagnosis, arrived at only when all other causes have been ruled out. Treatment consists of respiratory support with supplemental oxygen, continuous positive airway pressure (CPAP), or a ventilator in severe cases. **Caffeine** has largely replaced theophylline as the pharmacological treatment of choice for apnea of prematurity. Both are methylxanthines, but caffeine has a wider therapeutic index and a slower excretion rate than theophylline. Caffeine is a **central nervous system stimulant** that naturally occurs in tea, coffee, and chocolate. Give 10 mg CAFCIT to the infant orally. Side effects include irritability, tremors, tachycardia, tachypnea, vomiting, fever, and hyperglycemia. Peak blood levels will be reached in 30-120 minutes and should not exceed 6-10 mg/L. Toxicity is 50 mg/L. If seizures occur with caffeine overdose, give diazepam or pentobarbital sodium. Mean half-life is 3-4 days. Monitor trough levels periodically.

SURFACTANTS

Surfactants reduce surface tension to prevent collapse of alveoli. Beractant (Survanta) is derived from bovine lung tissue and calfactant (Infasurf) from calf lung tissue. Surfactant replacement therapy is used to prevent RDS for infants born at 27-30 weeks gestation. It is also used for infants showing signs of worsening lung disease. Surfactant has traditionally been given via the endotracheal tube (ETT) as an inhalant, but with advancing efforts to reduce mechanical ventilation in the context of RDS, other routes of administration are being considered, including minimally invasive surfactant therapy (MIST) through a thin catheter in the trachea while being oxygenated throug noninvasive means, or via nebulizer through a laryngeal mask. Both endoctracheal and MIST approaches have different protocol for determining the need of secondary doses, and facility policy for surfactant therapy should be followed closely.

STEROIDS

Steroids are commonly administered to mothers to promote fetal lung development for preterm births. These drugs include betamethasone and dexamethasone. Steroids may also be administered to the neonate, but they are associated with significant side effects:

- **Betamethasone** may be used for chronic lung disease (CLD) in the neonate and post-intubation airway edema, but high dose treatment has been associated with cerebral palsy, growth depression, hypertension, hyperglycemia, hypokalemia, and increased risk of infection. Airway edema is treated with 200 mcg/kg orally or IV every 8 hours beginning 4 hours before extubation. Dosages for other treatment vary widely with tapering of doses.
- **Hydrocortisone** may be used for physiologic replacement or acute hypotension. Replacement is begun with 1-2 mg orally every 8 hours and increased to 6-9 mg/m2/day. Hypotension is treated with 2 mg/kg IV loading dose and maintenance of 1 mg/kg IV every 8-12 hours.

VITAMIN K

Vitamin K deficiency in newborns may cause vitamin K deficiency bleeding (VKDB), also called **hemorrhagic disease of the newborn**. Vitamin K is a fat-soluble vitamin produced in the gut. Vitamin K is required by the liver to produce four of the clotting factors—II, VII, IX, and X. At birth, all infants are Vitamin K deficient because of limited transfer of vitamin K across the placenta. Newborns are injected with one intramuscular (IM) dose of vitamin K (AquaMEPHYTON), 0.5-1.0 mg within six hours of birth. The injection quickly raises the infant's vitamin K level to normal and maintains the normal level for several months. Vitamin K should be given prior to circumcision. Infants who do not receive vitamin K prophylaxis at birth will take several weeks (formula-fed) to several months (breastfed) to attain normal vitamin K levels. Formula contains higher levels of vitamin K than human breast milk. VKDB occurs in two forms:

- **Early-onset form** occurs within the first 24 hours after birth and is related to maternal medications that interfere with Vitamin K.
- **Late-onset form** occurs after two weeks of age, because of exclusive breastfeeding, diarrhea, hepatitis, cystic fibrosis, alpha 1-antitrypsin disease, or celiac disease.

NEONATAL ANALGESICS

SUCROSE ANALGESIA

Sucrose analgesia (Sweet-Ease) is used to relieve stress and discomfort in infants before and during medical procedures, such as heel sticks, IV insertion, injections, suctioning, and insertion of NG tubes. Sweet-Ease, a commercially prepared product, is 24% sucrose in an oral solution into which a standard pacifier is dipped and given to the infant, usually 2 minutes before a procedure. The pacifier may be re-dipped every 2 minutes for a total of 4 times. If the infant cannot suck, 0.1 mL of solution is placed on the anterior tongue with a medical syringe with the same frequency. For more painful procedures, such as lumbar puncture and circumcision, sucrose analgesia may be used in conjunction with other forms of analgesia to provide comfort. Contraindications include <32 weeks gestation, hyperglycemia, history of asphyxia or intolerance to feedings, critical illness, paralysis, opioid sedation, and infants NPO for surgery unless cleared by an anesthesiologist.

ACETAMINOPHEN

Acetaminophen (Tylenol) is used both for control of mild to moderate pain and fever. Acetaminophen can be administered orally and rectally, but absorption is less reliable with the rectal route. Acetaminophen has a half-life of 4 hours, is conjugated in the liver, and is excreted through the kidneys. **Oral dosage** is typically 24 mg/kg as a loading dose and 12 mg/kg every four hours (or 8 hours in infants <32 weeks); **rectal dosage** is 36 mg/kg (loading), followed by 24 mg/kg every 8 hours. Serum levels should be checked if treatment is to continue for >24 hours. Serum levels of 12-24 mg/L are required for adequate pain control. Acetaminophen is commonly used for control of pain after **circumcision**, although it is not sufficient for pain control during the procedure.

FENTANYL AND MORPHINE

Fentanyl and morphine are opioid analgesics/narcotics that treat moderate-to-severe pain:

- **Fentanyl** is for painful dressing changes or procedures. Duration of action is 1-2 hours and half-life is 2-4 hours. Dosage is 1-4 mcg/kg every 1-2 hours or by continuous infusion. Rapid tolerance develops, requiring higher doses to create the same relief, and increasing the chance of overdose. Fentanyl is metabolized by the liver and excreted by the kidneys. *Side effects of fentanyl include respiratory depression, peripheral vasodilatation, inhibition of intestinal peristalsis, and chest wall rigidity at higher doses, which compromises ventilation. Fentanyl is less likely to cause hypotension than morphine.
- **Morphine** is for postoperative pain. Duration of action is 3-4 hours, and half-life is 2-4 hours. Morphine is metabolized by the liver to an inactive metabolite and excreted by the kidneys; 2-12% is excreted unchanged in the urine. Dosage is 0.02-0.10 mg/kg every 1-4 hours or by continuous infusion. Side effects of morphine include respiratory depression, histamine release, and seizures.

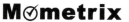

Management of the Drug Exposed Neonate

FETAL ALCOHOL SYNDROME

Fetal alcohol syndrome (FAS) is a syndrome of birth defects that develop as the result of maternal ingestion of alcohol. Fetal alcohol spectrum disorders (FASD) is an umbrella diagnosis that includes FAS along with infants impacted by alcohol in utero that do not meet the full FAS criteria. Despite campaigns to inform the public, women continue to drink during pregnancy, but no safe amount of alcohol ingestion has been determined. FAS includes:

- **Facial abnormalities**: Hypoplastic (underdeveloped) maxilla, micrognathia (undersized jaw), hypoplastic philtrum (groove beneath the nose), short palpebral fissures (eye slits between upper and lower lids).
- **Neurological deficits**: May include microcephaly, intellectual disability, motor delay, and hearing deficits. Learning disorders may include problems with visual-spatial and verbal learning, attention disorders, delayed reaction times.
- **Growth restriction**: Prenatal growth deficit persists with slow growth after birth.
- **Behavioral problems**: Irritability and hyperactivity. Poor judgment in behavior may relate to deficit in executive functions.

Indication of brain damage without the associated physical abnormalities is referred to as alcohol-related neurodevelopmental disorder (ARND).

FETAL EXPOSURE TO TOBACCO/NICOTINE

Tobacco smoke contains many substances known to be detrimental to a person's health. When a pregnant woman smokes, her fetus is exposed to carbon monoxide, nicotine, and hydrogen cyanide that all cross the placenta. Carbon monoxide displaces oxygen from hemoglobin, resulting in decreased oxygen delivery to the fetus. Exposure increases risk of miscarriage and perinatal death. Infants exposed *in utero* to tobacco may have the following problems:

- Decreased length, weight, and head circumference
- Increased rates of congenital birth defects, such as cleft palate or lip, limb reduction defects, and urinary tract anomalies
- Increased incidence of placenta previa, placental abruption, and preterm birth

If smoking continues after delivery, these further detrimental effects may occur:

- Sudden infant death syndrome
- Increased infant respiratory tract infections and childhood asthma
- Behavioral problems in later childhood

FETAL EXPOSURE TO MARIJUANA, PCP, AND MDMA

Marijuana, phencyclidine (PCP), and methylenedioxymethamphetamine (MDMA or ecstasy) are popular club drugs that may be used by some women during pregnancy:

- **Marijuana**: This is often used along with alcohol and tobacco, so effects are difficult to assess, but there do not appear to be teratogenic effects; however, some studies report exposure can result in fine tremors, irritability, and prolonged startle response for the first 12 months after birth.
- **PCP**: One of the biggest problems with PCP is that mothers may have an overdose or psychotic response that can result in hypertension, hyperthermia, and coma, compromising the fetus.
- **MDMA**: Ecstasy is frequently used by teenagers and young adults. There is no clear evidence regarding effects on the fetus although some research suggests it may cause long-term impairments in learning.

FETAL EXPOSURE TO AMPHETAMINES

Amphetamines are a class of drugs that cause CNS stimulation. The most commonly abused amphetamine is methamphetamine. Maternal use of these substances causes hypertension and tachycardia, which can cause miscarriage, abruptio placentae, and premature delivery. Vasoconstriction affects placental vessels, decreasing circulation, nutrition, and oxygen to the fetus. Methamphetamines can cross the placental barrier and cause fetal hypertension and prenatal strokes and damage to the heart and other organs. The neonate is commonly small for gestational age, often ≤5 pounds, full term but ≤10 percentile for weight, with shortened length and smaller head circumference. The neonate in withdrawal from maternal amphetamine use will suffer abnormal sleep patterns, often characterized by lethargy and excessive sleeping during the first few weeks, poor feeding, tremors, diaphoresis, miosis, frantic fist sucking, high-pitched crying, fever, excessive yawning, and hyperreflexia.

FETAL EXPOSURE TO HEROIN

Heroin is a highly addictive, opioid narcotic that is a common drug of abuse. Heroin users are at increased risk of poor nutrition, iron deficiency anemia, and preeclampsia-eclampsia, all negatively affecting the fetus. Infants with prenatal heroin exposure display symmetric intrauterine growth restriction (IUGR) and are often born prematurely. About 60-80% of these infants will undergo neonatal abstinence syndrome (NAS). Heroin has a relatively short half-life and symptoms of NAR typically begin 48-72 hours after delivery. Several different body systems are affected by NAS and include:

- **CNS Dysfunction**
  - High-pitched cry
  - Hyperactive reflexes
  - Irritability
  - Tremors

- **GI Dysfunction**
  - Poor feeding
  - Periods of frantic sucking or rooting
  - Vomiting
  - Loose or watery stools

- **Miscellaneous Signs**
  - Frequent yawning
  - Sneezing multiple times
  - Sweating
  - Fever
  - Tachypnea

FETAL EXPOSURE TO METHADONE

Methadone is commonly used to treat women who are addicted to opioids, such as heroin or prescriptive narcotics, as it blocks withdrawal symptoms and drug craving. An associated risk is that methadone crosses the placental barrier and exposes the fetus to the drug. Many female heroin users are of reproductive age, and methadone is often administered to pregnant women to decrease dangers associated with heroin, such as fluctuating levels of drug and exposure to hepatitis and HIV from sharing of needles. Exposure to methadone may result in miscarriage, stillbirth, intrauterine growth restriction, fetal distress, and low birth weight, although symptoms are usually less severe than with heroin. However, if the mother takes methadone and other drugs, this can compound the adverse effects. Additionally, sudden withdrawal from methadone may cause preterm labor or death of the fetus, so methadone should be monitored carefully.

FETAL EXPOSURE TO COCAINE

Cocaine/crack (freebase cocaine) is a nonopioid substance that readily crosses the placenta through simple diffusion. One of the most potent properties of cocaine is its ability to act as a vasoconstrictor. When a mother uses cocaine, the blood supply to the placenta is severely compromised when the vessels constrict, compromising blood flow and resulting in growth restriction and hypoxia. Cocaine also causes a programmed cell death (known as apoptosis) in the heart muscle cells of the fetus, resulting in cardiac dysfunction for the fetus. Maternal cocaine use increases the risk of premature birth and causes serious consequences for the neonate after birth. Maternal cocaine use can cause cerebral infarctions, non-duodenal intestinal atresia, anal atresia, NEC, defects of the limbs, and genitourinary defects. Cocaine stimulates the central nervous system by limiting the uptake of certain neurotransmitters, such as norepinephrine, serotonin, and dopamine. Cocaine has a direct toxic effect on the nervous system, so the infant will exhibit extreme irritability and tremors followed by sluggish, lethargic behavior.

FETAL EXPOSURE TO PRESCRIPTION/OTC DRUGS

Many OTC and prescription drugs have teratogenic effects on the developing fetus and can result in congenital abnormalities, growth restriction, intellectual disability, carcinogenesis, mutagenesis, and miscarriage. The degree of damage relates to multiple factors, such as the amount of drug reaching the fetus, the developmental period during which the drug is taken, and the duration for which the drug was taken. There are some recognizable syndromes:

- **Fetal warfarin (Coumadin) syndrome** (exposure 7-12 weeks): Nasal hypoplasia, laryngomalacia, atrial septal defects, patent ductus arteriosis, eye, ear, and skull abnormalities, intellectual disabilities and growth restriction, brachydactyly, and scoliosis. Exposure during 2nd and 3rd trimester may result in eye abnormalities (cataracts, optic atrophy), microphthalmia (eyes stop developing resulting in abnormally small eyes), fetal/maternal hemorrhage, and microcephaly.
- **Fetal hydantoin (Dilantin) syndrome** (exposure 1st trimester): Facial dysmorphism, microcephaly, underdeveloped nails (hands and feet), cleft left/palate, and developmental delays ranging from mild to severe.
- **Fetal valproate (Depakote) syndrome** (exposure 1st trimester): Facial dysmorphism, spina bifida, CNS and cardiac abnormalities, and delay in development.

Some drugs are classified as high risk (FDA classification D), but use is acceptable if the mother has a life-threatening illness or other drugs are not available, so neonates may exhibit adverse effects.

Drugs with high risk include and their adverse effects on the fetus/infant include:

- **ACE inhibitors** (2nd and 3rd trimesters): skull and pulmonary hypoplasia, renal tubular dysplasia, and oligohydramnios
- **Carbamazepine** (1st trimester): craniofacial defects, neural tube defects, restriction of growth, and hypoplasia of fingernails
- **Antineoplastic alkylating drugs** (1st to 3rd trimesters): eye disorders, including microphthalmia and cataracts, cardiac defects, renal agenesis, and cardiac abnormalities
- **Iodides** (3rd trimester): thyroid disorders, including goiter, and fetal hypothyroidism
- **Methimazole** (1st trimester): aplasia cutis
- **Lithium** (1st trimester): Ebstein anomaly, various cardiac abnormalities
- **Tetracycline** (2nd and 3rd trimesters): yellow discoloration of teeth, weakening of fetal bones, and dysplasia of tooth enamel

Some drugs are classified as extremely high risk (FDA classification X), and these drugs should not be used with women who are pregnant or might become pregnant because fetal risk outweighs benefits to mother:

- **Androgens** (1st trimester): Female fetus will become masculinized.
- **Retinoids**, such as isotretinoin, acitretin, tretinoin, and etretinate (1st trimester): Multiple deformities of heart, ears, face, limbs, & liver, cognitive impairment, thymic hypoplasia, microcephalus, hydrocephalus, microtia, and miscarriage.
- **Thalidomide** (days 34-60): Multiple facial, intestinal, cardiac, limb abnormalities, including lack of limbs and limb reductions, and deafness.
- **Vitamin A** (>18,000 IU/day): Multiple craniofacial deformities, microtia, cardiac abnormalities, atresia of bowel, limb reductions, and defects of urinary tract.

Neuroprotective and Neurodevelopmental Care

DEVELOPMENTAL CARE

Developmental care is neonatal nursing that acknowledges environmental conditions and behavioral cues. Minimize noises and bright lights to decrease excessive stimuli. Observe the patient for cues regarding his or her feeding requirements and emotional state. The goal is to provide the optimum environment and treatment modalities that are the least stressful to the neonate, allowing for positive growth and development. Encourage parental involvement to foster attachment and competence in caring for the neonate. **Key components of developmental care include:**

- Observe, interpret, and respond to infant cues during care.
- Alter care based on neonatal developmental changes (e.g., the needs of a neonate at 26 weeks gestational age are different from those of one at 38 weeks gestational age).
- Time, pace, and handle the infant based on observed cues during care.
- Position infants based on their needs.
- Modify the environment based on the infant's needs.
- Foster parental participation in the care of their infant.

NEUROBEHAVIORAL DEVELOPMENT

Terms related to neurobehavioral development:

- **Habituation**: A decreasing response to repeated stimuli. For example, if a child is exposed to repeated sounds, the child will over time become used to the sound and show less reaction.
- **Motor organization**: Motor organization involves 3 different levels:
  - The spinal cord (which mediates automatic movement and reflexes)
  - The brain stem (which includes the medial descending systems that control body movement and antigravity reflexes and the lateral descending systems that control voluntary limb movements)
  - The cerebral cortex (which regulates movement)
- **State organization**: The brain has the ability to respond differently in different states or conditions, suggesting that the neonate's brain is active and not just passive.
- **Sensory/Interaction capabilities**: The ability to respond to stimuli and to interact with the environment and others. The interactions the neonate has after birth with others (dyadic interactions) help the child to learn patterns of interactions and responses.

SLEEP STATES

Infants spend a high percentage of their time in **sleep states**. Sleep periods are divided into active sleep or quiet sleep by observing the infant's behavior:

- **Quiet sleep** is restorative and fosters anabolic growth. Quiet sleep is associated with increased cell mitosis and replication, lowered oxygen consumption, and the release of growth hormone. During quiet sleep, the infant appears relaxed, moves minimally, and breathes smoothly and regularly. The eyelids are still. The infant only responds to intense stimuli during quiet sleep.
- **Active sleep** is associated with processing and storing of information. Rapid eye movement (REM sleep) occurs during active sleep, but it is unknown if newborn infants are able to dream. During active sleep, the infant moves occasionally and breathes irregularly. Eye movements can be seen beneath the eyelids. Infants spend most of their sleep time in active sleep, and it usually precedes wakening.

AWAKE STATES

Infants have different levels of consciousness in the 4 **awake states**. Infants respond differently to outside stimuli and interaction from caregivers, depending on which state they are in:

- **Drowsy:** This is characterized by variable activity, mild startles, and smooth movement. There is some facial movement. Eyes open and close, breathing is irregular, and response to stimuli may be delayed.
- **Quiet alert:** The infant rarely moves, breathing is regular, and the infant focuses intently on individuals or objects that are within focal range, widening eyes. The face appears bright and alert, breathing is regular, and the infant focuses on stimuli.
- **Active alert:** The infant moves frequently and has much facial movement although the face not as bright and alert, eyes may have a dull glaze, breathing is irregular, and there are variable responses to outside stimuli.
- **Crying:** Characterized by grimacing, eyes shut, irregular breathing, increased movement with color changes and marked response to both internal and external stimuli.

BRAZELTON NEONATAL BEHAVIORAL ASSESSMENT SCALE

The Brazelton Neonatal Behavioral Assessment Scale is a multi-dimensional scale that is used to assess a neonate's state, temperament, and behavioral patterns. It includes the assessment of 18 reflexes, 28 behaviors, and 6 other characteristics. It is usually completed on day 3 with an attempt to elicit the most positive response, usually when the infant is comforted and in a quiet dim room. Scoring correlates to the child's awake or sleep state. Infants are scored according to response in many areas, including:

- **Habituation**: Ability to diminish response to repeat stimuli
- **Visual and auditory orientation**: Ability to respond to stimuli, fixate, and follow a visual object
- **Motor activity**: Assessment of body tone in various activities
- **Variations**: Changes in color, state, activity, alertness, and excitement during the exam
- **Self-quieting activities**: Frequency and speed of self-calming activities, such as sucking on their hand, putting their hand to mouth, and focusing on objects or sounds
- **Social behaviors**: Ability to cuddle, engage, and enjoy physical contact

STRESS RESPONSES

The neonate may exhibit a number of different stress responses:

- **Motoric responses:** Instead of normal and consistent muscle tone, the neonate may exhibit hypotonia with flaccid extremities and jaw. Some may exhibit hypertonicity with extremities hyperextended and/or hyperflexion of extremities. Some neonates may exhibit flailing, twitching, and tremors.
- **Attentional responses:** The neonate may react poorly to auditory, social, and visual stimuli and may exhibit poor sleeping, inability to be consoled, and staring or eye-roving behavior. The neonate may appear stressed and panicked or close eyes and withdraw.
- **Self-regulating/comforting responses:** The neonate may exhibit a number of behaviors to attempt to reduce stress. Motor activities may include grasping hands, moving hands toward the mouth, sucking, grasping blankets and tubing, moving about, and bracing feet against blankets or other barriers. The neonate may cry loudly and rhythmically to reduce stress and induce sleep. These tactics help the neonate to modulate responses to stimuli so that the newborn is not overwhelmed by the stress response.

AUTONOMIC STRESS RESPONSE

The autonomic nervous system is part of the peripheral nervous system and includes sympathetic nerves. The sympathetic nervous system (T1-L2 or L3) activates in times of stress and is implicated in pain. The nerves innervate deep structures, viscera, and skin. The autonomic nervous system mediates the body's organs and maintains homeostasis. When a neonate is stressed, the neonate typically responds by crying. Other signs of the **autonomic stress response** in the newborn include:

- **Change in skin color**: flushing, pallor, mottling rather than stable pink color
- **Respiratory changes**: when stable, respirations are regular and smooth; with stress, the neonate may exhibit gasping, sighing, apneic periods, and tachypnea
- **Cardiovascular changes**: heart rate and blood pressure increase
- **Visceral/GI response**: hiccups, gagging, coughing, vomiting, sneezing, passing flatus, choking, grunting

The caregiver must recognize the signs of stress, respond to the neonate's needs, and reduce stimuli. For example, a combination of stimuli, such as sound, lights, and touch, may overwhelm a newborn. Additionally, newborns may react to the stress of caregivers.

STRESS RELATED TO LIGHT

Light is a necessary component of caring for both sick and healthy neonates in the delivery room and nursery. Adequate lighting is required to evaluate the at-risk neonate, to assess color, to complete procedures such as intubation, or to give medications. Light also discourages the growth of pathogens. However, constant bright light interferes with the development of natural diurnal rhythms because it arouses the central nervous system and stresses the infant. Controlling light helps to stabilize the infant. Some simple methods to protect the neonate from light over-stimulation and to establish a normal sleep cycle include:

- Reducing overhead light levels when direct visualization is not necessary
- Covering incubator hoods to reduce light entering the incubator
- Dimming the lights at night to help establish a natural day/night pattern (circadian rhythm)

STRESS RELATED TO NOISE

Excessive **noise** causes agitation in all neonates, but especially in preterm neonates. The preterm neonate has less ability to self-calm, and over-stimulation results in decompensation, as demonstrated by increased oxygen requirements and increased apnea and bradycardia episodes. The American Academy of Pediatrics (AAP) recommends noise levels in the nursery and NICU be kept at **≤45 decibels**. A normal speaking voice is between 50-60 decibels. Noise levels above 80 decibels can damage the cochlea and cause hearing loss in adults. To keep noise acceptably low:

- Turn radios/TVs off or down.
- Designate a daily quiet time.
- Close incubator portholes gently, because closing a plastic porthole can spike the decibel level more than 80 dB.
- Whisper and, as much as possible, avoid speaking loudly.
- Remove bubbling water from ventilator tubing.
- Educate parents about the deleterious effects of over-stimulating their infant with loud noises.

ENVIRONMENTAL STRESSORS AND "TIME OUT"

Premature neonates have a very limited ability to deal with **environmental stressors,** but these stressors can affect all neonates. Signs of stress in neonates include:

- Color changes, such as mottling or cyanosis
- Episodes of apnea and bradycardia
- Activity changes, such as tremors, twitches, frantic activity, arching, and gaze-averting
- Flaccid posture (sagging trunk, extremities, and face)
- Easy fatigability

When the infant shows signs of stress, a **time-out** recovery period is indicated:

- Stop the activity causing the stress.
- Reduce unnecessary stimuli (e.g., lower the lights and postpone non-essential manipulation of the neonate).
- Give the neonate a chance to calm down or self-soothe.
- Bundle the neonate and place him/her in a comforting, side-lying position with the shoulders drawn forward and the hands brought to the midline.

NON-NUTRITIVE SUCKING

Non-nutritive sucking occurs when an infant sucks on an item such as a pacifier or his/her own fist. Non-nutritive sucking is not associated with nutritional intake, but it is an important method of self-quieting and begins in the uterus at about 29 weeks of gestation. Extremely premature infants often lack basic neurodevelopmental capabilities, and cannot coordinate sucking, swallowing, and breathing simultaneously. Typically, the ability to suck and swallow in a coordinated fashion is not present until 32-34 weeks of gestation. Premature infants should be encouraged to perform non-nutritive sucking during the gavage feeding process if they can accomplish it. Benefits of non-nutritive sucking include:

- Improved digestion of enteral feeds because digestive enzyme release is stimulated
- Facilitated development of coordinated nutritive sucking behavior
- Calming of the distressed infant

POSITIONING OF THE PREMATURE NEONATE

Correct positioning of the premature neonate minimizes outside stimuli and mimics the enclosed and calming environment of the womb, helping with the transition to extrauterine life:

- Place the neonate in a flexed position, with his hands close to midline and near his face.
- Create a nest of blankets or pillows to:
  - Help block out light and noise.
  - Give him the impression of a closed environment.
  - Minimize abnormal molding of the head from prolonged pressure on one side.
- Cover the incubator to further keep out sound and light.
- Place the neonate in the prone position (on his stomach) to help to stabilize the chest wall, improve ventilation, and increase the amount of time the infant is in quiet sleep. However, infants should be placed supine (on the back) most of the time, to decrease the chance of SIDS.

CLUSTERING CARE

The concept of clustering care for the premature neonate centers on allowing the neonate to have prolonged periods of rest or sleep in between required care procedures and manipulations. Long periods of rest and quiet simulate the uninterrupted and fairly constant environment of the womb. Clustering care means performing multiple tasks at the same time, such as feeding, bathing, wound care, drawing laboratory samples, or examining the infant. However, the premature infant may not be able to tolerate multiple manipulations and may show signs of decompensation before all the planned procedures are completed. The premature infant may need a time-out period to recover before performing more stressful procedures. Balance clustering care with observing the infant for cues of stress.

PROVISION OF SENSORY EXPERIENCES

While sensory interventions are important for neurobehavioral development, preterm neonates or those who are seriously ill may be able to tolerate only one or two types of sensory interventions, so each neonate must be assessed individually and carefully observed for signs of stress. **Sensory experiences** that benefit the neonate can include:

- **Auditory**: Talking to the neonates in a calm and soothing high-pitched tone of voice or providing toys that produce soft or low sounds (such as music) may be used, but loud or sudden noises should be avoided.
- **Tactile**: Gently massaging the neonate, starting from the head down to the extremities, abdomen, and back as the neonate can tolerate is highly beneficial for the neonate; however, light touch should be avoided. Neonatal hand-to-mouth activity should be encouraged.
- **Visual**: Keeping eye contact with the child during all interactions, providing other visual items (mirrors, bright red item, mobiles), and keeping lights low benefits the infant's visual development.
- **Vestibular** (middle ear/brain) **and proprioceptive** (position): Swaddling (legs flexed and hands near mouth), holding, and slowly rocking the neonate back and forth for at least 5 minutes benefits the neonate.

Infection and Immunology

IMMUNITY

Infants (especially preterm) have **increased susceptibility to infection** when compared to older children and adults because of immaturity or deficiencies in their immune systems:

- **Cellular immunity**: Neutrophils and macrophages in the neonate are deficient in chemotaxis and not as effective in killing invading bacteria. Reserves of neutrophils are easily depleted in neonates.
- **Humoral immunity**: Some passage of immunoglobulin G (IgG) occurs from the mother to the fetus, but mostly during the third trimester. In general, immunoglobulin levels are low. The neonate does not produce IgA until 2-5 weeks after birth. Complement activity is also immature in newborns, leaving them especially susceptible to Gram-negative organisms.
- **Barrier function**: The skin and mucous membranes, which normally act as barriers, are less effective in newborns. Prolonged invasive instrumentation (central lines or endotracheal tubes) associated with infants who are premature or those with complex congenital deformities are other routes for infection.

HUMORAL IMMUNITY

Humoral immunity in neonates is mainly mediated by maternal transfer of **Immunoglobulin G (IgG)** that greatly increases after 32 weeks of gestation. Infants born prior to 32 weeks have a significantly lower immunoglobulin level than term infants. Endogenous production of immunoglobulins does not begin until 24 weeks after birth, allowing serum immunoglobulin levels to trough until production begins. This trough further lowers the premature infant's ability to fight infections. The lower the infant's gestational age, the higher the incidence of neonatal sepsis. The risk of neonatal sepsis is 10 times higher in infants who weigh less than 2,500 grams, when compared to full term infants. Boost the premature infant's immunoglobulin level with intravenous IgG (IVIG) to prevent the acquisition of nosocomial infections or as adjunctive therapy in neonates with early onset sepsis. (Studies have shown mixed results with only minimal benefits.)

SOURCES OF NEONATAL INFECTION

For the neonate there are three main categories of sources of infection:

- **Transplacental (Intrauterine)** infection is a direct infection from the mother to the fetus prior to birth. Infections such as AIDS, Cytomegalovirus, Rubella, Syphilis and Toxoplasmosis are the most common types in this category.
- **Perinatal acquisition** during labor and delivery occurs at the time of birth rather than *in utero* and is a direct result of contact with a pathogen present on the mother at birth. Infections in this category include Chlamydia, Enterovirus, Group B *Streptococcus,* Hepatitis B and Herpes.
- **Hospital acquisition** in the neonatal period is the third category. This is an infection that the infant did not have at birth but acquired from hospital personnel, equipment, the mother, or visitors.

NOSOCOMIAL INFECTIONS IN NEONATAL UNIT

A nosocomial infection is acquired while in the hospital and is often responsible for late onset sepsis in neonates. The immature or compromised immune systems of premature neonates, combined with the frequent use of invasive ventilators, catheters, ventricular shunts, chest tubes, and IVs make neonates susceptible to nosocomial infections:

- **Peripheral IVs** are very common in neonates and often require restarting because of their small and fragile veins. Appropriate aseptic technique is essential to lessen infections associated with peripheral IVs.
- **Percutaneously inserted central catheters**, most commonly used in the NICU as they are more permanent than peripheral IVs, are also associated with nosocomial infections and should not be left in place longer than 21 days.

Pathogens commonly involved in nosocomial infections include coagulase-negative staphylococci (CoNS), *Klebsiella*, *Serratia*, *Enterobacter*, *Pseudomonas*, and *Candida*. Viral infections, such as respiratory syncytial virus (RSV), are usually introduced by parents and visitors. Frequent use of antibiotics contributes to the development of opportunistic bacteria and drug-resistant infections, such as Vancomycin-resistant *Enterococci* and methicillin-resistant *Staphylococcus aureus*.

GRAM-POSITIVE AND GRAM-NEGATIVE PATHOGENS IN THE NURSERY

The Gram stain is a rapid lab test that divides bacteria into two classes (gram-positive or gram-negative) depending on their staining characteristics. Gram staining narrows the range of likely pathogens so the doctor can choose an antibiotic, pending a culture and sensitivity, which requires several days.

- **Gram-positive**
  - Group B *Streptococcus* (most common)
  - *Staphylococcus aureus* and *S. epidermidis*
  - *Listeria monocytogenes*
- **Gram-negative**
  - *Escherichia coli* (most common)
  - *Klebsiella pneumoniae*
  - *Pseudomonas aeruginosa*
  - *Haemophilus influenzae*
  - *Enterobacter aerogenes*

Antibiotic resistance is increasing among gram-negative bacilli such as *Klebsiella pneumoniae*, *P. aeruginosa*, and *Enterobacter* spp. Organisms that are deemed significant may vary from one department to another, so that organisms that might prove fatal in the neonatal unit may pose less of a threat to adults.

CANDIDIASIS

Candida albicans is a fungus that can cause late onset sepsis and oral thrush in the neonate. Invasive **candidiasis** is a serious infection and has a mortality rate of 25-30%. The source of infection may be from the mother or from colonized health care workers. It is estimated that up to 30% of health care workers are colonized with *candida*. Immunocompromised patients, such as mothers with AIDS, are especially vulnerable to thrush. **Risk factors for the development** of candidiasis include:

- Birth weight less than 1,500 grams
- Prolonged use of broad-spectrum antibiotics
- TPN with infusion of lipids
- Prolonged urinary catheterization
- History of cutaneous or mucous membrane colonization or infection (thrush or candidal diaper rash)

Amphotericin B is the drug of choice for the treatment of candidiasis. Central lines and catheters may have to be removed.

ENTEROVIRUS

Enteroviruses include coxsackievirus, echovirus, and poliovirus (essentially eradicated in the United States). Most **enterovirus infections** (90%) in adults are asymptomatic or non-specific febrile illness with flu-like symptoms. There is no consensus regarding neonatal infections, but most researchers believe they are not acquired transplacentally but that infection occurs perineally (during delivery) or after birth (≥ 2 weeks) from exposure to a mother with the virus or another infected infant. Neonates are at increased risk of developing sepsis-like conditions, such as aseptic meningitis, myocarditis, and hepatitis. It may be difficult to differentiate enterovirus infection from bacterial sepsis. Because of lack of immune response, neonates <10 days are at increased risk from non-polio enteroviruses. Neonates may be lethargic, feverish, and exhibit signs of hypoperfusion (mottled skin, delay in capillary refill time, and cyanosis) and jaundice. They often feed poorly and cry inconsolably.

BACTERIAL INFECTIONS AFFECTING NEWBORNS

ESCHERICHIA COLI

Newborns who are preterm or low birth weight or whose mothers experienced prolonged labor or fever are at increased risk of ***Escherichia coli (E. coli)* infection**. Early recognition of **symptoms** and alerting the physician is critical. Contact precautions must be utilized.

- **GI infection:** Symptoms include green, watery, and bloody diarrhea, fever, and dehydration.
- **UTI:** Symptoms, such as fever pyuria, poor feeding, and irritability, usually occur in the 2nd to 3rd week but may be earlier in preterm neonates or secondary to bacteremia, so urine and blood cultures are usually done and antibiotics administered.
- **Neonatal sepsis:** Infection usually obtained intrapartum with symptoms within 6 hours of delivery. Symptoms include Low APGAR score, poor sucking, apnea, bradycardia, unstable temperature, vomiting, diarrhea, and dyspnea. Mortality rates are higher in low-birth weight and preterm neonates. Treatment is with antibiotics and supportive therapy.
- **Neonatal meningitis:** May progress from diarrhea or UTI. Onset after 48 hours usually includes neurological impairment, stupor, irritability, seizures, posturing, anterior fontanel bulging, and nuchal rigidity. Treatment is with antibiotics and supportive therapy.

STAPHYLOCOCCUS

Neonates may be exposed to *Staphylococcus* through contact with medical personnel or from contaminated equipment, such as ventilators. Risk factors include preterm birth, VLBW (<1500 g), prolonged hospitalization, and invasive procedures such as insertion of venous catheters. Indications of infection may include fever or hypothermia, cardiac changes (tachycardia, bradycardia), vomiting, lethargy, and skin rash or lesions. If the infection enters the bloodstream, the neonate may develop sepsis, which can progress to meningitis and to neurological compromise or death. *Staphylococcus aureus* is one of the most common infective agents and may be either methicillin-susceptible or methicillin resistant (MRSA), which is much more difficult to treat. *Staphylococcus epidermidis*, which is found on skin and mucosa, and coagulase-negative staphylococci both tend to colonize invasive devices, such as catheters, forming biofilms that lead to sepsis and are naturally resistant to antibiotics. Coagulase-negative staphylococci infections may also occur in preterm neonates receiving TPN.

BACTERIAL MENINGITIS

Bacterial meningitis is caused by a wide range of pathogenic organisms, varying with the infant's age:

- ≤1 month: *E.coli,* Group B *Streptococci, Listeria monocytogenes*, and *Neisseria meningitidis*
- 1-2 months: Group B *Streptococci*

Bacterial infections usually arise from the spread of distant infections but can enter the CNS from surgical wounds, invasive devices, or nasal colonization. The infective process includes inflammation, exudates, white blood cell accumulation, and tissue damage with the brain showing evidence of hyperemia and edema. Purulent exudate covers the brain and invades and blocks the ventricles, obstructing CSF and leading to increased intracranial pressure. Since antibodies specific to bacteria don't cross the blood-brain barrier, the body's ability to fight the infection is very poor.

DIAGNOSIS

Diagnosis of bacterial meningitis is based on examination of cerebrospinal fluid and symptoms. **Symptoms** may be very non-specific, such as hypo- or hyperthermia, jaundice, irritability, lethargy, irregular respirations with periods of apnea, difficulty feeding with loss of suck reflex, hypotonia, weak cry, seizures, and bulging fontanels (late sign). Nuchal rigidity does not usually occur with neonates. Meningitis is often difficult to diagnose in the neonate because it has early nonspecific clinical findings of irritability, lethargy, poor feeding, temperature instability, and hypotension. The more specific neurological symptoms of seizures or bulging fontanels are seen in late onset infection. Antibiotics given to the mother prior to delivery or to the neonate prior to performing a lumbar puncture inhibit bacterial growth in cerebrospinal fluid (CSF), making the diagnosis dependent on other CSF parameters. **CSF findings** suggestive of bacterial meningitis include:

- Decreased glucose
- Elevated protein
- White blood cells values in CSR greater than 100 WBC/dL

A polymerase chain reaction assay test for Group B strep antigen in CSF is available. Values may be more difficult to interpret in the premature neonate, as their blood brain barrier is more permeable.

HOSPITAL-ACQUIRED PNEUMONIA

KLEBSIELLA PNEUMONIAE

Klebsiella pneumoniae is a common cause of hospital-acquired infections of the urinary tract, surgical sites, and lower respiratory tract. *K. pneumoniae* is a gram-negative member of the Enterobacteriaceae family and is part of the normal body flora. It can infect children of all ages but is most common in infants who are premature and/or in neonatal intensive care. Infants with invasive devices, such as those with mechanical ventilation, are at increased risk. There have been a number of outbreaks in neonatal units, especially with multi-drugs resistant forms, with the hands of health staff and the gastrointestinal tract of the infants providing reservoirs of bacteria.

When the infection attacks the lungs, the **symptoms** include inflammatory changes that result in necrosis and hemorrhage, clogging the lungs with thick puro-sanguineous exudate. The disease spreads rapidly, with high fever and dyspnea. Mortality rates are high.

Treatment includes antibiotic therapy (such as 3rd generation cephalosporins or quinolones) based on cultures and sensitivities.

PSEUDOMONAS AERUGINOSA

Hospital-acquired pneumonias (HAP) are far more lethal than community-acquired pneumonias (CAP), with HAP death rates of 20-40% and up to 90% if the infant is on mechanical ventilation, with **Pseudomonas aeruginosa** one of the most lethal (40-60% mortality) because it can invade blood vessels, resulting in hemorrhage. Most infections are spread by contact with contaminated hands of healthcare staff or from invasive devices, such as endotracheal tubes and mechanical ventilators.

Symptoms include fever, cough, bradycardia, and elevated WBC counts.

Treatment includes:

- Antibiotic therapy: Usually combinations of 2 antibiotics are given, such as piperacillin or ceftazidime and gentamicin or ciprofloxacin (based on cultures). Vancomycin is generally avoided because of the rise of vancomycin-resistant organisms.
- Preventive measures include maintaining ventilated patients in 30° upright positions, universal precautions, and changing ventilator circuits as per protocol.

EARLY-ONSET SEPSIS

Early-onset bacterial sepsis usually occurs in the first 24 hours after birth, but may occur any time up to day 6 of life. Infants born prematurely have an increased rate of early-onset sepsis and more rapid onset of symptoms. In early onset sepsis, the source of infection is from the mother, either transplacentally, or a microorganism that colonized the mother's birth canal. Pathogens that most commonly cause early-onset sepsis are Group B *Streptococcus*, *E. coli*, *Haemophilus influenzae*, coagulase-negative staphylococci, and *Listeria monocytogenes*. **Risk factors** for the development of early onset sepsis include:

- Premature, preterm, or prolonged rupture of membranes
- Maternal colonization with Group B *Streptococcus*
- Fever in the mother greater than 38 °C during delivery
- Premature birth or low birth weight (<2500 g)
- Maternal urinary tract infection
- Chorioamnionitis
- APGAR score less than 6 at 1 minute or 5 minutes
- Delivery with birth asphyxia or meconium staining

CLINICAL MANIFESTATIONS AND DIAGNOSIS

The clinical manifestations for **early-onset sepsis** are often vague and nonspecific making it a particular challenge to diagnose early. Sometimes the only noticeable sign is that the mother or nurse will note that the infant just doesn't seem well—nothing that can be specified but general symptoms perhaps starting with a poor feeding or other seemingly minor event. Infection may localize or cause bacteremia and sometimes meningitis. Some **manifestations** that should be noted include:

- The inability of the infant to maintain a normal body temperature
- Apnea, tachypnea
- Vomiting
- Cyanosis
- Lethargy
- Jaundice
- Seizures
- Purpura

If sepsis is suspected, CSF examination is done to evaluate for possible meningitis, a frequent complication of sepsis, especially if the infant is exhibiting symptoms of sepsis, GBS sepsis, or late onset of infection.

LATE-ONSET SEPSIS

Late-onset sepsis occurs after day 6 of life and is more common in preterm infants and those with medical or surgical conditions. The infection is acquired from the environment after birth, rather than from the mother. Infants with indwelling catheters, nasal cannulas, continuous positive airway pressure (CPAP), intubation, ventricular taps, and any other type of prolonged instrumentation are at increased risk. Late onset sepsis generally has a more gradual onset than early onset sepsis, and the site of primary infection relates to the cause. For example, ventilation-associated infection results in pneumonia. **Likely organisms involved in late onset sepsis** include:

- Gram-positive organisms like *Staphylococcus aureus* and Group B *Streptococcus* in 2/3 of cases
- Gram-negative organisms such as *E coli, Klebsiella pneumoniae, Pseudomonas aeruginosa, Serratia, Enterobacter*, and *Acinetobacter*
- *Candida*

TREATMENT OF SEPSIS/MENINGITIS

Neonatal sepsis and meningitis are treated with **intravenous antibiotics**. Usually if sepsis is suspected, treatment with broad-spectrum antibiotics (IV aminoglycoside and penicillin) will be started while awaiting the culture results. Once culture results are obtained any adjustment to a more effective medication to treat the now identified organism may be made. Using antibiotics too liberally when not indicated by a confirmed bacterial infection can have serious consequences for the neonate, such as the development of antibiotic resistant strains of bacteria and the killing of the normal flora of organisms that inhabit the intestinal tract leading to digestive problems. These problems must be weighed with the need to quickly treat a suspected sepsis when cultures have not been completed as many of these take days to finish growing. If hydrocephalus occurs with meningitis, then a ventroperitoneal shunt may be inserted surgically. Enteral or parenteral feedings may be necessary to provide adequate nutrition during treatment. Radiant warmers or incubators may be needed for thermoregulation.

RANGE OF SEVERE INFECTIONS

There are a number of terms used to refer to the range of severe infections and often used interchangeably, but they are part of a continuum:

- **Bacteremia** is the presence of bacteria in the blood but without systemic infection.
- **Septicemia** is a systemic infection caused by pathogens (usually bacteria or fungi) present in the blood.
- **Systemic inflammatory response syndrome (SIRS)**, a generalized inflammatory response affecting many organ systems, may be caused by infectious or non-infectious agents, such as trauma, adrenal insufficiency, pulmonary embolism, and drug overdose. If an infectious agent is identified or suspected, SIRS is an aspect of sepsis. Infective agents for infants include a wide range of bacteria and fungi, including *Streptococcus pneumoniae* and *Staphylococcus aureus*. SIRS includes 2 of the following:
  - Elevated (>38 °C) or subnormal rectal temperature (<36 °C)
  - Tachypnea >60 for infants or $PaCO_2$ <32 mmHg
  - Tachycardia >160 for infants
  - Leukocytosis (>12,000) or leukopenia (<4000)
- **Sepsis** is the presence of infection either locally or systemically in which there is a generalized life-threatening inflammatory response (SIRS). It includes all the indications for SIRS as well as one of the following:
  - Hypoxemia (<72 mmHg) without pulmonary disease
  - Elevation in plasma lactate
  - Decreased urinary output <5 mL/kg/hr for ≥1 hour
- **Severe sepsis** includes both indications of SIRS and sepsis as well as indications of increasing organ dysfunction with inadequate perfusion and/or hypotension.
- **Septic shock** is a progression from severe sepsis in which refractory hypotension occurs despite treatment. There may be indications of lactic acidosis.
- **Multi-organ dysfunction syndrome** (MODS) is the most common cause of sepsis-related death. Cardiac function becomes depressed, acute respiratory distress syndrome (ARDS) may develop, and renal failure may follow acute tubular necrosis or cortical necrosis. Thrombocytopenia appears in about 30% of those affected and may result in disseminated intravascular coagulation (DIC). Liver damage and bowel necrosis may occur.

Assess and Manage Pathophysiologic States

Cardiovascular

CYANOTIC AND ACYANOTIC CONGENITAL CARDIAC DEFECTS

Congenital heart disease is one of the leading causes of death in children within the first year of life. There are two main types of congenital heart disease: acyanotic and cyanotic. They may also be classified according to hemodynamics related to the blood flow pattern.

Cyanotic defects includes those with decreased pulmonary blood flow or mixed blood flow.

- **Decreased pulmonary blood flow**
  - Tetralogy of Fallot
  - Tricuspid atresia
- **Mixed blood flow**
  - Ebstein anomaly
  - Hypoplastic left heart syndrome
  - Total anomalous pulmonary venous return
  - Transposition of great arteries
  - Truncus arteriosus

Acyanotic defects include those with increased pulmonary blood flow or obstructed ventricular blood flow.

- **Increased pulmonary blood flow**
  - Atrial septal defect
  - Atrioventricular canal defect
  - Patent ductus arteriosus
  - Ventricular septal defect
- **Obstructed ventricular blood flow**
  - Aortic stenosis
  - Coarctation of aorta
  - Pulmonic stenosis

CENTRAL AND PERIPHERAL CYANOSIS

Cyanosis results from lack of oxygen and desaturated hemoglobin level of at least 5 g/dL. The two primary types of cyanosis are central and peripheral:

- **Central cyanosis**: Results from desaturated blood (decrease in oxygen transport from the lungs to the bloodstream), often because of a heart lesion, heart failure, or respiratory disorder. Because the arteries carry insufficient oxygen, cyanosis is apparent in the tongue, conjunctiva, and mucous membranes.
- **Peripheral cyanosis**: Results from peripheral vascular constriction from various causes, including hypothermia, stress, hypovolemia, or from conditions that interfere with blood flow to the extremities, such as cardiogenic shock or sepsis. Because blood supply to the extremities is inadequate, cyanosis becomes evident in the distal hands (fingers, nailbeds) and feet as well as the lips, tip of the nose, perioral areas, periorbital areas, and earlobes. However, PaO_2 levels generally remain normal.

Note that cyanosis may be more difficult to assess in dark-skinned neonates and may appear as a gray "ashy" discoloration rather than blue. **Acrocyanosis** (about mouth and extremities) is often a normal finding in neonates for up to 48 hours.

CARDIAC AND PULMONARY CYANOSIS

Cyanosis can reflect underlying cardiac and pulmonary disease:

- **Cardiac cyanosis:** This generally presents as cyanosis without respiratory distress. Cyanotic heart disease is likely a factor if the neonate's PaO_2 remains <70 mmHg while the neonate breathes 100% oxygen. Typically, with cyanotic heart disease, central cyanosis is a diagnostic factor although the degree of cyanosis at onset may vary. With structural heart defects that result in right-to-left shunting, cyanosis is generally evident, often from birth, and heart murmurs or extra heart sounds are evident. In some cases, such as tetralogy of Fallot, the cyanosis is more noticeable during crying.
- **Pulmonary cyanosis:** The neonate often has obvious signs of respiratory distress, including grunting respirations and sternal retraction, as well as central cyanosis. PaO_2 usually remains >100 mmHg while on 100% oxygen. Pulmonary conditions that may cause cyanosis include pulmonary hypoplasia, pulmonary edema, pneumothorax, pleural effusion, pneumonia, phrenic nerve palsy, hypoventilation, and diaphragmatic hernia.

TETRALOGY OF FALLOT

Tetralogy of Fallot (TOF) is a combination of 4 different defects:

- **Ventricular septal defect** usually with a large opening
- **Pulmonic stenosis** with decreased blood flow to lungs
- **Overriding aorta** (displacement to the right so that it appears to come from both ventricles, usually overriding the ventricular septal defect), resulting in the mixing of oxygenated and deoxygenated blood
- **Right ventricular hypertrophy**

Infants with TOF are often acutely cyanotic immediately after birth, while others with less severe defects may have increasing cyanosis over the first year.

Symptoms include:

- Intolerance to feeding or crying, resulting in increased cyanotic "blue spells" or "tet spells"
- Failure to thrive with poor growth
- Clubbing of fingers may occur over time
- Intolerance to activity as child grows
- Increased risk for emboli, brain attacks, brain abscess, seizures, fainting, or sudden death

Treatment: Total surgical repair at ≤1 year is now the preferred treatment rather than the palliative procedures formerly used.

TRANSPOSITION OF THE GREAT ARTERIES

Transposition of the great arteries is a congenital heart defect in which the aorta is connected to the right ventricle instead of the left ventricle, and the pulmonary artery is connected to the left ventricle instead of the right ventricle. This transposition means that deoxygenated blood is being pumped back to the body and the oxygenated blood returns to the lungs instead of going to the body. Septal defects may also occur, allowing some mixing of blood, and the ductus arteriosus allows mixing until it closes.

Symptoms vary depending upon whether there is mixing of blood but may include:

- Mild-to-severe cyanosis
- Symptoms of congestive heart failure
- Cardiomegaly developing in the weeks after birth
- Heart sounds vary depending upon the severity of the defects

Treatment may include:

- Prostaglandin to keep the ductus arteriosus and foramen ovale open; balloon atrial septostomy to increase size of foramen ovale
- Surgical repair to transpose arteries to the normal position ("arterial switch") as well as to repair septal defects and other abnormalities

ACYANOTIC HEART DISEASE

PDA

Patent ductus arteriosus (PDA) is failure of the ductus arteriosus that connects the **pulmonary artery and aorta** to close after birth, resulting in left-to-right shunting of blood from the aorta back to the pulmonary artery. This increases the blood flow to the lungs and causes an increase in pulmonary hypertension that can result in damage to the lung tissue.

While some infants may be essentially asymptomatic, **typical symptoms** include:

- Cyanosis
- Congestive heart failure
- Machinery-like murmur
- Frequent respiratory infections and dyspnea, especially on exertion
- Widened pulse pressure
- Bounding pulse
- Atrial fibrillation/palpitations
- Increased risk for bacterial endocarditis, congestive heart failure, and development of pulmonary vascular obstructive disease

Treatment includes:

- Pharmacologic therapy: Nonselective COX inhibitors such as ibuprofen and indomethacin have proven effective in closing PDA. Ibuprofen has shown to equally effective as the traditional pharmacologic approach of indomethacin, and less-likely to induce necrotizing enterocolitis or renal dysfunction. Both of these options carry a risk for bleeding. For patients with contraindications to nonselective COX inhibitors, acetaminophen is a supported option, but requires high dosages for maximal effect which places the neonate at risk for liver damage.
- Surgical repair can be done with ligation of the patent vessel.

VENTRICULAR SEPTAL DEFECT

Ventricular septal defect is an abnormal opening in the **septum** between the right and left ventricles. If the opening is small, the child may be asymptomatic, but larger openings can result in a left-to-right shunt because of higher pressure in the left ventricle. This shunting increases in the 6 weeks after birth, with symptoms becoming more evident, but the defect may close within a few years.

Symptoms include:

- Congestive heart failure with peripheral edema
- Tachycardia
- Dyspnea
- Difficulty feeding
- Heart murmur
- Recurrent pulmonary infections
- Increased risk for bacterial endocarditis and pulmonary vascular obstructive disease

Treatment includes:

- Diuretics, such as furosemide (Lasix), may be used for heart failure.
- ACE inhibitor (Captopril) decreases pulmonary hypertension.
- Surgery, including pulmonary banding or cardiopulmonary bypass, can be performed to repair the opening with sutures or a patch, depending upon the size.

ATRIAL SEPTAL DEFECT

An atrial septal defect (ASD) is an abnormal opening in the **septum** between the right and left atria. Because the left atrium has higher pressure than the right atrium, some of the oxygenated blood returning from the lungs to the left atrium is shunted back to the right atrium, where it is again returned to the lungs, displacing deoxygenated blood.

Symptoms may be few or even absent depending upon the degree of the defect but can include:

- Congestive heart failure
- Heart murmur
- Increased risk for dysrhythmias and pulmonary vascular obstructive disease over time

Treatment may not be necessary for small defects, but larger defects require closure:

- Open-heart surgical repair
- Heart catheterization and placing of closure device (Amplatz device) across the atrial septal defect

COARCTATION OF THE AORTA

Coarctation of the aorta is a stricture of the aorta, proximal to the ductus arteriosus intersection. The increased blood pressure caused by the heart attempting to pump the blood past the stricture causes the heart to enlarge and also increases blood pressure to the head and upper extremities while decreasing blood pressure to the lower body and extremities. With severe stricture, symptoms may not occur until the ductus arteriosus closes, causing sudden loss of blood supply to the lower body.

Symptoms include:

- Difference in blood pressure between upper and lower extremities
- Congestive heart failure symptoms in infants
- Headaches, dizziness, and nosebleeds in older children
- Increased risk of hypertension, ruptured aorta, aortic aneurysm, bacterial endocarditis, and brain attack

Treatment includes:

- Prostaglandin (alprostadil), such as Prostin VR Pediatric, to reopen the ductus arteriosus for infants
- Balloon angioplasty
- Surgical resection and anastomosis or graft replacement (usually at 3-5 years of age unless condition is severe); infants who have surgery may need later repair

CONGESTIVE HEART FAILURE

TYPES

Congestive heart failure results from the inability of the heart to adequately pump the blood the body needs. In infants, it is usually secondary to cardiac abnormalities with resultant increased blood volume and blood pressure:

- **Right-sided failure** occurs if the right ventricle cannot effectively contract to pump blood into the pulmonary artery, causing pressure to build in the right atrium and the venous circulation. This venous hypertension causes generalized edema of lower extremities, distended abdomen from ascites, hepatomegaly, and jugular venous distension.
- **Left-sided failure** occurs if the left ventricle cannot effectively pump blood into the aorta and systemic circulation, increasing pressure in the left atrium and the pulmonary veins, with resultant pulmonary edema and increased pulmonary pressure. Symptoms include respiratory distress with tachypnea, grunting respirations, sternal retraction, rales, failure to thrive, and difficulty eating, often leaving the child exhausted and sweaty.

Children often have some combination of right and left-sided failure. Increased pressure in the lungs after birth may delay symptoms for 1-2 weeks.

MANAGEMENT

Management of congestive heart failure (CHF) in infants can be difficult. It is extremely important to establish the etiology and to treat the underlying cause. For infants with structural cardiac abnormalities, surgical repair may be needed to resolve the CHF. There are some medical treatments that can relieve symptoms:

- **Diuretics**, such as furosemide (Lasix), metolazone, or hydrochlorothiazide to reduce pulmonary and peripheral edema
- **Antihypertensives**, such as Captopril or Propranolol to decrease heart workload
- **Cardiac glycosides**, such as Lanoxin, may relieve symptoms if above medicines are not successful
- **High caloric feedings**, either by bottle or nasogastric feeding to provide sufficient nutrients
- **Oxygen** may be useful for some children with weak hearts
- **Restriction of activities** to reduce stress on the heart
- **Dopamine or dobutamine** may be given to increase the contractibility of the heart

HYPOTENSION

Hypotension is a systemic mean arterial blood pressure <2 standard deviations less that average values for gestational age. The lowest reading that is within normal limits for preterm infants is calculated as gestational age plus five. Thus, a 31-week preterm acceptable low BP would be 31-36 mmHg. Hypotension in the neonate most often relates to dysregulation of peripheral vascular tone and/or myocardial dysfunction. Hypotension may also occur as the result of hypocalcemia, hypovolemic, cardiogenic, or distributive shock, so determining the cause of hypotension is critical to planning appropriate intervention. Early signs of hypotension are those of compensated shock and later signs of decompensated shock. Tachycardia, respiratory distress, pallor, lethargy, and cyanosis may be evident. Dopamine (2-20 µg/kg/min) is the most commonly used drug to treat neonatal hypotension as it improves myocardial function and improves peripheral vascular tension without causing vasodilation. Oxygen is administered to combat hypoxia as well as saline bolus (10-20 mL/kg).

HYPERTENSION

Hypertension is a relatively rare finding in the neonate. Signs of elevated blood pressure include lethargy, increased apnea episodes, seizures, irritability, tachypnea, and intracranial hemorrhage. The nurse often discovers elevated blood pressure through a routine check of vital signs. Most **causes of hypertension** in the neonate are **renal** in origin and include:

- **Thrombus formation in the kidneys** from an umbilical artery catheter (the most common cause in the NICU)
- **Other vascular causes**, such as renal vein thrombosis, or renal artery stenosis, or coarctation of the aorta
- **Compression of renal artery** by a mass

Non-renal causes include:

- **Iatrogenesis**, due to administration of dopamine, Aminophylline, or glucocorticoids
- **Neurological**, secondary to seizures or intraventricular hemorrhage
- **Endocrine**, secondary to congenital adrenal hyperplasia or hyperthyroidism
- **Pulmonary**, secondary to pneumothorax or bronchopulmonary dysplasia

SHOCK

Shock is the result of circulatory failure in which there is inadequate perfusion to meet the metabolic needs of the body. There are a number of different causes, but the **physiologic responses** are essentially the same:

- Hypotension (which may not be present initially because of reactive vasoconstriction)
- Hypoxemia resulting in hypoxic tissue
- Metabolic acidosis

There are essentially **3 stages** in the progression of the shock response:

1. **Compensated shock**: The sympathetic nervous response causes vasoconstriction, which may mask essential underlying hypotension but serves to provide blood flow for vital organ functions, although there may be decreased circulation at the microvascular (small vessel) level.
2. **Decompensated shock**: The cardiovascular system is unable to adequately compensate and microvascular perfusion decreases.
3. **Irreversible/terminal shock**: Damage to internal organs, such as the heart and brain, is so extensive that therapeutic measures cannot reverse eventual death.

COMPENSATED SHOCK

During compensated shock, the blood pressure may remain normal initially as the compensatory sympathetic nervous response results in vasoconstriction and an increase in the heart rate and contractibility that combine to maintain cardiac output at a level adequate to supply the heart and brain while shifting circulation from other organs:

- **Skin:** Skin cold and clammy
- **Gastrointestinal tract**: Bowel sounds absent or decreased
- **Kidneys**: Urinary output decreased

Because of a decrease in tissue perfusion, lactic acid begins to build up, producing metabolic acidosis. The acidosis results in an increased respiratory rate, which serves to expel excess carbon dioxide. However, this also raises the pH of the blood and may result in respiratory alkalosis. Fluid replacement and medications to increase blood pressure and perfusion of the tissues are critical during this stage.

DECOMPENSATED SHOCK

Decompensated shock occurs as the body can no longer compensate, the blood pressure falls below normal, and all organ systems suffer from hypoperfusion. The heart is overworked and becomes dysfunctional, and chemical changes cause myocardial depression, so that the heart begins to fail. The permeability of the capillaries increases with fluid buildup in the interstitial tissues and decreased venous return to the heart. Multi-system effects occur:

- **Respiratory**: Respirations become rapid and shallow as the hypoxemia causes an inflammatory response and pulmonary edema, with collapse of alveoli and fibrotic changes in the lung tissue.
- **Cardiovascular**: Dysrhythmias and ischemia of the myocardium result in tachycardia. The myocardium is depressed and ventricles may dilate.
- **Neurological**: Hypoperfusion of the brain leads to changes in mental status, including lethargy and loss of consciousness. Pupils may dilate or react sluggishly.
- **Renal**: Acute renal failure occurs with decrease in urinary output, increase in BUN and creatinine, and electrolyte shifts.
- **Hepatic**: The liver loses the ability to filter and metabolize medications and metabolic waste products. Liver enzymes rise, and the skin becomes jaundiced.
- **Gastrointestinal**: Mucosal ulcerations may occur, causing bleeding and bloody diarrhea. Bacterial toxins may invade the lymphatic system where they are carried to the bloodstream, causing infection and increasing adverse cardiovascular responses.
- **Hematologic**: Disseminated vascular coagulation (DIC) may occur with both clotting and bleeding. The skin may show ecchymoses and petechiae. Clotting times are prolonged.

Treatment during this stage is dependent upon the underlying cause but includes intravenous fluids, medications to control blood pressure, cardiac function, infection, and gastrointestinal ulcerations and bleeding. Ventilatory support with oxygen and administration of sodium bicarbonate may be needed to treat metabolic acidosis. The infant must be monitored constantly, including hemodynamic monitoring, blood gases, urinary function, EKG, fluid and electrolytes, blood chemistries, enzyme levels, and neurological status.

IRREVERSIBLE/TERMINAL SHOCK

The irreversible/terminal stage of shock can be difficult to determine because the progression of shock is a continuum rather than clearly defined stages, so the usual strategy is to continue to treat the patient with fluids, vasoactive medications to improve cardiac function, and nutritional support. During this stage hypotension persists, and complete liver and renal failure occurs. As perfusion causes necrosis of tissue, the toxins created result in severe metabolic acidosis. There is also increased lactic acidosis. Adenosine triphosphate (ATP) levels are depleted and there are no mechanisms left to store energy. **Multiple organ dysfunction syndrome (MODS)** occurs. There is no specific treatment that can reverse MODS, so treatment at this point becomes supportive. The mortality rate for MODS ranges from 30-100%, depending upon the number of organ systems that are involved.

CARDIOGENIC SHOCK

Cardiogenic shock in infants usually relates to congenital heart disease (usually with systemic to pulmonary shunting), myocarditis, and dysrhythmias, such as AV block and paroxysmal atrial tachycardia. These disorders interfere with the pumping mechanism of the heart, decreasing oxygen perfusion. Cardiogenic shock has 3 **characteristics**:

- Increased preload
- Increased afterload
- Decreased contractibility

Together these result in a decreased cardiac output and an increase in systemic vascular resistance (SVR) to compensate and protect vital organs. This results in an increase of afterload in the left ventricle with increased need for oxygen. As the cardiac output continues to decrease, tissue perfusion decreases, coronary artery perfusion decreases, fluid backs up, and the left ventricle fails to adequately pump the blood, resulting in pulmonary edema and right ventricular failure.

CARDIAC DYSRHYTHMIAS

Cardiac dysrhythmias (abnormal heart beats), although more common in adults, can occur in infants and are frequently the result of damage to the conduction system during major cardiac surgery.

Bradydysrhythmias are pulse rates that are abnormally slow:

- Complete atrioventricular block (A-V block) may be congenital or a response to surgical trauma.
- Sinus bradycardia may be caused by the autonomic nervous system or a response to hypotension and decrease in oxygenation.
- Junctional/nodal rhythms often occur in post-surgical patients when absence of P wave is noted but heart rate and output usually remain stable, and unless there is compromise, usually no treatment is necessary.

Tachydysrhythmias are pulse rates that are abnormally fast:

- Sinus tachycardia is often caused by illness, such as fever or infection.
- Supraventricular tachycardia (200-300 bpm) may have a sudden onset and result in congestive heart failure.

Conduction irregularities are irregular pulses that often occur post-operatively and are usually not significant. Premature contractions may arise from the atria or ventricles.

CARDIOVERSION PROCEDURES FOR ARRYTHMIA TYPES

Cardioversion procedures for arrythmia types are as follows:

- **Stable tachyarrhythmia:** Vagal maneuver to increase parasympathetic input to the heart and slow it. Apply ice to the neonate's face, which triggers the diving response to slow the heart rate. If unsuccessful, try adenosine, digoxin, or propranolol.
- **Unstable arrhythmia with narrow QRS complex:** Synchronized electrical cardioversion is appropriate for atrial flutter or fibrillation, WPW, or PJRT. Set the defibrillator for 0.5-2.0 J/kg. Place two electrode pads on the infant's chest. Wait for the optimum moment in the cardiac cycle. Pass electrical current through the infant's heart.
- **Unstable arrhythmia with wide QRS complex:** Asynchronous cardioversion is appropriate for ventricular tachycardia or fibrillation, SVT with BBB, or antidromic SVT in WPW. Defibrillate because there is no R wave present to time the shock.
- **Stable arrhythmia with wide QRS complex:** Administer amiodarone or procainamide for rate control. If unsuccessful, consider adenosine (0.1 mg/kg, with a maximum of 6 mg, rapid IV push and up to 0.2 mg/kg or 12 mg for a second dose). If pharmacologic interventions are unsuccessful, consider cardioversion at 0.5-1.0 J/kg for the first attempt, and then 2 J/kg if the first attempt is unsuccessful.
- **Bradydysrhythmias:** For 1:1 sinus bradycardia, complete AV block, Wenckebach's phenomenon, and sinus exit block: Check airway, breathing, and circulation. Treat underlying cause. Give oxygen, atropine, and isoproterenol. Start transvenous pacing.

Respiratory

RESPIRATORY DISTRESS SYNDROME

Respiratory distress syndrome (RDS) (hyaline membrane disease) occurs in 14% of low-birth-weight infants. RDS is caused by the absence or deficiency of surfactant. Surfactant is a lipoprotein that reduces surface tension in the alveoli. Surfactant causes the lungs to be more compliant (alveoli expand with less effort) and the alveoli do not collapse on end expiration. Surfactant production begins at 22 weeks of gestation, but levels are inadequate until 36 weeks of gestation. Lack of surfactant produces alveolar collapse (atelectasis) and less compliant lungs that cause laborious breathing. Collapsed areas of lung may still receive blood flow, but no exchange of gases occurs (ventilation perfusion mismatch). If RDS is left untreated, hypoxemia and hypercarbia develop, leading to respiratory acidosis. Acidosis and hypoxemia lead to a cycle of increased pulmonary vascular resistance and vasoconstriction, causing increased hypoxemia.

AIR LEAK SYNDROMES

Premature infants have more fragile lung tissue and often require respiratory resuscitative measures, such as positive pressure ventilation (PPV), ventilator support, and administration of pulmonary drugs (e.g., surfactant) that make them more susceptible to air leak syndrome. **Air leak syndrome** occurs when an alveolus ruptures and air leaks into a space that it normally does not occupy. Different syndromes occur, depending on the area that air leaks into.

- **Pneumothorax**: Air leakage into the pleural cavity that surrounds the lungs
- **Tension pneumothorax**: One-way air flow into the pleural cavity, with pressure build-up and significant collapse of lung tissue, causing respiratory compromise
- **Pneumomediastinum**: Air traveling along the pulmonary blood vessels that enters the mediastinum
- **Pneumopericardium**: Air in the sac that surrounds the heart
- **Pulmonary interstitial emphysema**: Air trapped in the lung's interstitial spaces

PNEUMOTHORAX

Pneumothorax is the most common type of air leak syndrome. In infants, increased air pressure caused by the use of mechanical ventilation is the most common cause, but infants may develop spontaneous pneumothorax. Infants with fragile lung tissue are at especially high risk:

- Infants with lung disease, including hyaline membrane disease (HMD)
- Premature infants
- Infants with meconium aspiration

Symptoms vary according to the type of pneumothorax (spontaneous, traumatic, or tension) but can include:

- Increased respiratory distress with tachypnea and chest wall retractions
- Absence of breath sounds on auscultation
- Paradoxical chest movement in which the chest contracts during inhalation and expands during exhalation
- Shift in maximum intensity sounds of heart
- Bradycardia and cyanosis

Treatment includes:

- Evacuating air with needle aspiration or chest tubes to water seal drainage
- Correction of underlying cause

PNEUMOMEDIASTINUM

A pneumomediastinum is an air leak in the mediastinum, the area of the chest between the sternum and the spine, and between the lungs. Causes of neonatal **pneumomediastinum** vary. Often, this complication arises after or in conjunction with neonatal respiratory distress, pneumonia, mechanical ventilation use, meconium aspiration, or as a result of birth-related trauma. While pneumomediastinum is often asymptomatic, it can also present with cyanosis, diminished heart sounds or shallow respirations. The condition often resolves spontaneously, but the patient must be monitored closely for complications and may require mechanical ventilation despite this being a common cause of the condition. Diagnosis of pneumomediastinum is through chest x-ray, with ABG's to evaluate the impact of the condition on the newborn's gas exchange and oxygenation.

APNEA OF PREMATURITY

Premature infants (especially those <34 weeks) often exhibit **apnea of prematurity (AOP)**. AOP begins at birth and is believed to be caused by immaturity of the nervous system, and improves as the brain matures. It may persist for 4-8 weeks. There are 3 **types of apnea**:

- **Central**: no airflow or effort to breathe
- **Obstructive**: no airflow, but effort to breathe
- **Mixed**: both central and obstructive elements (75% of AOP)

Symptoms include:

- Swallowing during apneic periods
- Apnea >20 seconds
- Apnea <20 seconds with bradycardia 30 beats <normal
- Oxygen saturation <85% persisting ≥5 seconds
- Cyanosis

Treatment includes:

- Tactile stimulation (rubbing limbs or thorax or gently slapping bottoms of feet) or gently lifting the jaw to relieve obstruction
- Oxygen or bag/mask ventilation for bradycardia and decreased oxygen saturation
- Continuous positive airway pressure (CPAP) for mixed or obstructive apnea
- Aminophylline/theophylline or caffeine (for central apnea) may increase contractions of the diaphragm

TTN

Transient tachypnea of the newborn (TTN) occurs when fluid in the lungs is not adequately absorbed after birth. The neonate usually exhibits symptoms within 36 hours of birth, and the condition typically resolves within 3 days. TTN is most common in infants delivered by Cesarean section, but premature birth and having a mother who smokes or has diabetes increases risk to the infant.

Symptoms include:

- Dyspnea (>60/min)
- Sternal retraction (mild)
- Expiratory grunt
- Nasal flaring
- Poor feeding (because of increased respiratory rate)

Laboratory findings include:

- ABGs: hypoxemia
- Chest radiograph: fluid in lungs

Treatment includes:

- Monitor oxygen saturation levels
- Provide supplemental oxygen as indicated
- Provide intravenous fluids or nasogastric feedings if infant is unable to take oral feedings

MECONIUM ASPIRATION SYNDROME

Meconium aspiration syndrome (MAS) occurs when meconium, expelled in the amniotic fluid (occurring in about 20% of pregnancies), is aspirated by the fetus *in utero* or the neonate at first breath. Blood and amniotic fluids may be aspirated as well. Some infants may present with **symptoms** at birth, but sometimes symptoms are delayed for a number of hours:

- Tachypnea
- Lethargy, depressed state
- Hypoxemia and hypercapnia
- Metabolic acidosis may occur
- Hyperventilation may occur in early stages with hypoventilation in later stages

Symptoms are similar to transient tachypnea of the newborn (TTN) but they are more severe and the infant appears more compromised. Chest x-rays may show infiltrates, atelectasis, and hypoinflated areas as well as hyperinflated areas. Pulmonary hypertension may result. **Treatment** includes:

- Preventive suctioning of the oropharynx as soon as the head is delivered
- Intubation and suctioning of the trachea for infants with respiratory distress (weak respirations, bradycardia, hypotonia)
- Supplemental oxygen and/or mechanical ventilation as indicated

PPHN

Persistent pulmonary hypertension (PPHN) occurs when the high pulmonary vascular pressure that keeps fetal blood from circulating through the lungs fails to reduce after birth, so that blood continues to bypass the lungs, and the foramen ovale and ductus arteriosus are forced by pressure to remain open with venous blood shunting into systemic circulation instead of being oxygenated in the lungs. Infants are usually near or full-term, but present at birth with respiratory distress and cyanosis. PPHN is the cause of about 50% of neonatal deaths. There are 3 **classifications**:

- **Primary** is idiopathic with normal lung tissue but arterial hyperplasia and/or premature constricting of ductus arteriosus *in utero.*
- **Secondary** is precipitated by another disorder, such as meconium aspiration pneumonia (MAP), transient tachypnea of the newborn (TTN) or hyaline membrane disease. This is the most common form.
- **Hypoplastic** is related to pulmonary hypoplasia with anatomic changes in alveoli and vasculature in the lung.

PPHN has been linked to maternal use of SSRIs and NSAIDs.

Symptoms are usually evident within the first 12 hours of birth and progress over the next 24-48 hours:

- Cyanosis with poor cardiac perfusion, tachycardia
- Hypoxemia, persisting even with supplemental oxygen
- Systolic murmur with regurgitation of the tricuspid valve
- Tachypnea and general respiratory distress

TREATMENT

Treatment for persistent pulmonary hypertension (PPHN) will be specific for the underlying cause, and can include:

- Intubation and mechanical ventilation with HFV especially with parenchymal lung disease
- Central venous lines for administration of solutions, such as calcium gluconate
- Arterial line to monitor arterial blood gas
- Surfactants (beractant) to reduce surface tension in patients without primary PPHN
- High frequency ventilation (HFV) is used with underlying lung disease resulting in low volume
- Extracorporeal membrane oxygenation (ECMO) is used if other forms of support are not successful, and most often if the infant also has congenital diaphragmatic hernia
- Sodium bicarbonate is often used to correct metabolic acidosis in practice, however there is no evidence of short or long-term benefits
- Sedation (fentanyl) to reduce restlessness. Induced paralysis (pancuronium, vecuronium) has been used but is implicated in increased mortality rates, atelectasis, sensory hearing loss, and ventilation-perfusion mismatch
- Inhaled nitrous oxide

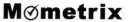

Pulmonary Hemorrhage

Pulmonary hemorrhage is bleeding within the alveoli. This usually is the result of some other event, such as intracranial hemorrhage, asphyxia, aspiration, heart disease, or sepsis. This can also be the result of a trauma from over-aggressive suctioning. **Pulmonary hemorrhage** presents as bright red blood from the trachea found with suctioning and as rapid, sudden respiratory deterioration. Pulmonary hemorrhage can cause rapid death if the bleeding is severe and is often only found during an autopsy. A more minor hemorrhage can be managed with blood transfusions and assisted ventilation. Pulmonary hemorrhage may result in hemothorax. In some cases, pneumothorax may also be present, resulting in mediastinal shift that increases the difficulty of identifying and repairing the bleeding vessel. If the infant is stabilized, computed tomography may provide accurate diagnosis to isolate the area of hemorrhage. The underlying cause of the hemorrhage must be discovered and treated.

Surfactant Therapy

Pulmonary hemorrhage is sometimes treated with **surfactant** although there are no adequate randomized studies at this time to show efficacy. However, preliminary reports appear positive. In some cases, pulmonary hemorrhage may be associated with the use of surfactant. The use of surfactant therapy is common in preterm infants to reduce morbidity and mortality related to respiratory distress syndrome. It is also sometimes used for infants receiving prolonged ventilatory support. Surfactant improves lung compliance, decreases pulmonary vascular resistance, and increases flow (right to left) through a patent ductus arteriosus or persistent foramen ovale. However, these very improvements in lung function can result in pulmonary hemorrhage, especially if ventilatory support is not adjusted with respect to the improved pulmonary function, so it's very important that ventilation be monitored carefully after administration of surfactant.

CDH

Congenital diaphragmatic hernias (CDH) may cause severe respiratory distress. The primary CDHs that affect infants are **posterolateral** (Bochdalek hernia).

- **Left-sided** in 85% of cases; includes herniation of the large and small intestine and intra-abdominal organs into the thoracic cavity
- **Right-sided** in 13% of cases; may be asymptomatic or involve only the liver and part of the large intestine herniate

Neonates with left CDH may exhibit **severe respiratory distress** and **cyanosis**. The lungs may be underdeveloped because of pressure exerted from displaced organs during fetal development. There may be a left hemithorax with a mediastinal shift, with the heart pressing on the right lung, which may be hypoplastic. Bowel sounds are heard over the chest area. Pulmonary hypertension and cardiopulmonary failure may occur. **Treatments** include:

- Immediate surgical repair
- HFOV and nitric oxide for pulmonary hypoplasia
- Extracorporeal membrane oxygenation (ECMO) for cardiopulmonary dysfunction

Despite treatment, mortality rates are 50%, and children who survive may have emphysema, with a larger volume but inadequate number of alveoli.

Hematopoietic

ABO INCOMPATIBILITY

About 20-25% of pregnancies involve ABO incompatibility, usually with the mother type O and the fetus A or B. **Anti-A and anti-B antibodies** occur naturally when a woman is exposed to A and B antigens in foods or bacteria, so these antibodies can cross the placenta and result in **hemolysis of fetal RBC**; however, the antibodies are relatively large and do not enter the fetal circulation easily. If fetal blood leaks into maternal blood (a common occurrence), then smaller antibodies form and these can cross the placenta more easily. There is no difference in effect between the first pregnancy and subsequent pregnancies. There are rarely serious complications for the fetus, although the neonate may develop hyperbilirubinemia, so the infant should be observed carefully. Only in severe cases of hemolysis (rare), does the child require exchange transfusions. Anemia may develop in the weeks after delivery because of increased rate of RBC breakdown, so the neonate should be monitored with blood counts.

MATERNAL RH ALLOIMMUNIZATION

Rh incompatibility occurs if the mother is Rh- and the father is Rh+, putting their infant at risk for hemolytic disease of the newborn (HDN) or Rh disease, (erythroblastosis fetalis). **Rh alloimmunization** (formation of antibodies against foreign antigens) can occur during abortion, abruptio placenta, amniocentesis, Cesarean section, chorionic villus sampling, cordocentesis, delivery, ectopic pregnancy, and toxemia. To prevent erythroblastosis fetalis, a woman who is Rh-with an Rh+ mate receives the serum **RhoGAM**, containing anti Rh+ antibodies. The purpose of the antibodies is to agglutinate any fetal red blood cells that pass over into the mother's circulatory system and thus prevent the mother from forming antibodies against them that will attack the infant and sensitize her for future pregnancies. Testing and administration of RhoGAM is as follows:

- Order Rh(D) tests. If the mother is Rh- and the father is Rh+, then their infant is at risk for hemolytic disease of the newborn (HDN).
- Order an antibody screen of the mother's blood to find out if she acquired anti-D antibodies from a previous blood transfusion or pregnancy.
- The mother receives 300 mcg RhoGAM (RhIg, Rh immunoglobulin) intramuscularly at 26-28 weeks of pregnancy and again within 72 hours after her delivery. Do not inject the infant or father. RhoGAM prevents Rh+ cells from the infant that have crossed over to the mother from causing her to create anti-D antibodies that will attack the infant and sensitize her for future pregnancies.
- Miscarriage, ectopic, abortion: At ≤12 weeks, the mother receives 50 mcg of MICRhoGAM. At ≥13 weeks, the mother receives RhoGAM as for pregnancy.

BLOOD-LOSS ANEMIA

Blood loss is the most common cause of anemia in the neonate. Anemia is hematocrit or hemoglobin level >2 standard deviations below the mean for age. For a term infant, anemia is a hematocrit <45%. The loss of blood may be internal or external, and may occur in utero, during delivery, or post-delivery. **Treatment** may include packed red blood cell transfusions. Common **causes** of neonatal blood loss include:

Antenatal

- Abruptio placentae or placenta previa
- Fetomaternal transfusion (passage of fetal blood to the mother)
- Twin-to-twin transfusion, resulting in one twin with polycythemia and the donor twin with anemia

Perinatal

- Trauma to the placenta or umbilical cord
- Rupture of anomalous cord vessels
- Fetoplacental transfusion that occurs when the infant is positioned above the level of the placenta after delivery

Postnatal

- Internal hemorrhage, such as intracranial hemorrhage or cephalohematoma
- Damage to internal organs, such as the adrenal gland or liver
- Iatrogenic blood loss secondary to frequent laboratory sampling, a major cause of anemia in premature infants

ANEMIA OF PREMATURITY

Anemia of prematurity (AOP) represents a pathologic exaggeration of the normal decrease in hematocrit that occurs in every newborn. AOP results from a combination of factors:

- **RBC production** decreases because the premature neonate's response to erythropoietin (EPO) has not matured. EPO is the main stimulus for RBC production. The normal progression of EPO production in the fetus is for the liver to initially be the primary site, with transfer to the kidney as the primary site of production in the full-term neonate. The liver is less responsive to hypoxia and allows for a lower threshold of anemia to progress until EPO production is increased. Lowest Hgb levels are usually at 2-3 months of age.
- **Premature RBCs have a shortened lifespan** when compared to the full-term neonate's because of decreased levels of intracellular ATP and enzyme activity.
- **Frequent blood draws** in premature neonates required for close monitoring deplete the blood supply.

Infants with signs of hypoxemia (poor feeling, tachypnea, tachycardia, pallor) may require transfusions.

ANEMIA OF RED BLOOD CELL DESTRUCTION

Causes of anemia of red blood cell destruction are discussed below:

- **Intrinsic causes**—continued production of abnormal red blood cells that have a decreased survival time because of rare hereditary disorders:
  - **RBC enzyme defects**, such as G6PD deficiency, where hemolytic crisis occurs in response to drugs such as sulfonamide antibiotics, or infections
  - **RBC membrane defects**, such as hereditary spherocytosis, where abnormally-shaped red cells are prone to hemolysis
  - **Hemoglobinopathies**, such as thalassemia, which results in the reduced production of one of the protein chains that make up hemoglobin
- **Extrinsic causes**—temporary RBC destruction caused by some external stimulus:
  - **Immune hemolysis** from transfusion of an incompatible blood product (wrong Rh, ABO, or a minor blood group incompatibility)
  - **Acquired hemolysis** from infection, vitamin E deficiency, or poisoning

POLYCYTHEMIA

Polycythemia is a hematocrit greater than 65%. An elevated hematocrit means that the blood has less plasma and more cellular elements, increasing the viscosity of the blood. Increased blood viscosity results in slowed blood flow and sludging of red blood cells. Small vessels become occluded with microthrombi, resulting in tissue or organ ischemia. **Clinical signs of polycythemia include:**

- **Dermatologic**: plethora and increased capillary refill time
- **CNS**: lethargy, irritability, abnormal cry, cerebrovascular hemorrhage, and seizures
- **Pulmonary**: respiratory distress, cyanosis, apnea, and the development of persistent pulmonary hypertension
- **Renal**: hematuria, oliguria, and renal vein thrombosis
- **Hematological**: thrombocytopenia secondary to the development of disseminated intravascular coagulation
- **Gastrointestinal**: abdominal distension, poor feeding, bloody stools, and necrotizing enterocolitis
- **Metabolic**: persistent hypoglycemia and hypocalcemia

RISK FACTORS

Polycythemia occurs in 4% of live-born infants. Its **etiologies** are divided into conditions that cause hypoxia and increased RBC production and those that cause abnormal transfer of RBCs to the neonate (hypertransfusion):

- **Hypoxia**
  - Disorders that disrupt normal placental function and decrease oxygen delivery to the fetus include preeclampsia, chronic placental abruption, maternal congenital heart disease, postdate pregnancy, and maternal smoking. Many of these are also associated with a growth-restricted neonate (IUGR).
  - Disorders that cause increased oxygen consumption by the fetus include infants of diabetic mothers and those with Beckwith-Wiedemann syndrome. Polycythemia occurs in 30 to 40% of neonates born to mothers with diabetes.
- **Hypertransfusion**
  - Delay in clamping the umbilical cord during delivery allows for increased blood volume to be transferred to the neonate.
  - Twin-twin transfusion creates one twin who is anemic and the second twin with an increased hematocrit in 10% of monozygotic twin pregnancies.

EXCHANGE TRANSFUSIONS

The infant with polycythemia requires a **partial exchange transfusion** with a plasma substitute in these situations:

- The hematocrit is greater than 65%, and the infant is symptomatic
- The hematocrit is greater than 70%, regardless of symptoms

Aliquots of the neonate's blood are replaced with isotonic saline to lower the hematocrit (Hct) to 50-55%. This formula calculates the volume of blood to be exchanged with an equal volume of saline:

$$\text{Exchange vol (mL)} = \frac{\text{initial Hct} - \text{desired Hct}}{\text{initial Hct}} \times \text{weight(kg)} \times 90\,\frac{\text{mL}}{\text{kg}}$$

The **procedure** is described below:

1. Withdraw no more than 5 mL of blood at a time from the umbilical artery or vein over 2-3 minutes.
2. Slowly infuse an equal amount of sterile normal saline.
3. Repeat the exchange until the desired volume of fluid is swapped.
4. Monitor the infant closely during the procedure.
5. Measure the hematocrit post procedure.

THROMBOCYTOSIS

Thrombocytosis is an increase in the platelet level >450,000/mcL; however, preterm infants often exhibit platelet levels of up to 600,000/mcL at 4-6 weeks. The normal reference range for platelets (thrombocytes) is 150,000-400,000/mcL. Thrombocytosis does not require specific treatment, but the underlying cause should be identified and treated. Neonates rarely have symptoms directly related to increased platelet count, but may experience cerebral ischemia with levels higher than 2,000,000/mcL. Treatment is aimed at the underlying cause. Almost all incidences of thrombocytosis in infants are secondary or reactive. **Common causes of thrombocytosis** in the neonate include:

- Infection
- Trisomy 21 (Down syndrome)
- Iron deficiency (often associated with chronic intrauterine blood loss from bleeding into a twin or GI bleeding)
- Congenital adrenal insufficiency
- Maternal abuse of narcotic drugs

THROMBOCYTOPENIA

Thrombocytopenia is a platelet count less than 150,000/mcL, caused either by decreased platelet production, increased platelet destruction, or a combination of both. Hematology labs use **mean platelet volume (MPV)**, a measure of the average platelet size, to differentiate the two. The MPV is normal if the cause is reduced production and elevated if the cause is accelerated destruction. Immature platelets are larger than normal and are released into circulating blood by the bone marrow when mature platelets are being destroyed. The lab may also differentiate the cause by a **retic count** (reticulated platelets are newly-produced platelets). If the retic count is elevated, then platelets are being destroyed, and if it is low, the production of platelets is suppressed. General guidelines for transfusing platelets depend on the clinical stability of the neonate. If the infant is stable, the attending physician considers a transfusion when the count is less than 25,000/mcL. If the infant is unstable, the attending physician considers a transfusion when the count is less than 50,000/mcL.

FETAL ONSET, EARLY ONSET, AND LATE ONSET

Causes of **fetal onset** include:

- Alloimmune thrombocytopenia: The mother produces antibodies specific to antigens on the neonate's platelets, which cross the placenta, causing thrombocytopenia.
- Autoimmune thrombocytopenia: Mothers with idiopathic thrombocytopenia purpura or lupus produce antibodies against fetal platelets.
- Congenital infection—mediated: CMV, rubella, toxoplasmosis. Neonates with trisomy 18 or 21.

Causes of **early onset** (<72 hours) include:

- Placental insufficiency occurs in infants who are small for gestational age or with intrauterine growth restriction
- Perinatal asphyxia
- Disseminated intravascular coagulation (DIC)

Causes of **late onset** (>72 hours) include:

- Late onset sepsis
- Necrotizing enterocolitis

HEMOPHILIA

Hemophilia is an inherited disorder in which the infant lacks adequate clotting factors. There are 3 **types**:

- Type A: Lack of clotting factor VII (90% of cases)
- Type B: Lack of clotting factor IX (about 5% of cases)
- Type C: Lack of clotting factor XI (affects both sexes, rarely occurs in the US)

Both Type A and B are usually X-linked disorders, affecting only males. The **severity** of the disease depends on the amount of clotting factor in the blood:

- Mild: >5% factor activity
- Moderate: 1-5% factor activity
- Severe: <1% factor activity

Severe neonatal hemophilia is often discovered when slow clotting is noted after circumcision or venipuncture. Approximately 1 to 2% of hemophiliacs have intracranial hemorrhage. Infants with severe hemophilia have a prolonged PTT, but normal PT values. Diagnosis is confirmed by Factor VIII and Factor IX tests.

Treatment includes:

- Desmopressin to stimulate production of clotting factor (if mild)
- Clotting factor or recombinant clotting factors (genetically-engineered)
- Plasma (Type C)

NEUTROPENIA

Reduced neutrophils (neutropenia) indicate infection or bone marrow suppression. In neonates, the most common reasons for neutropenia are infection or stresses, such as respiratory distress syndrome, although it may be associated with congenital disorders, such as Shwachman-Diamond and Kostmann's syndrome. A segmented neutrophil nucleus (seg) is a mature cell. A banded nucleus (band) is immature. To calculate the absolute neutrophil count (ANC), the percentage of segs is added to the percentage of bands and multiplied by the total white blood cell count. A low ANC is more specific for identifying sepsis than an elevated ANC, but ANC by itself is a poor indicator of sepsis. **Normal neutrophil counts**:

- At birth the lower limit of normal is 1,750 cells/mm^3
- At 12 hours it rises to 7,200 cells/mm^3
- At 72 hours it falls to 1,720 cells/mm^3

The immature to total neutrophil ratio (I:T) is a better indicator of sepsis than ANC. An I:T ratio greater than 0.2 indicates sepsis. The formula for calculating the I:T ratio:

$$\text{I:T} = \frac{\text{immature neutrophils}}{\text{immature neutrophils} + \text{mature neutrophils}}$$

HYPERBILIRUBINEMIA

Hyperbilirubinemia, excess of bilirubin in the blood, is characterized by jaundice. Hyperbilirubinemia is evaluated according to the levels of direct (conjugated) bilirubin and/or indirect (unconjugated) bilirubin:

- **Direct/conjugated bilirubin** levels increase with blockage of bile ducts, hepatitis, or other liver damage, including drug reaction.
- **Indirect/unconjugated bilirubin** levels increase with anemias (such as hemolytic disorders) and transfusion reactions.

Four basic **types** of hyperbilirubinemia and jaundice:

- **Physiologic**: Common in newborns and usually benign, resulting from immature hepatic function and increased RBC hemolysis. Infants have larger red blood cells with a shorter life than adults, leading to more RBC destruction and resulting in an increased load of serum bilirubin, which the liver of the newborn cannot handle. Premature infants have an even greater physiologic jaundice as their RBCs live even shorter lives than the term infant's. Onset is usually within 24-48 hours, peaking in 72 hours for full-term or 5 days for preterm infants and declining within a week. Phototherapy is the indicated treatment.
- **Hemolytic**: Caused by blood/antigen (Rh) incompatibility with onset in first 24 hours. Preventive treatment is RhoGAM prenatally or post-natal exchange transfusion. This type of hyperbilirubinemia may also result from ABO incompatibility but rarely requires treatment other than phototherapy.
- **Breastfeeding associated**: Relates to inadequate calories during early breastfeeding with onset on 2-3 days. This slows the excretion of stool and allows bilirubin levels to rise. More frequent feeding with caloric supplements is usually sufficient, but phototherapy may be used for bilirubin 18-20 mg/dL.
- **Breast milk jaundice**: May result from human breast milk breaking down bilirubin and its being reabsorbed in the gut. Characterized by less frequent stools and onset in 4-5 days, jaundice peaks in 10-15 days but may persist for a number of weeks. Treatment involves discontinuing breastfeeding for 24 hours.

KERNICTERUS

Kernicterus (also called bilirubin encephalopathy) occurs when elevated serum bilirubin levels cause damage to the brain. The exact serum bilirubin level at which damage occurs is unknown. Premature infants are more susceptible to the development of kernicterus at lower serum bilirubin levels because of the immaturity of their blood-brain barrier, causing it to be more permeable to bilirubin than in full term infants. Disease processes, such as acidosis or meningitis, further lessen the competency of the blood-brain barrier. **Early signs of kernicterus** are divided into three phases:

- **Phase I:** Occurs during the first few days of life and is characterized by decreased alertness, hypotonia, and poor feeding.
- **Phase II:** The onset and duration of this phase is variable. Hypertonia of the extensor muscles develops. Infants may display opisthotonos (extreme hyperextension or arching of the back) and/or retrocollis (extreme arching of the neck).
- **Phase III:** This occurs generally after one week with the recurrence of hypotonia.

> **Review Video: Jaundice Icterus**
> Visit mometrix.com/academy and enter code: 339680

PHOTOTHERAPY AND EXCHANGE TRANSFUSION

Hyperbilirubinemia is often treated with **phototherapy** to prevent the need for exchange transfusion. For phototherapy, the infant is placed under lights to decrease bilirubin levels in the blood. The lights usually consist of a single tungsten halogen lamp or 4-8 white or blue fluorescent lights and a Plexiglas shield. The infant is placed under these lights with a protective mask covering the eyes to prevent retinal toxicity. The lights should be 15-20 cm above the infant. The lights convert bilirubin into a water-soluble compound that can be excreted by the liver into bile and eventually into the infant's stool. The success of phototherapy is directly related to the quantity of body surface area that is exposed to the lights, so the infant is clad only in a diaper to expose the most skin to the light as possible. Indications:

Weight	Serum Bilirubin Level
500-750 g	5-8 mg/dL
750-1000 g	6-10 mg/dL
1000-1250 g	8-10 mg/dL
1250-1500 g	10-12 mg/dL

Exchange transfusions may be used for hyperbilirubinemia. Blood <72 hours old is used to maintain potassium levels. Indications include:

Weight	Serum Bilirubin Level
500-750 g	12-15 mg/dL
750-1000 g	>15 mg/dL
1000-1250 g	15-18 mg/dL
1250-1500 g	17-20 mg/dL

There are many risks associated with exchange transfusions, including vascular complications, such as emboli or thrombosis, often related to umbilical catheters. Cardiac complications include dysrhythmias and overload, leading to arrest. Clotting disorders may result from over-heparinization (reversed with protamine sulfate). Electrolyte and glucose abnormalities as well as infection may occur.

BLOOD COMPONENT THERAPY

Blood component therapy is described below:

- **Whole blood** has red blood cells (RBCs), white blood cells (WBCs), and platelets in their normal ratios. Whole blood is not a common neonatal blood transfusion product unless there is massive hemorrhage from trauma. Usually, its components are given individually to treat a specific condition.
- **Packed RBCs** are prepared by removing most of the plasma from blood, leaving a hematocrit of 70-90%. Use packed cells to treat anemia.
- **Leukocyte-poor RBCs** have more than 70% of WBCs removed by centrifuging, washing, or filtration. Much of the RBC mass is also lost. Leukocyte-poor blood products have less chance of passing on CMV infection or triggering a febrile reaction.
- **Washed RBCs** are cleaned with 0.9% sodium chloride to remove more than 95% of the nonviable RBCs and 80-90% of the WBCs. Washing is one method of producing leukocyte-poor RBCs.
- **Fresh frozen plasma** is comprised of 90-92% water, clotting factors, immunoglobulins, albumin, electrolytes, and enzymes and is used to add volume.

BLOOD PRODUCT ADMINISTRATION

In the NICU, **blood transfusions** are common, especially packed red blood cells. Blood should always be warmed to prevent hypothermia. Small volumes may be warmed passively by exposing to room temperature or heated isolette for 30 minutes prior to administration. Transfusions are given through peripheral IVs rather than umbilical lines except in extreme emergency. A filtered line should always be used for blood administration. During the transfusion, vital signs should be monitored and recorded every 15 minutes and the neonate carefully watched for any signs of a transfusion reaction. **Irradiated blood cells** are recommended for neonates <1200 mg and for those who are immunocompromised or receiving transfusions of granulocytes or exchange transfusions. Whole blood is not a common neonatal blood transfusion product unless there is massive hemorrhage from trauma. **Platelets** used for neonates to prevent cerebral hemorrhage with thrombocytopenia are collected from one donor instead of from pooled donations, suspended in plasma, and leukocyte depleted. Usual dose is 10-15 mL/kg given over 60-90 minutes.

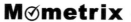

Gastrointestinal

DEVELOPMENT OF GI TRACT

The **gastrointestinal (GI) tract** is anatomically complete by about 24 weeks gestation but functional development continues through 36-38 weeks:

- Fetal swallowing of amniotic fluid begins at about 11 weeks gestation.
- Peristalsis begins at 28-30 weeks. In the preterm infant, it is bidirectional, so milk is not propelled toward the stomach. With normal peristalsis, meconium should pass within 24 hours of birth, but this is delayed in preterm infants.
- The cardiac sphincter and neural control of the stomach are immature at birth, resulting in frequent regurgitation.
- Coordination of sucking and swallowing begins at 33-36 weeks.
- Enzymatic activity and ability to transport nutrients matures by 36-38 weeks.
- Salivary glands are inactive until 3 months.
- Lactase deficiency causes poor carbohydrate digestion, pancreatic lipase deficiency causes poor fat digestion (10-20% excreted), but protein digestion is good.
- Bowel sounds are evident 30-60 minutes after birth. Stomach capacity is 50-60 mL, and emptying time is 2-4 hours.

SHORT BOWEL SYNDROME

The neonate's small bowel is approximately 250 cm long. Most absorption of nutrients and vitamins takes place in the first 100-150 cm of the jejunum while the ileum absorbs vitamin B_{12} and bile acids. Infants with less than 100 cm of jejunum after surgical removal have significant malabsorption and require aggressive nutritional support. Infants with **short bowel syndrome** (SBS) have diarrhea, steatorrhea, bloating, anemia, electrolyte imbalances, malnutrition, and poor weight gain secondary to decreased absorption of nutrients and vitamins. The severity and exact nature of their symptoms depend on the amount and type of bowel that has been removed. Removal of significant portions of the ileum results in steatorrhea and poor absorption of fat-soluble vitamins (K, A, D, E) and vitamin B_{12}. Removal of significant portions of the jejunum results in poor absorption of calories, proteins, carbohydrates, and fats. Infants require careful monitoring of serum electrolytes, multivitamins, and a combination of parenteral and enteral nutrition. Over time, the small bowel adapts, increases its absorption, and grows in length.

SUCKING AND SWALLOWING DISORDERS

Sucking and swallowing disorders are very common in the preterm infant because of immaturity (coordination of sucking and swallowing occurs at 33-36 weeks) but may be caused in term infants by a number of conditions, including trisomy 21, FAS, cleft palate, central nervous system disorders (anoxia, hydrocephalus), congenital infection (rubella, cytomegalovirus), respiratory disorders (apnea, pneumonia, RDS), and cardiac or ENT anomalies. Typical characteristics of swallowing disorders include:

- Silent aspiration (not associated with cough or clearing airway)
- Laryngeal penetration (associated with lack of pharyngeal response)
- Nasopharyngeal reflux (especially common in preterm infants and may trigger apnea)

Pneumonia frequently develops in infants with sucking and swallowing disorders, so diagnosing the cause is critical. Observation is not sufficient because of the frequency of silent aspiration. Feeding infants in the upright position can reduce nasopharyngeal reflux. Tests include radiographic (videofluoroscopy) or fiberoptic evaluation of swallowing.

HIRSCHSPRUNG'S DISEASE

Hirschsprung's disease (congenital aganglionic megacolon) is failure of **ganglion nerve cells** to migrate to part of the bowel, usually the distal colon, so that part of the bowel lacks enervation and peristalsis, causing stool to accumulate, leading to **distention** and **megacolon**. There is a genetic predisposition to the disease that affects more males than females and is associated with trisomy 21 (Down syndrome).

Symptoms include:

- Failure to pass meconium in 24-48 hours
- Poor feeding
- Bilious vomitus
- Abdominal distension

Delayed diagnosis includes:

- Chronic constipation
- Failure to thrive
- Periods of diarrhea and vomiting
- With infection—severe prostration, watery diarrhea, fever, and hypotension

Treatment includes:

- Resection aganglionic section and perform colorectal anastomosis
- There are a number of procedures—Swenson, Duhamel, and Soave—but recently, minimally invasive laparoscopic or transanal approaches have proven successful

GASTROESOPHAGEAL REFLUX

Gastroesophageal reflux (GER) is involuntary regurgitation of stomach contents into the esophagus, usually caused by decreased tone in the lower esophageal sphincter in neonates, especially preterm.

Symptoms include:

- Frequent non-bilious regurgitation (especially after feeding, usually not associated with respiratory distress)
- Some neonates may have colicky symptoms, and some may cough, choke, wheeze or have periods of apnea

Treatment includes:

- **Regulating feeding**: Small, more frequent amounts, thickened with rice cereal. Continuous gavage rather than bolus may reduce reflux.
- **Positioning**: Prone positioning after feeding/eating reduces regurgitation (although some concern remains about SIDS with neonates). Placing the neonate in an upright position (avoiding slumping) after meals or carrying the neonate upright can help, but placing in infant seat position may increase intraabdominal pressure.
- **Medications**: Medications are only recommended in severe cases. Histamine-2 receptor blockers (famotidine) or proton pump inhibitors (omeprazole) may be used short term.
- **Surgery**: Considered for severe or life-threatening symptoms.

MALROTATION/VOLVULUS

During weeks 4-8 of embryonic development, the GI tract is rapidly expanding and the abdominal cavity cannot accommodate it. Therefore, part of the intestinal loop buckles into the yolk stalk area, which will be the future umbilicus. As the intestinal loop buckles out of the abdomen, it begins a normal rotation of the bowel. As it continues to grow and returns to the abdomen during weeks 8-10, there is additional rotation occurring until it is situated into the anatomically correct position. Sometimes this rotation fails, and the result is a malrotation. **Malrotation** is a congenital defect in which the intestines are attached to the back of the abdominal wall by one single attachment, rather than a broad band of attachments across the abdomen, essentially suspending the bowels so they can easily twist, resulting in a **volvulus** (twisted bowel), cutting off blood supply. It may untwist but can lead to **bowel infarction.** Some children with malrotation have no symptoms, but most develop some of these **symptoms** by 1 year:

- Cycles of cramping pain about every 15-30 minutes
- Abdominal distension
- Diarrhea, bloody stools, or no stools
- Vomiting, occurring soon after crying begins, usually indicating small intestine obstruction; later vomiting usually indicative of large intestine blockage
- Tachycardia and tachypnea
- Decreased urinary output
- Fever

Treatment is by surgical repair.

MIDGUT VOLVULUS

A midgut volvulus is twisting of the bowel from the second portion of the duodenum to the mid-transverse colon around its mesenteric attachments. Signs depend on the extent of compromised blood flow to the bowel, blockage of lymphatic drainage, and obstruction of intestinal contents. **Signs** include bilious vomiting, gastric distension, rapid clinical deterioration, and shock. Midgut volvulus is usually secondary to congenital malrotation of the intestines. If this is the case, then it often presents during the first week of life, with complete obstruction and severe symptoms. Mortality rates range from 3-15%. The infant's prognosis depends on the amount of ischemic bowel and the length of time that elapsed before the volvulus was diagnosed and treated.

IMPERFORATE ANUS

Imperforate anus (anorectal malfunction) is a congenital abnormality in which the **rectum is absent, malformed, or displaced** from normal position. It may include disorders of the urinary tract. Imperforate anus occurs in 1 in 5000 births, more commonly in males than females. Imperforate anus may include stenosis or atresia of the anus. There are 3 main **categories,** classified according to the relationship of the rectum to the puborectalis musculature:

- **Low anomalies:** no external opening, but rectum otherwise in normal position through the puborectalis muscle, with normal function and no connection to the genitourinary tract.
- **Intermediate anomalies:** rectum at or below the level of puborectalis muscle, anal dimple evident, and external sphincter in normal position.
- **High anomalies:** rectum ending above the puborectalis muscles, internal sphincter absent often with a rectourethral fistula in males or a rectovaginal fistula in females, and sometimes fistulas to the bladder or perineum.

DIAGNOSIS, SYMPTOMS, AND TREATMENT

Imperforate anus is **diagnosed** by physical examination, digital or endoscopic examination, and contrast radiography with the infant inverted. An opaque marker at the anal dimple will outline the location of a pouch in relation to the normal position of the anus.

Symptoms include:

- Absence of anal opening, no meconium in 24-48 hours, Abdominal distension, and vomiting
- Rectovaginal fistula or rectourethral fistula (may not be evident at first because stool passes through fistula)
- Fistula between the rectum and the bladder with gas or fecal material possibly expelled through the urethra
- Displacement of the anus, with chronic constipation developing over time

Treatment includes:

Surgery performed in most cases, type depending upon extent of abnormality:

- With low anomalies, simple excision of anal opening
- Two- or three-step procedure for higher anomalies; colostomy first, with later reconstruction of the anus in the proper position, involving anoplasty and pull-through procedures
- Manual dilation to treat stenosis

INTESTINAL ATRESIA

When a portion of the bowel comes to a stop and then starts back up again forming a discontinuous or segmented bowel, this is called **intestinal atresia.** This condition usually relates to failures during the 5th to 10th week of fetal development, so it is often associated with other anomalies. The most common site for atresia to occur in the neonate is the duodenum. Atresia can also occur in the ileum, jejunum, colon, and even rarely the stomach. An atresia that occurs anywhere in the intestine except the duodenum is not associated with any other disorders. However, an atresia that occurs in the duodenum (the most common type) is usually (30% of the time) associated with other disorders such as trisomy 21, congenital heart disease, and VACTERL association. (VACTERL stands for **v**ertebral defects, **a**nal atresia, **c**ardiac defects, **t**rachea-**e**sophageal fistula, **r**enal anomalies, and **l**imb abnormalities.) The only treatment for intestinal atresia is surgical reconnection of the bowel.

DUODENAL ATRESIA

Duodenal atresia occurs when the duodenum fails to correctly form in the fetus. Often, duodenal atresia is discovered prenatally via ultrasound examination. Neonates with **duodenal atresia** vomit within hours after birth. The vomitus may or may not be bilious, depending on the exact location of the defect. The infant may have a scaphoid abdomen and usually passes meconium. X-rays often show the "double-bubble" sign: The distended stomach is the first bubble and the distended duodenum proximal to the defect is the second bubble. One-third of all patients with duodenal atresia also have Down syndrome. An orogastric tube is immediately placed to relieve the Abdominal distension, and IV fluids and TPN nutrition are administered. When IV hydration is delayed, infants with duodenal atresia often develop hypokalemia, hypochloremia, and metabolic alkalosis. Definitive treatment is surgical repair.

ESOPHAGEAL ATRESIA AND TRACHEOESOPHAGEAL FISTULA

Esophageal atresia often occurs with tracheoesophageal fistula (TEF). In esophageal atresia, the esophagus has a blind pouch and does not completely pass to the stomach. In TEF, an abnormal connection is present between the trachea and the esophagus. A congenital tracheoesophageal fistula (TEF) is present in 1 out of every 2,000-4,000 live births. There are 5 different **types of TEF**:

- **Esophageal atresia with distal TEF** (87%) is the most common type. The proximal esophagus ends in a blind pouch and the distal esophagus is connected to the trachea.
- **Isolated esophageal atresia without TEF** (8%), where the proximal esophagus ends in a pouch and there is no connection with the trachea.
- **Isolated TEF** (4%), where the esophagus is patent, traveling to the stomach with a fistula from the esophagus to the trachea. It is also called "H" type because of its resemblance to the letter H.
- **Esophageal atresia with proximal TEF** (1%), where the proximal esophagus connects with the trachea and there is no connection to the distal esophagus.
- **Esophageal atresia with proximal and distal TEF** (1%), where both the proximal and the distal esophagus connect with the trachea.

Infants born with tracheoesophageal fistula (TEF) are often diagnosed prenatally with ultrasound. TEF is often associated with polyhydramnios, as esophageal atresia prevents the fetus from swallowing amniotic fluid. Infants born with TEF have **symptoms** that include:

- Fine, white, frothy bubbles of mucous in the mouth and nose
- Copious secretions, despite suctioning
- Episodes of coughing, choking, and cyanosis that worsen with feeds
- Associated genetic anomalies, such as trisomy 13, 18, or 21
- Other digestive tract problems, heart problems, or kidney and urinary tract problems

Bowel Obstructions

Bowel obstruction occurs when there is a mechanical obstruction of the **passage of intestinal contents** because of constriction of the lumen, occlusion of the lumen, or lack of muscular contractions (paralytic ileus). Obstruction may be caused by congenital or acquired abnormalities/disorders:

Small Bowel Obstructions:

- Duodenal atresia
- Malrotation and volvulus
- Jejunoileal atresia
- Meconium ileus
- Meconium peritonitis

Large Bowel Obstructions:

- Hirschsprung disease
- Anorectal malformations
- Meconium plug syndrome

Symptoms include:

- Abdominal pain, distention, and rigidity
- Vomiting and dehydration
- Diminished or no bowel sounds
- Severe constipation (obstipation)
- Respiratory distress from diaphragm pushing against pleural cavity
- Shock, as plasma volume diminishes and electrolytes enter intestines from bloodstream
- Sepsis, as bacteria proliferate in the bowel and invade the bloodstream

Hypertrophic Pyloric Stenosis

Hypertrophic pyloric stenosis (PS) is obstruction of the pyloric sphincter between the gastric pylorus and small intestine, caused by hypertrophy and hyperplasia of the circular muscle of the pylorus so the enlarged tissue obstructs the sphincter. PS is more common in boys than girls and has a genetic predisposition. Onset of **symptoms** is usually >3weeks:

- Projectile vomiting (1-4 feet) usually shortly after eating but may be delayed for a few hours. Emesis may be blood-tinged but non-bilious
- Infant is hungry and eats readily, but shows weight loss and signs of dehydration
- Upper Abdominal distension with palpable mass in epigastrium (to right of umbilicus)
- Visible left to right peristaltic waves

Diagnosis is based on ultrasound. Decreased sodium and potassium levels may not be evident with dehydration.

Treatment includes:

- Intravenous fluids to restore hydration and electrolyte balance
- Surgical pyloromyotomy: longitudinal incisions through the circular muscle fibers down to the submucosa to release the restriction and allow the muscle to expand

MECONIUM PLUG SYNDROME

Meconium plug syndrome (also called functional colonic obstruction) occurs when the first stool obstructs the intestinal tract and no other pathology is present. This will be evident in the first 24 to 48 hours of life, when the infant fails to pass the first meconium stool. Meconium plug syndrome usually occurs in full-term infants, infants of diabetic mothers, or infants with hypermagnesemia. The infant may have abdominal distension, poor feeding, and vomiting (often bilious in nature). An x-ray of the abdomen will show dilated loops of bowel. A contrast enema is diagnostic and helps differentiate from other causes of intestinal obstruction. It may also be therapeutic, causing the plug to pass. Infants usually do well after the plug has passed. A small percentage of infants initially identified as having meconium plug syndrome (5 to 10%) have Hirschsprung disease. The cause of meconium plug syndrome is thought to be immaturity of the ganglion cells of the colon.

MECONIUM ILEUS CAUSED BY CYSTIC FIBROSIS

Cystic fibrosis is a congenital disease associated with the collection of thick mucus in the **lungs and intestines**. **Meconium ileus** is obstruction of the ileum with inspissated (thick) mucilaginous meconium that clings to the side of the narrowed lumen of the intestine and forms hard pellets (usually the first clinical sign of cystic fibrosis). The mucus interferes with the absorption of fat, protein, carbohydrates, and other nutrients, leading to malabsorption syndromes. **Diagnosis** is by abdominal x-rays to show air-to-fluid levels and contrast enemas to show obstruction.

Symptoms include:

- **Uncomplicated**: Abdominal distension, vomiting, no meconium in the first 24-48 hours
- **Complicated** (may include volvulus, gangrene, perforations, or bowel atresia): pain, fever, erythema, and edema of abdominal wall consistent with peritonitis

Treatment includes:

- Contrast enema with water-soluble contrast (may relieve obstruction by emulsifying fecal material)
- 10-15 mL small volume enemas to flush stool, especially after contrast enema
- Enterotomy, with proximal instillation of wetting agent
- Resection of colon/fecal diversion for perforated or gangrenous bowel
- High protein diet with pancreatic enzyme supplementation

NECROTIZING ENTEROCOLITIS

Necrotizing enterocolitis (NEC) is the most common gastrointestinal emergency in premature neonates. Seventy-five percent of neonates who develop NEC are less than 37 weeks gestation and weigh less than 2,000 grams. NEC is rare in healthy, full-term infants. NEC is an acute necrosis (death of cells) in a bowel segment anywhere from the stomach to the rectum. Inflammation, bacterial invasion, and perforation often occur. NEC is fatal in up to 30% of cases. Risk factors other than prematurity and size should trigger careful observation. These risk factors include:

- **Prenatal**
  - Maternal age >35 years
  - Maternal cocaine use
  - Maternal infection requiring antibiotics

- **Perinatal**
  - Birth asphyxia
  - Respiratory distress syndrome
  - Systemic hypotension
  - Depressed 5-minute Apgar score

- **Postnatal**
  - Congestive heart failure
  - Use of hyperosmolar formula
  - Patent ductus arteriosus
  - Umbilical artery catheterization

The causes of necrotizing enterocolitis (NEC) are not completely understood, but it appears to be related to an ischemic episode, colonization by bacteria, and excess/rapid enteral feedings.

Symptoms include:

- Gastric retention, Abdominal distension, and vomiting (bilious)
- Periods of apnea
- Occult or frank blood (25%) in stool
- Pneumatosis intestinalis (gas in intestinal wall) (75%)
- Portal venous gas (10-30%)
- Decrease in urinary output
- Jaundice
- Unstable temperature

Treatment includes:

- Cessation of oral feeding
- NG decompression
- Systemic antibiotics
- Correcting fluid and electrolyte imbalance
- Surgical repair with bowel resection may be necessary

DIASTASIS OF RECTI MUSCLES

Diastasis of the recti muscles is a postnatal maternal condition in which the abdominal muscles, specifically the rectus abdominis muscles (that have separated during pregnancy) remain separated. The pressure of the expanding fetus causes the connective tissue to stretch between the vertically running muscles and often after birth, the tissue slowly heals and the separation closes. When the connective tissue does not heal fully within 6 months, the gap can become permanent. This condition can lead to lower back pain, pain during intercourse, incontinence, or constipation in the mother. Diastasis of the recti muscles can be treated with specific physical therapy. Traditional abdominal crunches are avoided as a treatment because they may worsen the condition by making the muscles tighter in the separated position. Abdominal exercises during pregnancy are recommended as preventative measures. Surgical closure is a treatment option for extreme cases.

NEONATAL UMBILICAL HERNIA

Umbilical hernia is a skin-covered herniation of intestine and omentum through an abdominal wall defect near the umbilicus caused by an incomplete closure of the umbilical ring. The herniation may range from 1-5 cm in size and may be obvious on physical examination or felt on palpation. It may appear flat when the infant is supine but protrude when the infant is upright or crying. Approximately 1 in 6 infants are born with umbilical hernias. Symptoms are usually absent unless strangulation of the hernia occurs, and then the infant may cry with pain, feed poorly, vomit, and have an increase in temperature. The abdomen may become distended. In this case, emergency surgical repair must be done. Treatment usually involves just observing the hernia for complications as, in most cases, it will reduce on its own. If the hernia is still present at 3-4 years, a simple surgical repair of the hernia may be done.

GASTROSCHISIS

Gastroschisis is extrusion of the non-rotated midgut through the abdominal wall to the right of umbilicus with no protective membrane covering matted, thickened loops of intestine. The abnormality is usually small, but the stomach and almost all of the small and large intestines can protrude. Because the intestines float without protection in amniotic fluid, there may be severe damage to the intestines with bowel atresia and ischemia. Gastroschisis is usually diagnosed with fetal ultrasound and is obvious at birth. These infants lose body temperature, fluids, and electrolytes and receive intravenous fluids. The exposed organs are covered with sterile plastic film for protection and to prevent fluid loss and a nasogastric feeding tube is inserted. Primary closure is done when the infant stabilizes for small abnormalities. Larger abnormalities may require stages with only part of organs returned to the cavity and the remaining covered with a Silastic pouch until the abdominal cavity grows and surgical repair can be completed.

OMPHALOCELE

Omphalocele is a congenital herniation of intestines or other organs through the base of the umbilicus with a protecting amniotic membrane but no skin. The sac may contain only a loop or most of the bowel and the internal abdominal organs. This sac differentiates gastroschisis from omphalocele. Diagnosis is usually with fetal ultrasound.

Symptoms vary widely. Maintaining integrity of tissues by keeping exposed sac or viscera moist and providing intravenous fluids is important. Small omphaloceles are repaired immediately, but more extensive repair is usually delayed until the infant is stable if sac is intact. Silvadene cream toughens the sac, which is usually covered with a Silastic (plastic) pouch to protect the tissue. The abdomen may be unusually small, making correction difficult, so surgeons may wait 6-12 months while the abdominal cavity grows. Surgical repair may be done in stages over 8-10 days.

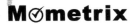

Genitourinary

RENAL VEIN/ARTERY THROMBOSIS

A thrombosis that is not catheter-related, occurring predominantly in the neonatal period, is **renal vein thrombosis (RVT).** Upon diagnosis, the presence of a palpable abdominal mass, macroscopic hematuria, and thrombocytopenia are typically noted. Risk factors associated with RVT may include perinatal asphyxia, dehydration, maternal diabetes, as well as hereditary prothrombotic risk factors, though studies have shown the absence of the first three underlying factors in neonatal history. Therefore, it is considered good practice to screen children with thromboembolic diseases for prothrombotic risk factors. The diagnosis of RVT can also be confirmed with renal ultrasound, demonstrating enlarged and echogenic kidneys with loss or attenuation of corticomedullary differentiation, and the presence of calcification and thrombus outside of the kidneys, extending to the inferior vena cava. In addition, Doppler studies evaluate blood flow resistance, either venous or arterial, caused by intrarenal venous thrombosis. Finally, radionuclide scans can identify renal scarring and atrophy.

TREATMENT

Treatment of renal vein thrombosis (RVT) varies greatly among neonatal centers. Heparin therapy, with the use of low molecular weight heparin (LMWH), as opposed to unfractionated heparin, is likely to be initiated, often with the presence of inferior vena cava involvement and bilateral RVT. In contract, approximately 40 percent of neonates will be managed supportively without heparin therapy. Studies do not show a more favorable outcome in the prevention of renal atrophy or irreversible damage with or without heparin therapy. Supportive management in the acute phase of RVT by the multidisciplinary team of neonatologists, hematologists, nephrologists, and radiologists includes the maintenance of electrolyte and fluid balance, and renal replacement therapy, thereby treating acute renal failure (ARF). In addition, anticoagulant or fibrinolytic treatment may be initiated. On an ongoing basis, the need for monitoring of renal complications is imperative, to include hypertension, renal atrophy and functional loss, and chronic renal insufficiency.

ACUTE RENAL FAILURE/INSUFFICIENCY IN NEONATES

Acute renal failure (ARF) or insufficiency is commonly found in the neonatal intensive care unit. Most neonates experience pre-renal failure due to underlying disease, recent heart surgery, or less commonly a congenital renal malformation. ARF is characterized by a sudden decrease in glomerular filtration rate (GFR), resulting in progressive retention of nitrogenous waste products and creatinine, and the loss of fluid and electrolyte homeostasis regulation. Early diagnosis of neonatal ARF is vital in order to preserve the neonate's renal function. At birth, a very low GFR is maintained in the kidney by the baby's own vasoconstrictor and vasodilator forces. This is normally sufficient for the newborn's growth and development of the kidney. However, the low GFR limits the newborn's ability to functionally adapt to endogenous and exogenous stresses, such as is seen with a low-birth-weight infant (less than 2.5 kg), predisposing the infant to ARF.

TREATMENT

Treatment of acute renal failure or insufficiency involves a conservative approach of adequate fluid and caloric intake in the neonatal intensive care unit, with ongoing daily monitoring and reevaluation of the fluid regimen, maintenance of acid-base balance and nutrition, and renal replacement therapy, if indicated. The latter is achieved by peritoneal dialysis, intermittent hemodialysis, or hemofiltration with or without a dialysis circuit. Although it is considered by some providers to be controversial, acute peritoneal dialysis (APD) may be initiated in the treatment of progressive renal failure, and is considered safe and effective by some recent studies. APD is reportedly successful in controlling hyperkalemia, fluid overload, and metabolic acidosis. Rapid

176

exchanges during a short dwell time promoted maximum peritoneal permeability and transport. APD aids in managing the metabolic and hemodynamic imbalance present with ARF. Neonates can achieve a full recovery of renal function, but there may be complications such as peritonitis, leakage, hemoperitoneum, and hernia.

POLYCYSTIC DYSPLASTIC KIDNEYS

Polycystic or multicystic dysplastic kidneys in the neonate refers to a condition in which the kidney has been replaced by multiple cysts due to abnormal fetal development, resulting in little to no normal kidney function. This condition can typically be detected via a prenatal ultrasound, and most likely occurs on the left side. Occasionally, this condition occurs bilaterally, which is grave as the kidney produces the amniotic fluid needed for developing the fetus' lungs in utero. The presence of one multicystic dysplastic kidney with a properly functioning other kidney will likely ensure that the required amount of amniotic fluid is maintained. However, there is approximately a 51 percent risk of an associated abnormality, such as vesicoureteral reflux, uretero-pelvic junction obstruction, or uretero-vesical junction obstruction, with the normal functioning kidney. Therefore, consultation with a pediatric urologist is necessary following birth to determine the treatment regimen.

TREATMENT OPTIONS FOR COMPLICATIONS

The three **complications** commonly found in the non-polycystic-dysplastic kidney (vesicoureteral reflux, uretero-pelvic junction obstruction, and uretero-vesical junction obstruction) are all surgically correctable via laparoscopic surgery, with a reduction in incision size and recovery time. Occasionally, these complications can have self-resolution. Prior to determining the proper treatment plan, radiological studies will be performed. These include a voiding cystourethrogram (VCUG), intravenous pyelogram (IVP), and a renal ultrasound (RUS). Currently, the majority of pediatric urologists recommend the monitoring of the kidney with serial RUS versus nephrectomy to remove the diseased kidney, as the diagnostic studies can help to pinpoint the exact diagnosis. Additionally, the risk of developing hypertension and malignancy is fairly low even if the kidney is not removed.

URINARY OUTFLOW TRACT OBSTRUCTION

In utero, the fetal urine forms the amniotic fluid, which is crucial for healthy lung development as it is swallowed by the fetus. If there is a blockage in the urinary system, a backup of urine results in dilation, which can be detected on the prenatal ultrasound. Various types of **blockage** preventing or slowing the urine from leaving the body include:

- Bladder outlet or urethral obstruction, most commonly due to an abnormal flap or tissue, or a posterior urethral valve.
- Bladder inlet or ureterovesical junction obstruction, or where the ureter connects the kidneys to the bladder.
- Kidney outlet or ureteropelvic junction obstruction, found between the kidney pelvis and the ureter, dilating the kidney's collection tubules.
- Ectopic ureter, an abnormal position of the ureter exiting the kidney or entering the bladder.
- Ureterocele, or a cyst that may cause obstruction at the end of the ureter.

DIAGNOSTIC TESTS AND TREATMENT

As **blockage of urine** can ultimately result in kidney damage, careful monitoring is prudent. Most often, one kidney is affected, leaving the undamaged kidney to function. Should both kidneys be affected, the decrease in urine production will likely result in decreased amniotic fluid and impaired lung development. Prenatal ultrasounds will monitor for amniotic fluid level changes, urinary system dilation, and any kidney changes. In addition, an amniocentesis with genetic counseling may be performed for mild hydronephrosis, which does not typically require surgery. Approximately half of babies with mild hydronephrosis will have resolution after birth. For severe and rare cases of urinary tract obstruction, such as the result of a posterior urethral valve, a catheter may be inserted into the fetal urinary system to aid in draining the urine into the amniotic sac. Early intentional delivery has not proven successful, but some neonates will undergo corrective surgery.

HYDRONEPHROSIS

Hydronephrosis is a dilated kidney that is swollen with urine. It most commonly results from a narrowed or blocked ureter, which under normal circumstances drains the urine into the bladder. This condition is more prevalent in male neonates than in females. **Prenatal hydronephrosis** is rarely diagnosed before it resolves by itself, or before the kidneys begin to compensate for the blockage. Prenatal ultrasounds can identify these cases that normally might not be detected until three or four years later when symptoms become obvious. Symptoms include nausea, vomiting, fever, swelling, and urinary difficulties. The presentation of symptoms depends on the severity of the case, as mild and occasionally moderate hydronephrosis may not present with symptoms at all. Severe hydronephrosis, if left untreated, is always accompanied by complications, such as kidney damage, infections, bleeding, and pain.

TREATMENT

The first action should be a prophylactic treatment to prevent a kidney infection that can result from the urine not adequately draining from the kidney. The preferred antibiotic selection is typically a low-dose with limited side effects. The pediatric urologist will determine the length of prophylactic treatment based on the results of diagnostic imaging studies, such as renal ultrasound. Surgical intervention is most likely considered for children with grade IV hydronephrosis. The overall goal of surgery is to relieve the uretero-pelvic junction (UPJ) obstruction. Pyeloplasty, or renal pelvic reconstruction\revision, is performed to decompress and drain the kidney to prevent recurrent infection and ultimately kidney damage. However, grades I, II, and III of hydronephrosis, as well as non-obstructive hydronephrosis, are not surgical candidates as these conditions will most likely resolve by themselves. The presentation of megaureters, or dilation due to ureterovesical junction abnormalities, typically does not require surgery either.

HYDROCELE

A hydrocele is fluid in the scrotum or inguinal region. It co-occurs with an inguinal hernia in 10-20 infants per 1,000 live births. During fetal development, the testicles migrate from the abdominal cavity through the inguinal canal to the scrotum. A piece of peritoneum called the process vaginalis travels with the testicle into the scrotum. Normally, this extension of peritoneum closes and becomes a fibrous chord (tunica vaginalis), so there is no connection between the peritoneal cavity and the scrotum. If closure does not occur (patent process vaginalis), fluid accumulates in the scrotum. If the fluid collection comes and goes, then it is termed a communicating hydrocele. A non-communicating hydrocele is one where fluid is trapped in the scrotum after the process vaginalis closes. Physical examination reveals a bulge in the scrotum that may or may not be reducible. No bowel sounds should be audible with auscultation, which indicates a hernia. Transillumination of the scrotum reveals fluid retention.

TESTICULAR TORSION

Two types of testicular torsion, or the twisting of the spermatic cord structures, are **extravaginal torsion**, which develops in the prenatal period and presents at birth, also associated with a high birth weight; and **intravaginal torsion**, which typically presents in older children, also referred to as a bell-clapper with its anomalous testicular suspension. Normally, the testes freely rotate within the scrotum via the tunica vaginalis. Extravaginal torsion occurs proximally to the tunica vaginalis, while intravaginal torsion occurs within the tunica vaginalis. Upon physical examination of the neonate, an affected testis will exhibit swelling, tenderness, and may appear to be high-riding. There may also be an absence of the cremasteric reflex. When torsion occurs, blood flow to the testis and epididymis may be interrupted. Salvage is more likely within 6-8 hours of noted torsion. However, testicular necrosis often develops when the torsion duration increases to 24 hours or longer.

TREATMENT

Discussion regarding the **treatment of perinatal testicular torsion (PTT)** can lead to increased anxiety for the surgeon and the parents, as this condition occurs infrequently, and research does not compare success rates between non-surgical and surgical intervention. For the neonate born with testicular torsion, surgical exploration with contralateral orchidopexy, or anchoring, is indicated following stabilization of the overall physiological status of the neonate, since imaging studies of neonatal bilateral torsion provide limited information. If the neonate born with a normal testis develops torsion, immediate exploration is warranted, with the preferred method being scrotal incision. Once the testis is examined for viability, any necrotic testis is removed, as the presence of necrotic tissue may trigger an autoimmune phenomenon and subsequent infertility. During surgery, any viable gonads are attached to the scrotal wall, to prevent recurrence of the torsion. Surgical exploration will also lend to ruling out additional possible diagnoses.

UNDESCENDED TESTICLES IN PREMATURE INFANT

Cryptorchidism occurs when one or both of the testicles in the male infant fail to migrate from the abdominal cavity into the scrotum. Migration normally occurs sometime during 28-40 weeks gestation. Up to 30% of males born prematurely and 3% of those born full term, have an undescended testicle. When cryptorchidism is discovered on physical exam, it should be noted on the infant's chart. The parents should be reassured that it is not an immediate concern, as most testes will descend without therapy by 6 months of age. Those infants whose testes have not descended by 6 months of age may be treated medically with human chorionic gonadotropin or with surgery. A testicle that is allowed to remain in the abdominal cavity is at increased risk for malignancy, and adult men with undescended testicles have increased rates of infertility.

HYPOSPADIAS/EPISPADIAS

The congenital defect with the urethral opening on the underside of the penis is **hypospadias**. The urethral opening typically presents near the tip of the penis; however, it may be located at the midshaft or base of the penis, or behind the scrotum. The penis is positioned in a downward curve, otherwise noted as ventral curvature or chordee. As a result, infants may commonly experience erections, as well as abnormal spraying of urine, the presence of malformed foreskin with the appearance of a "hooded" penis, and the necessity to sit down to urinate when older. Imaging studies may be indicated to rule out other associated congenital defects. In contrast, **epispadias** is much less common than hypospadias, with the urethral meatus dorsally displaced, and may be associated with exstrophy of the bladder in its severe form. Routine circumcision is contraindicated, as the penis appears splayed open lengthwise on the dorsal surface.

TREATMENT

In preparation for **surgical repair**, the foreskin should be preserved. Surgery is routinely performed prior to the beginning of elementary school, and can be performed as early as four months of age, typically at approximately eighteen months. Multiple surgeries may be required, with the straightening of the penis and the use of tissue grafts from the foreskin. Repeat or multiple surgeries may be indicated for correction of a returned abnormal curve of the penis, or to correct a fistula. If left untreated, urethral strictures and fistulas may form, and the growing boy will experience difficulty with toilet training and, in adulthood, difficulty with sexual intercourse. For the treatment of epispadias, surgical correction is also required. Parental education is imperative as parents must contact a pediatrician if they notice the presence of a curved penis with erection or an abnormal location of the urethral opening.

VAGINAL DISCHARGE

Neonatal vaginal discharge, or physiologic leukorrhea, is a normal occurrence in female newborns immediately after birth due to the drop in exposure to hormones that were present in the uterus. This discharge may be blood-tinged and should subside after a few months. The external genitalia (labia and surrounding area) can be cleaned with warm water (but without soap).

Vaginal discharge is concerning if it is accompanied by a foul odor or yellow/green coloration (which could indicate infection). Perfuse bleeding that continues after several months should also be investigated.

Neurological/Neuromuscular

NEONATAL NEUROSENSORY CAPABILITIES

A neonate is born with the following neurosensory capabilities:

- **Hearing**: The neonate's crying after birth clears middle ear mucus and the eustachian tubes, and hearing becomes acute with hearing thresholds similar to adults and children. Because hearing deficit is one of the most common congenital abnormalities, all infants should be assessed for hearing.
- **Vision**: The neonate's vision is about 10-30 times less acute than that of an adult, but the infant has peripheral vision, can fixate at 8-14 inches, and can accommodate to large objects. The neonate is able to perceive shapes, colors, and faces.
- **Tactile sense**: The neonate has a good sense of touch and reacts emotionally to tactile stimulation.
- **Smell**: The neonate has a strong sense of smell after nasal passages clear and will react to the smell of milk or turn away from strong smells.
- **Pain**: Neonates experience pain, and pain prevention/management should be part of neonatal care.

BIRTH ASPHYXIA

Birth asphyxia is the cause of many problems after birth. **Birth asphyxia** is defined as an event that alters the exchange of gas (oxygen and carbon dioxide). This interference with gas exchange leads to a decrease in the amount of oxygen delivered to the fetus along with an increase in the level of carbon dioxide the fetus is exposed to. This gas imbalance causes the fetus to switch from normal aerobic metabolism to anaerobic metabolism. Fetal distress results, which then leads to increased fetal heart rate, release of meconium into the amniotic fluid, and lowered pH. Infants experiencing birth asphyxia will often present at birth with APGAR scores that are less than 5. Symptoms of birth asphyxia include:

- **Mild**
  - Overly alert for the first 45 minutes to one hour following birth (infants are normally sleepy after about 15 minutes following birth)
  - Pupils dilated
  - Respiratory rate and heart rate both slightly increased
  - Newborn reflexes and muscle tone normal
  - Oxygen may be administered
- **Moderate**
  - Hypothermia as evidenced by low body temperature
  - Hypoglycemia as glucose stores are used up trying to supply organs needed energy
  - Pupils are constricted
  - Signs of respiratory distress evident
  - May experience seizure activity at 12-24 hours of age
  - Lethargy (floppy infant)
  - Bradycardia
- **Severe** (Requires close monitoring in a NICU)
  - Pale color related to the inability of the heart to perfuse the body
  - Cerebral edema related to apnea episodes and/or intracranial hemorrhage

Resuscitation will vary according to the infant's condition, but warming the infant, stabilizing the glucose level, and providing oxygen or EMCO (in severe cases) may be indicated.

HIE

Hypoxic-ischemic encephalopathy (HIE) results when oxygen supply to the brain is impaired. A common cause of HIE is perinatal asphyxia. The degree of insult to the neonate depends on the severity of the ischemic event. HIE is typically divided into three categories:

- **Mild HIE**: Characterized by increased muscle tone with brisk deep tendon reflexes. The infant may also exhibit poor feeding, irritability, and excessive sleepiness. These abnormalities generally resolve after 3-4 days.
- **Moderate HIE**: Characterized by significant hypotonia and lethargy with diminished deep tendon reflexes. Moro and grasp reflexes may be absent. Seizures may occur. Full recovery may still occur after 1-2 weeks.
- **Severe HIE**: Generalized hypotonia with depressed deep tendon reflexes and coma. The infant may not respond to physical stimulus. Breathing may be irregular and the infant requires ventilatory support. Basic neonatal reflexes may be absent. Pupils may be dilated and fixed. Generalized seizure activity is present and may be difficult to treat.

RISK FACTORS AND TREATMENT OPTIONS

Neonatal **risk factors** for hypoxic-ischemic encephalopathy include:

- Cardiac arrhythmias
- pH <7.10 (umbilical artery), indicating acidosis during delivery
- Meconium-stained amniotic fluid
- Apgar <7 at 5 minutes after birth or <4 for more than 5 minutes
- Seizures during the first 24 hours
- Neurological dysfunction as demonstrated by coma, lethargy, irritability, hypotonia, and/or altered reflexes
- Symptoms of multiple organ damage: Cardiac damage, indicated by reduced contractility with hypotension; renal damage, indicated by oliguria; and damage to the intestinal tract, indicated by poor peristalsis, delayed gastric emptying, and the development of necrotizing enterocolitis

Identifying infants at risk and instituting treatment may decrease neurological impairment. **Treatment** may include:

- Phenobarbital given in high doses after birth decreases seizures and improves long-term outcome.
- Calcium channel blockers may improve cerebral blood flow during ischemia.
- Mild to moderate hypothermia for 5-72 hours may decrease damage; studies are in progress.
- Allopurinol (40 mg/kg) 4 hours after birth reduces mortality rates.

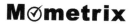

SUBDURAL AND SUBARACHNOID CRANIAL HEMORRHAGES

Subdural hemorrhage between the dura and the cerebrum, usually from tears in the cortical veins of the subdural space, tends to develop more slowly and can result in a subdural hematoma. If the bleeding is acute and develops within minutes or hours of injury, the prognosis is poor. Subacute hematomas that develop more slowly cause varying degrees of injury. Subdural hemorrhage is a common injury related to birth trauma and child abuse, although it can result from coagulopathies or aneurysms. Symptoms of acute injury may occur within 24-48 hours, but subacute bleeding may not be evident for up to 2 weeks after injury. Symptoms may include bradycardia, tachycardia, hypertension, and alterations in consciousness. Subdural taps may suffice for infants, but some infants will require surgical evacuation of the hematoma.

Subarachnoid hemorrhage may result from childbirth (one of the most common causes) or from shaken impact syndrome. The presenting symptom may be seizures, and other symptoms are similar to those of subdural hematoma. Symptoms worsen as ICP rises.

INTRAVENTRICULAR HEMORRHAGE

Intraventricular hemorrhages (IVH) are common in premature neonates less than 32 weeks estimated gestational age. IVH presents within the first 72 hours of life in 90% of affected neonates, and within the first 24 hours in 50% of cases. Infants less than 35 weeks gestational age or who weigh less than 1500 grams have a 50% incidence rate of IVH; however, this rate is declining due to improvements in obstetrical care and nursing management of fluids and respiration. Depending on the amount and location of bleeding seen on cranial ultrasound, IVH is **graded** as follows:

	Anatomy	Severity
Grade I	The hemorrhage is limited to the germinal matrix (subependymal region).	Mild (5% death rate; 5% motor or cognitive impairment)
Grade II	The hemorrhage extends 10-40% into the lateral ventricles on sagittal view, but has not dilated them significantly.	Moderate (10% death rate; 30-40% motor or cognitive impairment)
Grade III	The hemorrhage extends 50% or more into the lateral ventricles with significant ventricular dilation.	Severe (27-50% death rate; 35% motor or cognitive impairment)
Grade IV	The hemorrhage extends into brain tissue.	Periventricular hemorrhagic infarction (80% death rate; 90% motor or cognitive impairment)

SYMPTOMS AND TREATMENT

IVH is also categorized based on **symptoms**:

- **Asymptomatic**: 25-50% of IVH infants are asymptomatic or have only a fall in hematocrit and anemia, but ultrasound shows an IVH.
- **Saltatory**: Infants are pale or ashen and have gradual neurological deterioration (attention, movements, level of consciousness, eye movements).
- **Catastrophic**: Acute onset of decreased level of consciousness, bulging fontanel, cranial nerve abnormalities, decerebrate posturing, and hypotension with drop in hematocrit.

IVH **treatment** must be approached with extreme caution. The pediatrician orders one of the following to suppress CSF production:

- **Indocin** 0.1 mg/kg/dose IV when the baby is 6 hours old, 24 hours old, and 48 hours old

  OR

- **Diamox** 5 mg/kg/dose PO or IV every 6 hours, which is increased by 25 mg/kg/day (with a maximum dosage of 100 mg/kg/day)

HYDROCEPHALUS

Hydrocephalus occurs when there is an imbalance between production and absorption of cerebrospinal fluid in the ventricles, resulting from impaired absorption or obstruction, which may be congenital or acquired. There are **primarily 2 types** of hydrocephalus that affect infants:

- **Communicating**: CSF flows (communicates) between the ventricles but is not absorbed in the subarachnoid space (arachnoid villi).
- **Noncommunicating**: CSF is obstructed (non-communicating) between the ventricles with obstruction, often stenosis of the aqueduct of Sylvius but it can occur anywhere in the system.

In early infancy, before closure of cranial sutures, head enlargement is the most common presentation while brain damage occurs later as pressure causes damage to the central nervous system. **Early infancy symptoms** include bulging, non-pulsating fontanels (usually anterior) with increasing head circumference, dilated scalp veins, separating sutures, and positive Macewen sign (resonance on tapping near the frontal-temporal-parietal juncture), irritability, seizures, vomiting, and setting-sun sign (the upper eyelids retract and the eyes turn downwards due to pressure on the mesencephalic tegmentum and paralysis of upward gaze).

CAUSES

Hydrocephalus can be acquired or congenital. Approximately 75% of neonates with intraventricular hemorrhage (IVH) develop hydrocephalus. **Congenital hydrocephalus** is present at birth and can occur due to:

- **Aqueductal stenosis**, the most common cause, when the cerebral aqueduct connecting the third and fourth ventricles is blocked by an infection (toxoplasmosis, mumps, syphilis, or cytomegalovirus), tumor, hemorrhage, or developmental narrowing, and fluid accumulates in the third ventricle
- **Spina bifida**, where 80-90% of infants born with meningocele or myelomeningocele also have hydrocephalus.
- **Arnold-Chiari malformations** in the base of the brain where the spinal column joins the skull, characterized by parts of the cerebellum protruding through the foramen magnum into the spinal canal, which interferes with the normal flow of CSF.

TREATMENT

Hydrocephalus is diagnosed through CT and MRI, which help to determine the cause. Treatment may vary somewhat depending upon the underlying disorder, which may also require treatment. For example, if obstruction is caused by a tumor, surgical excision to directly remove the obstruction is required. Generally, however, most hydrocephalus is treated with **shunts**:

- **Ventricular-peritoneal shunt**: This procedure is the most common and consists of placement of a ventricular catheter directly into the ventricles (usually lateral) at one end with the other end in the peritoneal area to drain away excess CSF. There is a one-way valve near the proximal end that prevents backflow but opens when pressure rises to drain fluid. In some cases, the distal end drains into the right atrium.
- **Third ventriculostomy**: A small opening is made in the base of the third ventricle so CSF can bypass an obstruction. This procedure is not common and is done with a small endoscope.

NEURAL TUBE DEFECTS

The neural tube is the embryonic structure that eventually forms the brain and spinal cord. **Neural tube defects** (NTD) are a spectrum of congenital disorders involving the meninges covering the spinal cord. Mild forms are asymptomatic. Severe cases are incompatible with life. Diagnosis is often made in pregnancy by ultrasound or by an elevated level of alpha-fetoprotein in the amniotic fluid or in the mother's serum. Causes are multifactorial, with both genetic and environmental components. **Risk factors** for NTD include:

- Poor diet lacking in folic acid
- Family history of a NTD in a parent or sibling
- Maternal obesity with poorly controlled diabetes
- Maternal use of valproic acid or carbamazepine during pregnancy
- Increasing core temperature 3-4 °F (2 °C) through saunas, hot tubs, or fever

Studies have shown that if the mother ingests 400 micrograms of folic acid daily before and during pregnancy, it protects the fetus from developing an NTD.

TYPES

The neural tube defects, spina bifida and myelomeningocele, are often used interchangeably, but there is a distinction. Spina bifida is a neural tube defect with an incomplete spinal cord and often missing vertebrae that allow the meninges and spinal cord to protrude through the opening. There are **5 basic types**:

- **Spina bifida**: Defect in which the vertebral column is not closed with varying degrees of herniation through the opening.
- **Spina bifida occulta**: Failure of the vertebral column to close but no herniation through the opening, so the defect may not be obvious.
- **Spina bifida cystica**: Defect in closure with external sac-like protrusion with varying degrees of nerve involvement.
- **Meningocele**: Spina bifida cystica with meningeal sac filled with spinal fluid.
- **Myelomeningocele**: Spina bifida cystica with meningeal sac containing spinal fluid and part of the spinal cord and nerves.

MYELOMENINGOCELE

Myelomeningocele, which involves spina bifida cystica with a meningeal sac containing spinal fluid and part of the spinal cord and nerves, comprises about 75% of the total cases of spina bifida. There are numerous **physical manifestations**:

- **Exposed sac** poses the danger of infection and cerebrospinal fluid leakage; so surgical repair is usually done within the first 48 hours although it may be delayed for a few days, especially if the sac is intact.
- **Chiari type II malformation** comprises hypoplasia of the cerebellum and displacement of the lower brainstem into the upper cervical area, which impairs the circulation of spinal fluid. It may result in symptoms of cranial nerve dysfunction (dysphonia, dysphagia) and weakness and lack of coordination of upper extremities.
- **Neurogenic bladder** is common and may require the Credé maneuver for infants and later intermittent clean catheterization.
- **Fecal incontinence** is common and is controlled with diet and bowel training as the child gets older.
- **Musculoskeletal abnormalities** depend upon the level of the myelomeningocele and the degree of impairment but often involve the muscle and joints of the lower extremities and sometimes the upper. Dysfunction often increases with the number of shunts. Scoliosis and lumbar lordosis are common. Hip contractures may cause dislocations.
- **Paralysis/paresis** may vary considerably and be spastic or flaccid. Many children require wheelchairs for mobility although some are fitted with braces for assisted ambulation.
- **Seizures** occur in about a quarter of those affected, sometimes related to shunt malfunction.
- **Hydrocephalus** is present in about 25-35% of infants at birth and 60-70% after surgical repair with ventriculoperitoneal shunt. Untreated, the ventricles will dilate and brain damage can occur.
- **Tethered spinal cord** occurs when the distal end of the spinal cord becomes attached to the bone or site of surgical repair and does not move superiorly with growth, causing increased pain, spasticity, and disability and requiring surgical repair.

ANENCEPHALY

Anencephaly is a neural tube defect in which the **embryological neural tube**, which forms the brain and spinal cord, fails to close at the **cephalic (head) end**, resulting in an infant without most of the brain, skull, or scalp, so that the top of the head is open. The eyes bulge forward. Because the forebrain is missing, the child has no cognitive ability or sensation of pain. A rudimentary brain stem may be present, supporting reflexive breathing and cardiac function, but the child's condition is not compatible with life. Most are stillborn, and others live a few hours or days. There is no treatment possible other than supportive care until death. The condition is often diagnosed with ultrasound. An ethical dilemma exists about the use of these infants' organs for donation, with some authorities believing that viable organs should be harvested before brain death.

ENCEPHALOCELE

Encephalocele is a neural defect that involves a bony defect and herniation of the brain and/or cerebrospinal fluid through part of the skull in a skin-covered sac. In the United States, most commonly the mass is midline in the occipital and occasionally the frontal area. The **encephalocele** may be as large as the skull or may look like a small nasal polyp. In many cases, other abnormalities may exist, so thorough examination, including angiography and MRI, are usually required. Often, the part of the brain that herniates is disorganized, so the condition may be associated with cognitive impairment, although in mild cases the child has normal mentation. Surgical repair to place the herniated mass inside the skull and to repair the bony defect is the standard treatment. If the sac is left in place, the skin can erode, resulting in meningitis.

NEONATAL SEIZURES

CAUSES

Causes of neonatal seizures are listed below, roughly in order of frequency:

- **Hypoxic-ischemic encephalopathy** after a difficult or traumatic delivery
- **Metabolic abnormality**:
  - Low levels of glucose, calcium, or magnesium
  - Elevated or low levels of sodium
- **Infections**:
  - Bacterial meningitis caused by Group B strep, *E. coli, S. pneumoniae*, or Listeria
  - Viral encephalitis caused by herpes simplex, cytomegalovirus, or enterovirus
- **Cerebrovascular accidents**:
  - Intraventricular hemorrhage
  - Subarachnoid hemorrhage
  - Subdural hematoma
  - Sinus thrombosis
- **Seizure syndromes**:
  - Epileptic encephalopathies (early myoclonic or early infantile)
  - Benign neonatal seizure syndromes, such as benign familial neonatal convulsions, benign idiopathic neonatal seizures, or benign sleep myoclonus

TYPES

Seizures indicate an abnormality of the central nervous system and are differentiated by their associated abnormal movements:

- **Subtle seizures** are more common in full-term infants, who present with feet pedaling, chewing, apnea, eye movements, or a blank stare.
- **Tonic seizures** are more common in preterm infants, who present with tonic flexion or extension of the limbs, which may be focal (one limb) or generalized.
- **Clonic seizures** occur primarily in full-term infants, indicate a focal cerebral injury, and involve slow, clonic movements (1-3 movements per second), often in one extremity or on one side of the body.
- **Myoclonic seizures** are rare in neonates and may be focal, multi-focal, or generalized, with rapid jerking movements of the extremities.

Treatment depends upon identifying underlying cause but may include glucose (if related to hypoglycemia), phenobarbital (drug of choice), fosphenytoin, and phenytoin.

> **Review Video: Seizures**
> Visit mometrix.com/academy and enter code: 977061

INITIAL MANAGEMENT

Seizures in the neonate require immediate treatment to avoid brain injury from hypoxia and hypoglycemia:

- Glucose (10% solution) if indicated for hypoglycemia with bolus 2 mL/kg and maintenance ≤8 mL/kg.
- Provide supplemental oxygen and ventilation.
- Give a loading dose of phenobarbital (20 mg/kg IV); if the initial loading dose is ineffective, give an additional 10-20 mg/kg IV.
- Draw STAT blood glucose and electrolyte levels.
- Correct electrolyte abnormalities such as low calcium, magnesium, and sodium.
- Give a maintenance dose of 4-6 mg/kg of phenobarbital IV every 12-24 hours.
- Monitor blood pressure and respiratory status frequently, because large doses of phenobarbital cause respiratory and cardiac depression.
- Give fosphenytoin, phenytoin, and lorazepam per order if seizures are uncontrolled.

JITTERINESS

Jitteriness (tremor of chin and extremities) occurs in about half of neonates within the first few days of life and may persist intermittently when the child is excited or crying for ≤2 months. Jitteriness may also be present with drug withdrawal, hypoglycemia, hypocalcemia, and encephalopathy. Jitteriness must be differentiated from seizures, which may have a similar appearance. **Characteristics of jitteriness** include:

- There is a lack of ocular deviation or other abnormalities.
- Gentle restraint halts jitteriness.
- Stimulation elicits jitteriness.
- Clonic jerking has both fast and slow elements.
- Autonomic changes involving the heart rate, respirations, and blood pressure are not present.
- EEG is normal.

Jitteriness is distinct from shuddering, a 10-15 second period of fast tremors that may recur ≤100 times daily. Both jitteriness and shuddering are benign conditions that require no treatment.

THERAPEUTIC HYPOTHERMIA

Therapeutic hypothermia for the neonate is used for neuroprotection to prevent neonatal asphyxia leading to severe hypoxic-ischemic encephalopathy. The temperature of deep brain structures is lowered to 33-34 °C through the whole body, hypothermia or head cooling only (CoolCap). **Therapeutic hypothermia** should be initiated within 6 hours after resuscitation for neonates ≥35 weeks with moderate to severe HIE. Other indications include fetal heart disorders, fetal anemia, meconium in amniotic fluid, SGA, LGA, and maternal prenatal hypoxemia. Criteria includes asphyxia as evidenced by Apgar ≤5 after 10 minutes. The goal of hypothermia is to reach the target temperature within 60 minutes. Cooling is typically carried out for about 72 hours followed by 12 hours of rewarming. The neonate must receive sedation and ventilatory support to ensure oxygen levels and ventilation are adequate. The neonate must be monitored carefully (ECG, BP, oxygen saturation, $ETCO_2$). The heart rate normally decreases about 15 bpm per 1 °C decrease, so bradycardia may occur. Temperature must be constantly monitored and temperature alarms set. EEG and neurological monitoring may be necessary because almost half of infants with HIE have seizures during cooling, especially during the first 48 hours. Fluids are limited to 40-60 mL/kg/day.

BIRTH-RELATED NERVE TRAUMA

CRANIAL NERVE TRAUMA

Injury to cranial nerves can occur during birth (most commonly the recurrent laryngeal nerve) and is caused by compression of the head against the sacrum during birth or from the use of forceps. Symptoms relate to the specific type of nerve injury but may present as temporary or permanent paralysis. Often asymmetry, drooping of the eye or mouth, or failure of the eyelid to close is noted, especially when the infant cries. Traumatic injury to nerves usually resolves over time, beginning by the end of the first week but symptoms may persist to some degree for months. An open eye must be protected by the use of synthetic tears and patching to prevent damage. Those with injury to the laryngeal nerve may have dyspnea and dysphagia and may require small frequent feedings or enteral feedings until the condition resolves. In most cases, treatment is symptomatic with careful observation so that complications can be treated promptly.

BRACHIAL PLEXUS TRAUMA

Trauma to the brachial plexus may cause a full-term infant to hold his or her arm adducted and internally rotated after a delivery complicated by shoulder dystocia. There is movement in the hands. About 1-3 infants per 1,000 live births suffer **trauma to the brachial plexus**. The brachial plexus is a collection of nerve tissue located in the shoulder area that is the pathway for nerves traveling from the spine to the arm and shoulder. These nerves control the movement of the shoulder and arm. Most commonly, the upper portion of this plexus is damaged, leading to weak arm muscles (Erb's palsy). When examined, the infant holds the arm adducted and internally rotated. The startle reflex is abnormal on the affected side, but the grasp reflex is normal. If the lower portion of the plexus is damaged, the hand is paralyzed also, and the grasp reflex is absent (Klumpke's paralysis). Most infants recover fully, but recovery depends on the degree of damage to the brachial plexus (complete tear vs. stretching).

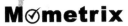

BIRTH INJURIES

CONGENITAL MUSCULAR TORTICOLLIS

Congenital muscular torticollis occurs when the infant's sternocleidomastoid muscle is shortened or excessively contracted secondary to trauma. The sternocleidomastoid muscle has its origin on the sternum and the clavicle and inserts at the mastoid process of the temporal bone. It flexes the neck and rotates the head. Torticollis occurs in 0.5-2.0% of live births. Damage to the muscle may occur *in utero* or if the birth process was difficult or traumatic. The muscle may tear, causing fibrosis or scarring. Symptoms of torticollis may not present for several weeks, especially if the trauma occurred during birth. Physical exam shows a head tilt away from the affected side, with limited range of motion. Face and skull asymmetry may be present from lack of position changes. A palpable mass may be felt within the sternocleidomastoid muscle. Treatment involves physical therapy to stretch the tight muscle and strengthening exercises to stimulate symmetry. Torticollis is rarely associated with malformations of the cervical vertebrae.

FRACTURES

Clavicular fracture is the most common injury during a vaginal birth. They are most commonly seen with high birth weight babies, shoulder dystocia, and forceps delivery. Newborns with a fractured clavicle often exhibit fussiness or crying with movement of the affected arm due to pain in the clavicle. The infant may not be able to move the arm at all if nerve injury occurred. An x-ray or ultrasound image of the clavicle is needed to confirm the fracture. In most cases, birth fractures of the clavicle usually heal in 7 to 10 days without any problems. Usually no treatment is required, but the parent may need to pin the infant's sleeve of the affected arm to the front of their clothing to immobilize the arm while it heals.

Rib fractures from birth trauma are rare, but may have the same origin as clavicle fractures, caused by the shoulder compression forces to the chest from a high birth weight infant or shoulder dystocia. These fractures may not cause any noticeable symptoms. If there are multiple rib fractures, the infant will show signs of pain when moved or picked up and may develop difficulty breathing that could indicate atelectasis from the fracture. Premature infants can also develop rib fractures after birth from simple handling and chest physiotherapy due to the extremely fragile nature of these bones. A chest x-ray is needed to diagnose a rib fracture.

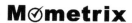

Genetic

AUTOSOMAL INHERITANCE PATTERNS

Autosomal inheritance patterns involve genetic **abnormalities in chromosome pairs 1-22**:

- **Autosomal recessive:** This occurs when two parents (without active disease) each have a copy of the same abnormal recessive gene, and both pass the abnormal copy to offspring. The **recurrence risk** (the chance to have affected offspring) for two carrier parents with the same abnormal gene mutation is 25% for each pregnancy and 50% chance the child will become a carrier. Autosomal recessive disorders, such as cystic fibrosis, Tay Sachs, and sickle cell anemia, are seen more frequently among certain ethnic groups and in offspring of related parents.
- **Autosomal dominant:** This means that only one abnormal dominant gene needs to be inherited to cause the condition. Autosomal dominant diseases include Huntington's disease and Marfan syndrome. The recurrence risk for an affected parent to pass the disease to a child is 50% with each pregnancy, but there is no carrier state.

SEX-LINKED INHERITANCE

Sex-linked inheritance involves the sex chromosomes (**chromosome 23**). Y-linked disorders such as Klinefelter syndrome are rare, but they will be passed from the father to all male children. X-linked diseases, such as hemophilia and Duchenne muscular dystrophy, usually occur in males because males have only one X chromosome, so a single recessive gene on that X chromosome causes the disease. Females have two X chromosomes, so the normal gene on an unaffected X chromosome can usually compensate. Although the Y chromosome is the other half of the XY chromosome pair in the male, the Y chromosome is much smaller than the X chromosome and doesn't contain most of the genes of the X chromosome—it's not a complete match—so there is no compensating gene to protect the male. Thus, females carry the disease and males inherit the disease. A man with an X-linked recessive disorder will not pass the disease to his sons (because they don't inherit his X chromosome), but his daughters will inherit the mutated gene, so they have one abnormal X (from the father) and one normal (from the mother). These daughters then have a 50% chance of having sons who are affected and a 50% chance of having daughters who carry one copy of the mutated gene. X-linked dominant inheritance also differs depending upon whether the mother or father carries the defective gene. There is no carrier state with X-linked dominant disorders. If the father has the disease, such as Rett's syndrome, all daughters will inherit. If the mother has the disease, each child, regardless of gender, has a 50% chance of inheriting.

MULTIFACTORIAL INHERITANCE

Complex or multifactorial inheritance relates to an interaction of many different genes, as well as the environment and lifestyle choices. Thus, a genetic disorder may depend upon genes inherited from both parents as well as unidentified environmental factors (smoking, drug use, diet) interacting in such a way as to produce an abnormality. This type of inheritance pattern is much less predictable than the others. Neural tube defects, for example, are caused by multifactorial inheritance. In some cases, an infant may inherit only a tendency toward a disease, such as diabetes type 2, but development of the disease may depend up weight, diet, smoking, and other factors as the child matures. Complex diseases include such things as asthma, heart disease, and osteoarthritis. Multifactorial traits often run in families, with risk 50% in first-degree relatives (parents), 25% in second-degree (grandparents, aunts, uncles), and 12.5% in third-degree (cousins).

NEWBORN SCREENING

Screening of the newborn to detect genetic diseases varies somewhat from one state to another. Because about 1 in 200 newborns has chromosomal abnormalities, screening is an important tool, although many birth defects, such as defects caused by maternal alcohol abuse or vitamin deficiency, are not genetic in origin. Screening tests for these genetic diseases are available:

- Biotinidase deficiency (autosomal recessive)
- Congenital adrenal hyperplasia (autosomal recessive)
- Congenital hearing loss (autosomal recessive, autosomal dominant, or mitochondrial)
- Congenital hypothyroidism (autosomal recessive or autosomal dominant)
- Cystic fibrosis (autosomal recessive)
- Galactosemia (autosomal recessive)
- Homocystinuria (autosomal recessive)
- Maple syrup urine disease (autosomal recessive)
- Medium-chain Acyl-CoA dehydrogenase (autosomal recessive)
- Phenylketonuria (autosomal recessive)
- Sickle cell disease (autosomal recessive)
- Tyrosinemia (Two types are autosomal recessive; a third type is unclear)

CYSTIC FIBROSIS

Cystic fibrosis (mucoviscidosis or CF) is a progressive congenital disease that particularly affects the pancreas and lungs, causing digestive and respiratory problems. It is caused by a genetic defect that affects sodium chloride movement in cells, including mucosal cells that line the lungs, causing the production of thick mucus that clogs the lungs and provides a rich medium for bacteria. While most patients with cystic fibrosis at one time died in childhood, the life expectancy is now about 30 years. About 15-20% of neonates with CF have meconium ileus (obstruction of small intestine with meconium) at birth. Other infants have no symptoms at first but show failure to thrive in the first 4-6 weeks and may develop a cough and wheezing. Cystic fibrosis patients usually suffer from recurrent respiratory infections of the lower respiratory tract. The most common infective agents are *Pseudomonas aeruginosa* and *Burkholderia cepacia* complex. The screening test for CF is IRT/DNA. If the IRT/DNA is positive, the infant is scheduled for a sweat test and buccal swab.

G6PD DEFICIENCY

Glucose-6-phosphate dehydrogenase (G6PD) deficiency is an X-linked recessive disease and can often present as, or similar to, hyperbilirubinemia. Because female infants inherit two X chromosomes, it's rare that both are defective, and the normal chromosome compensates, so X-linked recessive disorders affect primarily male children (who get the X chromosome from the mother, not the father) but are passed on by the mother. G6PD is an enzyme utilized to process carbohydrates and to protect red blood cells. G6PD results in premature destruction of red blood cells and hemolytic anemia, which can be triggered by infection, some medications (antimalarial drugs, sulfa, ASAS, NSAIDS, quinidine, quinine, and nitrofurantoin), and eating or inhaling the pollen of fava beans (favism). Infants may be asymptomatic, although some may exhibit increased jaundice. In the United States, G6PD is most common in African American males (1 out of 10) and those with Middle Eastern heritage. Treatment includes avoiding triggers, treating infections, and transfusions if necessary.

CHROMOSOME ABNORMALITIES

TRISOMY 13

Trisomy 13 (Patau syndrome) may occur with complete trisomy, mosaicism, or partial trisomy, so symptoms may vary depending upon the amount of extra genetic material in **chromosome 13**. Diagnosis can be made prenatally with amniocentesis. This disorder occurs in 1 of every 20,000 live births in both males and females. **Indications** include:

- Cleft lip/palate
- Polydactyly and clenched fists
- Microcephaly, abnormal brain structure, profound intellectual disability, seizures
- Small or absent close-set eyes (may be fused into one eye), vision impairment
- Coloboma (split or hole in iris)
- Low-set ears and deafness
- Umbilical/inguinal hernias
- Cardiac abnormalities with heart on right side of chest and congestive heart disease (80%)
- Rocker-bottom feet
- Micrognathia
- Multiple system disorders

Treatment is supportive and symptomatic, but despite interventions, about 80% die ≤1 month. Infants may have profound dyspnea, seizures, and difficulty feeding.

TRISOMY 18

Trisomy 18 occurs when the infant has **three number 18 chromosomes**, instead of the normal two. Trisomy 18 is an aneuploidy second only to Down syndrome (trisomy 21) for frequency. Trisomy 18 occurs in 1 of every 6,000-8,000 live births, and is associated with severe malformations and high infant mortality. Only 5-10% of affected children survive beyond the first year of life. **Malformations** include:

- **Neurological**: Microcephaly, anencephaly, hydrocephaly, Arnold-Chiari malformation, hypoplasia of the corpus callosum, wide occipitoparietal skull diameter with narrow frontal diameter, called "strawberry sign" because of its appearance on ultrasound.
- **Facial**: Epicanthal folds, short palpebral fissures, cataracts, short nose with upturned nares, micrognathia, narrow palate, cleft palate, and low-set ears.
- **Skeletal**: Clenched fists, radial hypoplasia, rocker-bottom feet, hypoplastic nails, and short neck with excessive skin folds.
- **Cardiac**: Ventricular septal defect is most common, but some heart problem is present over 90% of the time.
- **Other**: Pulmonary hypoplasia, omphalocele, esophageal atresia, multicystic kidneys, cryptorchidism, and intrauterine growth restriction.

TRISOMY 21

Trisomy 21 (**Down syndrome**) occurs in 1 out of every 800 live births. Trisomy 21 is the most common chromosomal disorder in humans. Advanced maternal age is a risk factor. The definitive diagnosis is made by cytogenetic examination of the infant's DNA from amniocentesis or chorionic villi sampling. Common **physical characteristics** of infants born with Down syndrome are listed below in decreasing order of incidence:

- Low birth weight
- Brachycephaly (head is short in diameter from front to back and disproportionately broad)
- Upslanting palpebral fissures (openings between the eyelids)
- Wide gap between first and second toes
- Small, low set ears
- Hypotonia
- Epicanthic skin folds (redundant skin folds in the upper eyelid from the nose to the inner side of the eyebrow)
- Brushfield's spots (small white or gray spots on the periphery of the iris)
- Short, wide hands
- Single transverse palmar crease
- Heart disease (40-50%); murmur may be heard on physical exam

DiGEORGE SYNDROME

DiGeorge syndrome is a series of congenital defects that results from a deletion of part of the long arm of **chromosome 22**. This same area of the chromosome is also missing in infants with velo-cardio-facial syndrome and conotruncal anomalies face syndrome, so use the preferred name **22q11 deletion syndrome** to describe all three syndromes. The basic **defects** in 22q11 deletion syndrome are:

- Conotruncal heart defects: Tetralogy of Fallot, ventricular septal defect, or interrupted aortic arch (80%)
- Cleft lip or palate (70%)
- Hypocalcemia secondary to hypoparathyroidism (20-60%), which causes seizures
  - Note: Hypocalcemia is often temporary; many children do not require calcium supplementation after their first year of life
- Microcephaly, small ears, hooded eyelids, small mouth, and small chin
- Mild to borderline intellectual disability, with IQs in the 70-90 range (40%)
- Hypoplastic or absent thymus, resulting in T-cell dysfunction, recurrent infections secondary to immune deficiencies, and rarely, severe immune deficiency

TURNER SYNDROME

Turner syndrome is one of the most common chromosomal abnormalities, occurring in approximately 1 in 2,000 live female births (male fetuses die). **Turner syndrome** is caused by the absence of a set of genes that form the short arm of one of the X chromosomes. Most infants are missing the entire second chromosome (45X). Most pregnancies in which the infant has Turner syndrome end in spontaneous abortions. **Clinical signs** present at birth include:

- Webbed neck from fetal lymphedema; after the swelling resolves, loose folds of skin are still present on the neck
- Broad chest with wide spaced nipples (shield chest)
- Swollen hands and feet
- Short 4th or 5th metacarpals or metatarsals
- Increased incidence of congenital hip dislocation
- Increased incidence of coarctation of the aorta and bicuspid aortic valve

The **diagnosis** of Turner syndrome is confirmed by a karyotype. All infants with Turner syndrome must have their hearts evaluated.

SKELETAL DYSPLASIA

Skeletal dysplasias are a large group (450+) of genetic disorders affecting the bones and cartilage, one bone, or a group of bones, and the mode of inheritance can vary. Some disorders may result from spontaneous mutations or exposure to toxins. For example, X-linked disorders may affect males and not females. Often parents have mild symptoms but the child has a more severe disorder. Some of these disorders, such as osteogenesis imperfecta, may be diagnosed in the fetus by screening or ultrasound during the first trimester, but others may not be diagnosed until the third trimester or birth of the infant. Common dysplasias include thanatophoric, campomelic, achondroplasia, and achondrogenesis. About half of infants with skeletal dysplasias are stillborn or die within a few weeks of birth. If the dysplasia is lethal, then the neonate is provided comfort care, but if the dysplasia is consistent with life, then the infant must be stabilized, consultation with genetic specialists conducted, and non-skeletal complications assessed.

OSTEOGENESIS IMPERFECTA

Osteogenesis imperfecta (OI) is a genetic disorder of collagen synthesis that results in brittle, easily fractured bones. OI occurs in 1 in 20,000 live births. Collagen is a major component of bone that gives it both strength and flexibility. Infants with OI either produce defective collagen or deficient amounts of collagen. Four different types of OI have been identified, with symptoms ranging from very mild to lethality in the neonatal period. **Common features** of OI include:

- Brittle bones that fracture easily (fractures may be present at birth)
- Bowing of long bones
- Shortened limbs
- Discolored, brittle teeth
- Blue sclera
- Skeletal deformities, including scoliosis
- Respiratory difficulties
- Weak muscles

Generally, OI is inherited in a dominant fashion, but a new mutation may cause the disorder in approximately 25% of cases. Parents of children diagnosed with OI must be instructed on correct methods of handling and bathing their child and placing the child in the crib to minimize trauma and the development of fractures.

OSTEOPENIA OF PREMATURITY

Osteopenia of prematurity (OOP) is a disorder of decreased bone mineralization seen in premature infants. Infants born extremely premature are at greatest risk for developing OOP. During the last trimester of pregnancy, large amounts of calcium and phosphorus are provided to the developing fetus to aid in bone mineralization. Clinical findings that may not be apparent until 2 to 4 months of age are craniotabes and impaired linear growth. Pediatricians diagnose rickets (vitamin D deficiency) when the preterm infant shows thickening of wrists and ankles, rachitic rosaries, and cupping of bone metaphysics in x-rays, and elevated alkaline phosphatase in blood serum. **Risk factors** for the development of OOP include:

- Preterm (less than 34 weeks of gestation)
- Weight less than 1,500 grams
- Delayed onset of enteral feeds
- Chronic use of steroids or diuretics by the mother or infant, which increase excretion of minerals
- Feeding unfortified human milk or full term formulas to preterm infants

Treatment includes supplementing calcium, phosphorus, and vitamin D.

Endocrine and Metabolic

HYPOTHYROIDISM

Hypothyroidism is caused by a deficiency in production of the thyroid hormones (TH) T_4 and T_3. All newborns are screened for congenital hypothyroidism because of the severe consequences associated with lack of treatment and the ease of treatment with exogenous thyroid hormone. It may be congenital or acquired. **Congenital hypothyroidism** (formerly called cretinism) may manifest at birth or be delayed for years, but severe early onset can result in profound neurological deficit and intellectual disability if undiagnosed and treated:

- **Neonates**: Widened posterior fontanel, hypothermia ≤95 °F, edema, respiratory distress, feeding difficulties, lethargy, delayed passage of meconium, prolonged physiologic jaundice, and vomiting
- **≤3 months of age**: Umbilical hernia, dry skin, constipation, enlarged tongue, lethargy, and minimal crying

Treatment includes oral TH replacement therapy. Prompt initiation of therapy is critical for congenital hypothyroidism in order to prevent developmental abnormalities. If symptoms of hypothyroidism are severe, therapy to reach appropriate levels of TH is initially given gradually over 3-4 weeks to avoid hyperthyroidism.

HYPERTHYROIDISM

Hyperthyroidism is caused by excess production of T3 and T4 thyroid hormones. Suppression of TSH may be present in neonates born to thyrotoxic mothers or those with genetic disorders, such as McCune-Albright syndrome. Hyperthyroidism may develop during the fetal stage, resulting in IUGR, fetal hydrops (non-immune), and fetal death. **Symptoms** of neonates include:

- Hyperkinesis
- Diarrhea
- Vomiting
- Failure to thrive or gain weight
- Tachycardia with increased pulse pressure
- Hypertension (systemic and pulmonary)
- Hepatosplenomegaly
- Thrombocytopenia
- Hyperviscosity syndrome
- Ophthalmic abnormalities
- Craniosynostosis

Treatment includes the use of antithyroid medications, such as Propacil or Tapazole, β-adrenergic blockers, and iodine. Digoxin may be necessary as well as glucocorticoids. Remission usually occurs in 20-48 weeks. In rare cases, thyroid ablation (thyroidectomy) may be necessary.

INBORN ERRORS OF METABOLISM

Inborn errors of metabolism comprise a wide range of genetic metabolic disorders, usually related to defects in gene coding for enzymes, resulting in toxic accumulations that interfere with metabolism. Disorders are classified according to the type of metabolic disorder and include:

- **Carbohydrates** (glycogen storage disease, fructose intolerance)
- **Proteins** (clotting defects, sickle cell, thalassemia, osteogenesis imperfecta, Marfan's)
- **Amino acids** (phenylketonuria, hyperammonemia)
- **Organic acid** (alcaptonuria)
- **Cholesterol/lipoprotein** (hyperlipoproteinemias, hypoproteinemias)
- **Mitochondrial** (Kearns-Sayre syndrome)
- **Porphyrin** (porphyria)
- **Defective DNA repair** (xeroderma pigmentosum)

Symptoms relate to the specific defect. Some symptoms are present in the neonate but others appear in childhood or adulthood, with some diseases life-threatening and others slowly progressive. Symptoms common to many disorders may include:

- Encephalopathy with poor feeding, lethargy, tachypnea
- Metabolic acidosis and/or hyperammonemia
- Hypoglycemia, hepatic dysfunctions with jaundice
- Dysmorphism (structural anomalies)
- Abnormal body odor or urine odor

PHENYLKETONURIA

Phenylketonuria (PKU) is an inborn error of metabolism that results from a deficiency of the liver enzyme that changes phenylalanine to tyrosine (phenylalanine is a product that results when protein is digested). These infants are unable to digest protein. The symptoms of this disorder will show up sometime before 3 months if not caught in a screening. The first symptoms will be vomiting, poor feeding effort, and irritability. Later, if not treated, the infant will develop eczema and will have urine that smells musty. Once this condition is diagnosed, the infant must be put on a strict diet that restricts phenylalanine. Extensive family training must take place to educate the family about the diet. If the infant does not follow this diet restriction, intellectual disability will result. PKU screening within 7 days of birth is required in all 50 states.

GALACTOSEMIA

Galactosemia, an autosomal recessive disorder, is the most common inborn error of metabolism. In this disorder, the infant is lacking the enzyme that converts galactose to glucose. Because lactose is made up of galactose and glucose, the infant who cannot convert the galactose in lactose to glucose cannot tolerate lactose. Usually, the neonate is asymptomatic but develops symptoms rapidly. The clinical manifestations seen with galactosemia include jaundice, vomiting, diarrhea, inability to gain weight, and hypoglycemia. An infant with this condition that does not receive treatment can contract a serious gram-negative infection related to damage to the intestinal lining, and death may occur at 1-2 weeks. This condition must be treated by removing all lactose products and replacing the formula with soy or lactose-free formula. If left untreated, severe intellectual disability can result.

CONGENITAL ADRENAL HYPERPLASIA

Congenital adrenal hyperplasia (CAH) is an autosomal recessive defect that results in a cortisol deficiency, and is often accompanied by an aldosterone deficiency. 90 to 95% of CAH cases are due to a deficiency in 21-hydroxylase, the enzyme responsible for catalyzing two reactions in the adrenal glands:

- 17-Hydroxyprogestorne → 11-deoxycortisol → cortisol
- Progesterone → deoxycorticosterone → aldosterone

The cortisol deficiency results in shock, hypoglycemia, and circulatory collapse. The infant becomes dehydrated when CAH is accompanied by aldosterone deficiency (salt wasting), because of excessive loss of urinary sodium. Symptoms do not usually occur until the infant is 2 to 4 weeks old. Metabolic abnormalities of hyperkalemia, hyponatremia, hypoglycemia, and metabolic acidosis are present shortly after birth. Some infants have milder forms of CAH and are not diagnosed until later in life. Elevated levels of ACTH cause hypertrophy of the adrenal glands and increased production of androgens. Elevated androgens *in utero* virilize the female infant, so she has ovaries and uterus but external genitalia are often ambiguous.

HYPOGLYCEMIA

Hypoglycemia is low blood sugar of 30 mg/dL or less during the first day after birth, or below 45 mg/dL thereafter. One neonate in every 25,000 experiences persistent **hypoglycemia**. Half of hypoglycemic neonates develop brain damage. The hypoglycemic patient may be asymptomatic or may have these symptoms: apnea, tachypnea, respiratory distress, vomiting, diminished oral intake, tachycardia, bradycardia, jitteriness, lethargy, brisk Moro reflex, seizures, coma, and temperature instability. Suspect hypoglycemia in these circumstances:

- Elevated insulin levels in the infant with a brittle diabetic mother
- Premature or SGA baby
- KATP-HI diffuse or focal disease, GDH-HI, or GK-HI genetic disorders
- Septic shock
- Hyperthyroidism
- Inadequate glucose stores in malnourished infants and poor feeders
- Hypoxemia or ischemia
- Ingestion of alcohol, beta blockers, or salicylates

Treatment is 5-20 mg/kg/day oral diazoxide, 2-3 times per day. The doctor may also order hydrochlorothiazide, nifedipine, octreotide, and glucagon. Partial pancreatectomy is required if drugs are ineffective.

CAUSES AND RISK FACTORS

Causes and risk factors for hypoglycemia include the following:

- **Decreased glucose availability**—Risk factors include preterm birth, glycogen storage diseases, intrauterine growth restriction, and prolonged fasting.
- **Increased glucose utilization**—Risk factors include cold stress and hypothermia, sepsis, labored breathing, perinatal asphyxia, Rh incompatibility, persistent neonatal hyperinsulinism, and maternal tocolytic drugs.
- **An umbilical artery catheter placed with the tip right above the pancreas**—delivers glucose directly to the pancreas and can stimulate too much insulin production.
- **Elevated insulin levels**—Risk factors include infant of diabetic mother (elevated glucose levels trigger increased insulin production), islet cell hyperplasia, abrupt cessation of IV glucose, exchange transfusion, and Beckwith-Wiedemann syndrome.

ACUTE HYPOGLYCEMIA/HYPERINSULINISM

Acute hypoglycemia/hyperinsulinism can cause damage to the central nervous and cardiopulmonary systems, interfering with development of the brain and causing neurological impairment. **Causes** may include:

- Persistent hyperinsulinemic hypoglycemia of infancy (PHHI) in infants of diabetic mothers, usually apparent in the first 3 months
- Genetic defects in chromosome 11 (short arm)
- Severe infections, such as Gram-negative sepsis and endotoxic shock
- Maternal tocolytic administration

Symptoms in infants include:

- Blood glucose <40 mg/dL
- Central nervous system: seizures, altered consciousness, lethargy, and poor feeding with vomiting, myoclonus, respiratory distress, diaphoresis, hypothermia, and cyanosis

Treatment includes:

- Glucose/Glucagon administration to elevate blood glucose levels.
- Diazoxide (Hyperstat) inhibits release of insulin.
- Somatostatin (Sandostatin) to suppress insulin production.
- Nifedipine.
- Careful monitoring. Surgical removal of 85-90% of pancreas may be needed for infants to reduce insulin but poses risk of diabetes.

HYPOGLYCEMIA SECONDARY TO GLYCOGEN STORAGE DISEASE

Glycogen storage diseases (GDS) are inherited enzyme deficiencies that prevent/inhibit glycogenolysis and release of glycogen. There are 10 different types, but I, III, and IV are most common. All are autosomal recessive defects. Glycogen is stored in the liver and muscles but cannot be accessed and builds up, eventually resulting in cirrhosis of muscles and organs (heart, liver, kidney). Infants present with hypoglycemia that does not respond to the administration of glucagon, enlarged liver, and failure to thrive. GSD infants require almost continuous enteral feeds to maintain their blood glucose levels. They are susceptible to episodes of damaging hypoglycemia that can cause seizures, apnea, hypothermia, hypotonia, and cyanosis. Some types can be treated with diet, monitoring of symptoms, and medications, but others have no effective treatment. Uric acid may accumulate, so medications to lower uric acid levels may be needed.

HYPERGLYCEMIA

Hyperglycemia is a value greater than 100 mg/dL glucose in the newborn and is often iatrogenic (caused by glucose infusion). Premature and very low birth rate infants receiving IV glucose are at greatest risk for developing **hyperglycemia** because these infants often have decreased insulin production or decreased insulin insensitivity. Congenital diabetes mellitus is rare and may either be transient or permanent in nature. One of the main dangers of hyperglycemia is dehydration from osmotic diuresis. The neonate's urine will contain glucose (glucosuria). Intracranial hemorrhage is associated with hyperglycemia. Decreasing the amount of IV glucose usually resolves hyperglycemia. Dehydration must be corrected with IV fluids, if necessary. Enteral feeds stimulate insulin production by the pancreas, so exogenous insulin is rarely required to control the infant's elevated blood sugar levels.

EXCESS IV GLUCOSE

If excessive IV glucose is administered to a newborn, it will cause hyperglycemia to develop. Newborns utilize glucose at a rate of 4-8 mg/kg/min. Premature infants have a lower glucose tolerance, so start them at 4 mg/kg/min. Full term infants are started at 8 mg/kg/min. At levels greater than 150-180 mg/dL, osmotic diuresis occurs (glucose in the urine). The infant develops dehydration. Dextrose is the d isomer of glucose (d-glucose). In order to supply a 2-kg infant with 7 mg/kg/min of glucose using a solution of D10 (10% dextrose solution, 100 mg dextrose per mL) the following calculations are used:

$$\text{Required dextrose} = \left(7\,\frac{\text{mg}}{\text{kg}\cdot\text{min}}\right) \times (2\text{ kg}) = 14\,\frac{\text{mg}}{\text{min}}$$

$$14\,\frac{\text{mg}}{\text{min}} \times \frac{1\text{ mL}}{100\text{ mg}} = 0.14\,\frac{\text{mL}}{\text{min}}$$

$$0.14\,\frac{\text{mL}}{\text{min}} \times \frac{60\text{ min}}{1\text{ hr}} = 8.4\,\frac{\text{mL}}{\text{hr}}$$

IDM

Infants of diabetic mother (IDM) are exposed to elevated levels of glucose during their intrauterine development, as glucose freely crosses the placenta; the blood glucose level of the developing fetus mirrors that of the mother. The fetus increases production of insulin at around 20 weeks of gestation in response to the mother's elevated blood glucose. When the umbilical cord is cut, it abruptly disrupts the neonate's supply of glucose. The infant's greatest risk for hypoglycemia occurs 30-90 minutes after delivery. Because insulin levels are elevated in the fetus, the newborn may have an increased glucose need for several days to prevent hypoglycemia—as high as 10-15 mg/kg/min. Glucose is given as a continuous infusion to prevent the newborn from developing rebound hypoglycemia after a bolus of glucose. IDM infants show fewer symptoms of hypoglycemia when compared to other neonates and may also suffer from hypocalcemia, hypomagnesemia, and hyperbilirubinemia. Hypoglycemia is an easily treatable condition that, when left untreated, causes long-term neurological damage.

Infants of diabetic mother (IDM) often **present** with:

- Birth trauma secondary to cephalopelvic disproportion, including shoulder dislocation
- Hypoglycemia from sudden withdrawal of maternal glucose and elevated insulin in the infant
- Respiratory distress syndrome because elevated insulin inhibits surfactant production
- Polycythemia (excessive red blood cell production) and hyperviscosity because of elevated insulin and glucose increase the metabolic rate and oxygen consumption
- Iron deficiency because polycythemia leaches iron from the heart and brain
- Hyperbilirubinemia because of increased red blood cell destruction after birth
- Cardiovascular malformations, such as intraventricular hypertrophy with outflow tract obstruction, transposition of the great arteries, ventral septal defects, and coarctation of the aorta
- Congenital malformations, such as anencephaly, spina bifida, renal agenesis, and duodenal atresia
- Electrolyte abnormalities, including hypocalcemia and hypomagnesemia

COMPLICATIONS

There are several complications resulting from IDM, including:

- **Seizure activity** can occur in some of these infants due to the lack of sufficient fuel for the brain when the infant becomes hypoglycemic. Glucose is the fuel the brain needs to function properly, and when it is in short supply, the brain is essentially starved.
- **Shoulder dystocia** is a condition that is directly related to an infant that is large for gestational age (LGA) because of diabetes. Large babies will often experience shoulder dislocation at birth as they try to fit through the birth canal.
- **Thrombosis** sometimes forms in the kidneys (venous or arterial) as a result of a high hematocrit and increased viscosity of blood.
- **Increased diabetic risk**—2% of female and 6% of male IDMs will go on to develop juvenile type 1 diabetes.

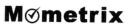

Head, Eyes, Ears, Nose, and Throat

CATARACTS

Cataracts, partial or complete opacity of the lens of one or both eyes preventing refraction of light onto the retina, can be either congenital or acquired and are associated with prenatal infections, such as rubella and CMV, hypocalcemia, or drug exposure. It can be related to trauma, systemic corticosteroids, genetic defects (albinism, Down syndrome), and prematurity. Clouding of the lens is not always obvious to the naked eye, so careful visual evaluations should be done for those children at risk.

Treatment depends upon the extent of the cataracts and whether they are unilateral or bilateral. Early diagnosis is important because surgical repair ≤2 months is the most successful with visual acuity in 55% at 20/40. The opaque lens is removed and the child uses corrective lenses or a lens is implanted. Antibiotic or steroid drops may be used after surgery.

GLAUCOMA

Glaucoma is an increase in intraocular pressure (IOP) caused by abnormal circulation of fluid in the eyes: the ciliary body of the eyes produces aqueous fluid that flows between the iris and lens to the anterior chamber where it collects and increases pressure, which can result in blindness. Normal is 10-21 mmHg. Increased IOP is >21 mmHg. Glaucoma may affect one eye or both, but 75% of primary congenital glaucoma is bilateral. Congenital glaucoma includes an abnormality of structures that drain aqueous humor. Treatment is often unsuccessful.

Symptoms include:

- Photophobia
- Tearing
- Clouding of cornea
- Eyelid spasms and enlargement of eyes

Treatment considerations include:

- Eye drops used for adults are relatively ineffective for children.
- Surgical reduction of pressure is treatment of choice, and the infant may require multiple procedures.
- Surgery does not cure the condition and the child must continue to be monitored.

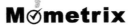

RETINOPATHY OF PREMATURITY

Retinopathy of prematurity (ROP), an abnormal vascular proliferative disease of the immature retina, is associated with infants born ≤31 weeks and <1500 g (50-70% of infants whose birth weight is <1250 grams), especially those receiving oxygen therapy, and is a preventable cause of blindness in neonates. Retinal vascularization begins at around 16 weeks' gestation and is not complete until the infant is full term. Premature birth interrupts this normal progression. Exposure of these infants to hyperoxia causes reduction in their production of retinal vascular endothelial growth factor and vasoconstriction. Initially, oxygen can be supplied to the retina from the underlying choroid capillary bed. Over time, the retina becomes thicker and outgrows this blood supply. Hypoxia of the retina triggers neovascularity (disorganized growth of new blood vessels) and is accompanied by scar tissue. Contracting scars can cause retinal detachment. ROP may regress or progress and require treatment, such as cryotherapy, photocoagulation, or scleral buckling. Untreated ROP causes acuity defects, refractive errors, strabismus, glaucoma, retinal detachment, or blindness.

INTERNATIONAL CLASSIFICATION

The international classification of retinopathy of prematurity was initially developed in 1984 as a method to standardize the diagnosis of retinopathy of prematurity (ROP):

The **five stages of ROP** are as follows:

- Stage 1: A line of demarcation is present separating the leading edge of abnormal vascularization from the anterior avascular area
- Stage 2: The demarcation line is elevated rather than flat
- Stage 3: Vessels have grown into the ridge and into the vitreous humor
- Stage 4: Partial retinal detachment
- Stage 5: Total retinal detachment

The **zones of disease** are as follows:

- Zone 1: Posterior zone defined as a circle centered on the optic nerve with a radius double the distance to the macula
- Zone 2: Ring with the inner edge bordering zone 1 and the outer edge defined by a radius centered on the optic nerve and extending to the nasal-oral serrata
- Zone 3: Remaining crescent area on the peripheral temporal edge

If the vessels are extremely tortuous (may be present at any stage) the term 'plus disease' is used.

STRABISMUS

Strabismus occurs when the muscles of the eyes are not coordinated so that one eye deviates from the axis of the other. Strabismus may be congenital or acquired or associated with other disorders, such as albinism.

Deviations include:

- **Phoria** is intermittent deviation, but the child can focus their eyes and maintain alignment for periods when looking at an object.
- **Tropia** is consistent or intermittent deviation in which the child is unable to maintain alignment of the eyes.
- Both phorias and tropias may be *hyper* (up), *hypo* (down), *exo* (out), *eso* (in toward nose), or *cyclo* (rotational).
- **Esotropia** is both eyes turning inwards (cross eyes) and *exotropia* is both eyes turning outward (wall eyes).

Treatment <24 months reduces *amblyopia* (reduced vision):

- Occlusion therapy: patching or eye drops to blur vision in one eye
- Surgical repair of rectus muscle

NYSTAGMUS AND BLEPHAROPTOSIS

Nystagmus is involuntary rhythmic movements of one or both eyes, with horizontal, vertical, or circular movements, sometimes accompanied by rhythmic movements of the head. Nystagmus is common in neonates and should resolve in a few weeks, but may indicate pathology if it persists. It is often associated with albinism, CNS abnormalities, or diseases of the ear or retina, and sudden onset is cause for concern. There is no specific treatment other than to identify and treat underlying causes.

Blepharoptosis is drooping of one or both upper **eyelids** and may be congenital (autosomal dominant), with defective development of the levator muscles or cranial nerve III, or acquired as the result of trauma or infection. If vision is affected, surgical repair is done early to avoid amblyopia. If vision is unaffected, surgical repair is deferred until the child is 3 or older.

CONJUNCTIVITIS

Conjunctivitis is inflammation of the conjunctiva of the eye from bacteria, viruses, or chemical irritants. If infectious conjunctivitis occurs <30 days of birth, it is referred to as **ophthalmia neonatorum** and is commonly acquired during delivery:

- Pathogenic agents include *Chlamydia trachomatis, Neisseria gonorrhea,* and herpesvirus. It can also be caused by chemical irritants, such as silver nitrate (this is why silver nitrate is no longer routinely used for eye prophylaxis).
- Antibiotic drops or ointment (typically erythromycin ointment) is applied to the newborn's eyes to prevent conjunctivitis. Intravenous acyclovir is given to infants exposed to herpesvirus.

Untreated, gonococcal conjunctivitis usually develops in ≤5 days of birth and is characterized by purulent discharge and inflammation. It is treated with IV antibiotics (benzylpenicillin or cefotaxime). Chlamydial conjunctivitis develops at 3-14 days and is characterized by watery discharge and less inflammation that gonococcal conjunctivitis. It is treated with IV erythromycin and topical tetracycline.

CORNEAL ABRASION

Cutting or scratching the ocular epithelium can cause **corneal abrasion**, resulting in pain, tearing, extended crying, and photophobia. The most common cause in infants is scratching by the infant's fingernails. Neonates receiving mask ventilation may develop pressure on the eye orbit, causing an abrasion. Bacterial infection (such as with *Pseudomonas*) may occur as a result of the abrasion. The masks of mask-ventilated neonates should be examined for evidence of discharge and infants routinely screened for corneal abrasions. Diagnosis is by symptoms and slit-lamp examination. Topical antibiotics are routinely given with corneal abrasion to prevent secondary infection from occurring. Studies indicate that patching the eye has no beneficial effect and may slow healing. Superficial abrasions usually heal within a few days, but deeper abrasions or cuts are more likely to develop infection and require prolonged treatment.

COLOBOMA

Coloboma is a congenital abnormality of eye development that most often results from a spontaneous mutation, although it can also be inherited as an autosomal recessive, X-linked dominant, or X-linked recessive congenital disorder. Coloboma results from failure of the optic fissure (which forms the eyes structures) to close during the second month of gestation. Colobomas may be unilateral or bilateral and may or may not affect vision, depending on the severity of the condition. With colobomas, various parts of the eye may be affected. Notches or gaps may be obvious in some parts of the eye (such as the iris) giving a keyhole appearance, but disorders of the optic nerve may be hidden. Some neonates may exhibit microphthalmia, or one or both eyeballs may be completely missing. Additional disorders (such as photophobia, amblyopia, glaucoma, cataracts, nystagmus, retinal detachment, visual acuity abnormalities, and facial nerve palsy) may occur. Treatment over time may include surgical repair, glasses, occlusive patching, artificial tears, and low-vision aids.

NASOLACRIMAL OBSTRUCTION

The nasolacrimal duct system is usually mature by the eighth month of gestation, but in some cases, abnormalities such as fistula of the lacrimal sac, atresia, or lack of valves can cause malfunction or **nasolacrimal obstruction.** Nasolacrimal obstruction occurs in only 2-4% of newborns, but incidence is much higher in those with trisomy 21 (Down syndrome) at 22-36%. Nasolacrimal obstruction is often associated with eye anomalies (20%) or systemic anomalies (25%). Diagnostic tests include a dye disappearance test (most effective) and fluorescein drops in each eye (should clear in 5 minutes). Most cases (90%) of congenital obstruction resolve within a year without treatment, although some physicians recommend digital massage. If infection occurs, topical antibiotics are indicated. If obstruction persists, surgical repair (probing, intubation, dilatation) may be indicated.

DEVIATED SEPTUM

A deviated septum occurs when the cartilage that divides the nasal cavity is shifted off center, often the result of birth trauma. If the deviation is mild, it poses little problem, but if more severe, it can result in occlusion. Bilateral obstruction is an emergent condition. If the nose appears deformed externally, then anterior dislocation is likely. Since neonates breathe primarily through the nose (although they can breathe through the mouth to some degree), nasal obstruction can result in increased pulmonary resistance, periods of apnea, and cyanosis progressing to respiratory failure. The Strut test (inserting acrylic strips into the nares) can determine if deviation and obstruction are, present on either side. For positional deformities that are not obstructing airflow, surgical tape may be used to hold the nose in correct position. For more severe deviations, surgical septoplasty may be indicated.

CYSTIC HYGROMA

A cystic hygroma is the presence and growth of a fluid-filled cyst in the newborn's head or neck caused by a blockage of the lymphatic system due to the fetal exposure to infection or drugs/alcohol in utero. This cyst can become evident in the womb (developing in the 9th-16th week of pregnancy) or after birth. In instances where the cyst is not noticeable at birth, it will grow over time, and is most often noticeable by age 2. Most commonly, a cystic hygroma presents as a spongy soft bump in the neck, but it can also appear in the armpit or groin. If it noticed by ultrasound during pregnancy, the diagnosis is confirmed with amniocentesis. There is a 50% chance of association with chromosomal abnormalities (such as Turner's Syndrome; Trisomy 13, 18, or 21; or Noonan syndrome) and this can increase the risk of miscarriage or be life threatening to the newborn. Surgery is generally scheduled immediately if the cyst is noticeable in the newborn. If the cyst arises later surgery may not be an option, but the cyst may be shrunk with steroids, chemotherapy, or radiation therapy.

CRANIOSYNOSTOSIS

Craniosynostosis is a condition caused by the premature closing of the cranial sutures while the newborn brain is still growing, resulting in a misshapen head. Complex craniosynostoses involves more than one suture closing prematurely. In some cases, craniosynostosis has genetic/inherited origins, but this condition may also occur spontaneously. Surgery is required to correct the misshapen head and is also necessary to provide space for the neonate's brain to continue to grow. Generally, this condition does not affect the cognitive ability of the child.

CHOANAL ATRESIA

If the nurse is unable to pass a suctioning tube through the nares, the infant may have **choanal atresia,** a rare condition that occurs in approximately 1 in 10,000 live births. It occurs in females twice as often as males. The choana are the two openings in the posterior nares that connect the nasal passages with the nasopharynx. Newborns are obligate nasal breathers. Successful nose breathing requires air to pass through the choana, so if these openings fail to form during fetal development, the infant must become a mouth breather. If atresia occurs only on one side (unilaterally), the infant may have no symptoms. The infant with bilateral choanal atresia has periods of respiratory distress and cyanosis that are alleviated by crying. Bilateral choanal atresia often becomes a medical emergency requiring intubation.

OROFACIAL CLEFTS

Cleft lip (CL), **cleft lip with cleft palate** (CLP), and **cleft palate** (CP) are orofacial clefts, which can be a part of a more complex syndrome or isolated anomalies:

- **CL** occurs when the medial nasal and maxillary processes fail to merge during the fifth week of embryological development. The cleft is generally at the junction of the central and lateral parts of the upper lip and may be on the left or right side. If the cleft extends into the maxilla, it may be accompanied by a cleft palate and be deemed a CLP. Surgical repair is usually at 10 weeks.
- **CP** occurs when the palatal shelves of the maxillary bone fail to fuse. Fusion usually begins at the eighth week and continues until the twelfth week of embryological development. A spectrum of CP exists. Bifid uvula is the mildest form. Clefting of the soft palate is more severe. A complete CP (most severe form) involves clefting of the uvula, soft palate, and hard palate. Surgical repair usually begins at about 4 months.

ROBIN SEQUENCE

Robin sequence (RS) was previously called Pierre Robin syndrome. RS is associated with the following anomalies:

- Micrognathia (small lower jaw)
- Glossoptosis (the tongue tends to fall back in the throat, causing airway obstruction)
- Horseshoe-shaped cleft palate

RS sequence may occur as part of a more complex syndrome or as an isolated defect. Infants with RS should have a full genetic evaluation. The immediate concern is maintaining the airway, especially during feeds. Lay the infant prone and allow gravity to pull the tongue away from the back of the throat. Use a nasopharyngeal airway if positional changes are inadequate. If this does not work, ask the surgeon for a lip-tongue plication (the tongue is attached to the lower lip temporarily) to alleviate the obstruction and to allow the infant to breathe while feeding, or a tracheotomy. Because of increased work of breathing and feeding difficulties, RS infants require increased calories for adequate growth.

NATAL TEETH

Natal teeth are teeth present at birth in the newborn, generally erupting above the gum line. Normal neonatal teeth begin growing after the first 30 days after birth. While uncommon, natal teeth are generally found along lower gum line and can cause irritation and interfere with the baby's ability to nurse. These teeth may also be uncomfortable to the mother during nursing. Natal teeth are often removed at birth due to the risk of the neonate aspirating (breathing in) the tooth.

LARYNGOMALACIA AND TRACHEOMALACIA

Laryngomalacia results from a congenital shortening of the aryepiglottic folds that open and close the vocal cords. This shortening causes an omega-shaped curling of the epiglottis that causes respiratory obstruction, characterized by inspiratory stridor, usually not associated with other symptoms. Stridor may be absent at birth but increase over the first few weeks. This condition usually resolves by 2 years, but may require surgical repair in severe cases.

Tracheomalacia is a congenital abnormality of the trachea in which the supporting cartilage is weak and the posterior membranous wall is widened. The distal third of the trachea is most commonly affected, and the condition may be associated with other congenital defects, such as cardiovascular abnormalities. Tracheomalacia may be associated with tracheoesophageal fistula. Symptoms include expiratory stridor, cough (especially during feeding), recurrent respiratory infections, and reflex periods of apnea. Treatment includes humidified air, antibiotics, and care in feeding. This condition usually resolves as the infant grows, but surgery may be indicated in rare cases.

MOUTH/THROAT ABNORMALITY

MICROGNATHIA

Micrognathia (mandibular undergrowth) is fairly common and often resolves as the child grows over 6-12 months; however, marked micrognathia can result in respiratory obstruction, including obstructive sleep apnea, gastric reflux, and difficulty feeding. Micrognathia may be associated with other genetic abnormalities, such as cleft lip and cleft palate, Robin sequence, trisomy 18 (Edwards syndrome), trisomy 22, and Stickler's syndrome. Interventions may include:

- **Prone positioning** to relieve respiratory distress as this causes the base of the tongue to move forward, preventing obstruction of the airway; however, the neonate must be carefully supervised because of the risks of prone positioning.
- **Nasopharyngeal or oral airway** placement to open the airway.
- **Endotracheal tube** and ventilation in more severe cases.
- **Tracheostomy** is rarely required unless other abnormalities present.
- **Surgical repair**, such as mandibular distraction, tongue-lip adhesion, or other repair, may be done if more conservative approaches are ineffective.
- **Feeding** the neonate may require some modifications, such as the use of special nipples and positioning the child upright, to prevent aspiration.

RETROGNATHIA AND MACROGLOSSIA

Retrognathia refers to a facial deformity with abnormal positioning of the mandible, resulting in a receding chin (overbite). Retrognathia is associated with congenital disorders, such as Treacher Collins syndrome, Robin sequence, and Nager syndrome. Neonates with retrognathia may have poor feeding because of difficulty latching on and may have obstructive sleep apnea. If the condition is interfering with the ability to feed or breathe, the neonate may undergo surgical repair. If not severe, the condition may be corrected with orthodontia during childhood.

Macroglossia is a condition in which the tongue is abnormally large because of muscle hypertrophy or vascular malformation, often associated with congenital disorders, such as trisomy 21 (Down syndrome) and Beckwith-Wiedemann syndrome. Pseudo-macroglossia is a condition in which the tongue only appears enlarged because of other factors, such as abnormalities in the shape of the mouth or displacement of the tongue. If the tongue interferes with breathing or swallowing, then surgical reduction is carried out, sometimes with a tracheostomy done prior to surgery.

MICROTIA

Microtia (from the Latin for *tiny ears*) is a congenital deformity of the outer ear that ranges from a slightly small pinna to complete absence of the external ear and the external auditory canal. Microtia can involve one or both ears, and is usually not seen on prenatal ultrasound, but is discovered at birth. Microtia has four grades:

- **Grade I**: The ear is smaller but still has identifiable structures (pinna, helix, and antihelix). The external ear canal is present but is often narrowed.
- **Grade II:** The pinna is smaller and less developed than in Grade I. The external auditory canal is closed off.
- **Grade III**: The external ear is essentially absent, except for a small remnant of tissue. This is the most common type of microtia.
- **Grade IV**: Total absence of the external ear and external auditory canal, also called anotia.

Infants with microtia usually have conductive hearing loss in the affected ear. Reconstruction of the affected ear is generally begun when the child is 4-6 years old, and will require a hearing aid if conductive hearing loss is present.

HEARING LOSS
TYPES

The neonate may have a number of different types of hearing loss:

- **Sensorineural** hearing loss may be mild or severe and occurs when the cochlea is impaired by a genetic syndrome or *in utero* infections like rubella, postnatal meningitis, or ototoxic medication, such as aminoglycoside antibiotics or the diuretic furosemide, which damage the cochlea.
- **Conductive** hearing loss occurs from an abnormality in the sound conduction system in the outer and middle ears (external ear canal, tympanic membrane, and auditory ossicles). Congenital cholesteatoma is an example of conductive hearing loss.
- **Mixed** hearing loss occurs when an infant has a component of both sensorineural and conductive hearing loss.
- **Central** hearing loss is rare and occurs when defects or damage of the auditory nervous pathway or auditory brain centers are present in infants with kernicterus, episodes of hypoxia, or intraventricular hemorrhage.

OTOACOUSTIC EMISSION EXAMINATION AND AUDITORY BRAINSTEM RESPONSE SCREENINGS

Otoacoustic emissions (OAE) are sounds generated by the cochlea. They are a measure of the integrity of the middle and inner ear, or more specifically, the outer hair cells of the cochlea. The audiologist measures OAE by inserting a probe into the infant's external auditory canal and stimulating the cochlea with several clicking noises. The audiologist uses a microphone to measure the OAE sent off by the cochlea.

Auditory brainstem response (ABR) examination measures the brain's reaction to sound (middle and inner ear and nerve pathway). The audiologist places electrodes on the infant's scalp, positions a device that makes sounds outside the ear, and measures the brain's response to the sound. Measured waveforms are compared to the normal, expected pattern. Both of these hearing examinations are scored as pass or fail. If the infant fails an audiology screening examination, further testing should be conducted by an **otorhinolaryngologist** to confirm if a problem truly exists and if so, the nature of the hearing loss.

Psychosocial Support

General Discharge Planning and Parent Teaching

PRINCIPLES OF ADULT LEARNING

Adults have a wealth of life and/or employment experiences. Their attitudes toward education may vary considerably. There are, however, some **principles of adult learning** and typical characteristics of adult learners that an instructor should consider when planning strategies for teaching parents, families, or staff.

- Practical and goal-oriented:
  - Provide overviews or summaries and examples.
  - Use collaborative discussions with problem-solving exercises.
  - Remain organized with the goal in mind.
- Self-directed:
  - Provide active involvement, asking for input.
  - Allow different options toward achieving the goal.
  - Give them responsibilities.
- Knowledgeable:
  - Show respect for their life experiences/education.
  - Validate their knowledge and ask for feedback.
  - Relate new material to information with which they are familiar.
- Relevancy-oriented:
  - Explain how information will be applied.
  - Clearly identify objectives.
- Motivated:
  - Provide certificates of professional advancement and/or continuing education credit for staff when possible.

> **Review Video: Adult Learning Processes and Theories**
> Visit mometrix.com/academy and enter code: 638453

LEARNING STYLES

Not all people are aware of their preferred **learning style.** A range of teaching materials and methods that relate to all three major learning preferences (visual, auditory, and kinesthetic) and that are appropriate for different ages should be available. Part of assessment for teaching involves choosing the right approach based on observation and feedback. Often, presenting learners with different options gives a clue to their preferred learning style. Some people have a combined learning style.

Visual learners learn best by seeing and reading:

- Provide written directions or picture guides, or demonstrate procedures. Use charts and diagrams.
- Provide photos or videos.

Auditory learners learn best by listening and talking:

- Explain procedures while demonstrating and have the learner repeat.
- Plan extra time to discuss and answer questions.
- Provide audio recordings.

Kinesthetic learners learn best by handling, doing, and practicing:

- Provide hands-on experience throughout teaching.
- Encourage handling of supplies and equipment.
- Allow the learner to demonstrate.
- Minimize instructions and allow the person to explore equipment and procedures.

APPROACHES TO TEACHING

There are many approaches to teaching, and the educator must prepare, present, and coordinate a wide range of educational workshops, lectures, discussions, and one-on-one instructions on any chosen topic. All types of classes will be needed, depending upon the purpose and material:

- **Educational workshops** are usually conducted with small groups, allowing for maximal participation. They are especially good for demonstrations and practice sessions.
- **Lectures** are often used for more academic or detailed information that may include questions and answers but limits discussion. An effective lecture should include some audiovisual support.
- **Discussions** are best with small groups so that people can actively participate. This is a good method for problem solving.
- **One-on-one instruction** is especially helpful for targeted instruction in procedures for individuals.
- **Online learning modules** are good for independent learners.

Participants should be asked to evaluate the presentations in the forms of surveys or suggestions, but ultimately the program is evaluated in terms of patient outcomes.

READINESS TO LEARN

The patient/family's readiness to learn should be assessed because if they are not ready, instruction is of little value. Often, readiness is indicated when the patient/family asks questions or shows an interest in procedures. There are a number of factors related to readiness to learn:

- **Physical factors:** There are a number of physical factors that can affect ability. Manual dexterity may be required to complete a task, and this varies by age and condition. Hearing or vision deficits may impact a person's ability to learn. Complex tasks may be too difficult for some because of weakness or cognitive impairment, and modifications of the environment may be needed. Health status, age, and gender may all impact the ability to learn.
- **Experience:** People's experience with learning can vary widely and is affected by their ability to cope with changes, their personal goals, motivation to learn, and cultural background. People may have widely divergent ideas about what constitutes illness and/or treatment. Lack of English skills may make learning difficult and prevent people from asking questions.
- **Mental/emotional status:** The external support system and internal motivation may impact readiness. Anxiety, fear, or depression about one's condition can make learning very difficult because the patient/family cannot focus on learning, so the nurse must spend time to reassure the patient/family and wait until they are emotionally more receptive.
- **Knowledge/education:** The knowledge base of the patient/family, their cognitive ability, and their learning styles all affect their readiness to learn. The nurse should always begin by assessing what knowledge the patient/family already has about their disease, condition, or treatment and then build from that base. People with little medical experience may lack knowledge of basic medical terminology, interfering with their ability and readiness to learn.

BLOOM'S TAXONOMY

Bloom's taxonomy outlines behaviors that are necessary for learning and that can be applied to healthcare. The theory describes three types of learning.

Cognitive: Learning and gaining intellectual skills to master six categories of effective learning.

- Knowledge
- Comprehension
- Application
- Analysis
- Synthesis
- Evaluation

Affective: Recognizing 5 categories of feelings and values from simple to complex. This is slower to achieve than cognitive learning.

- **Receiving phenomena**: Accepting need to learn
- **Responding to phenomena**: Taking active part in care
- **Valuing**: Understanding the value of becoming independent in care
- **Organizing values**: Understanding how surgery/treatment has improved life
- **Internalizing values**: Accepting the condition as part of life, being consistent and self-reliant

Psychomotor: Mastering 7 categories of motor skills necessary for independence. This follows a progression from simple to complex.

- **Perception**: Uses sensory information to learn tasks
- **Set**: Shows willingness to perform tasks
- **Guided response**: Follows directions
- **Mechanism**: Does specific tasks
- **Complex overt response**: Displays competence in self-care
- **Adaptation**: Modifies procedures as needed
- **Origination**: Creatively deals with problems

TEACHING TECHNIQUES

There are many teaching techniques the nurse can utilize when educating patients. The nurse can demonstrate skills repeatedly when teaching and then allow the patient as much time as needed to practice the skill. The nurse should use equipment that will be available in the home and provide written instructions that can be referred to later if needed. Encouraging discussion of the information helps the patient understand and clarify. Discussion also allows the patient to vent emotions about the disease and the learning process, and to assimilate the information so that a change in behavior can result. Discussion provides feedback to the patient and encouragement to continue learning. Teaching groups of people may be appropriate when there are others who require the same information. The members can support each other with encouragement, empathy, and camaraderie, although some patients will not learn well in groups and will need individual teaching. Groups must be followed up with on an individual basis to give the chance to clarify information, to evaluate the level of learning and goal achievement, and to alter the learning plan as needed for each person.

INSTRUCTION GROUP SIZES

Both one-on-one instruction and group instruction have a place in patient/family education.

- **One-on-one instruction** is the most costly for an institution because it is time intensive. However, it allows the patient and family more interaction with the nurse instructor and allows them to have more control over the process by asking questions or having the instructor repeat explanations or demonstrations. One-on-one instruction is especially valuable when patients and families must learn particular skills, such as managing dialysis, or if confidentiality is important.
- **Group instruction** is the less costly because the needs of a number of people can be met at one time. Group presentations are more planned and usually scheduled for a particular time period (an hour, for example), so patients and families have less control. Questioning is usually more limited and may be done only at the end. Group instruction allows patients/families with similar health problems to interact. Group instruction is especially useful for general types of instruction, such as managing diet or other lifestyle issues.

RESOURCES TO USE WHEN TEACHING PATIENTS AND THEIR FAMILIES

Many hospitals that find the need to repeatedly teach the same information to patients and families prepare brochures or other written materials or teaching videos that are available for use. The nurse should review material first and make notes specific to the patient. The nurse should also watch the video with the patient and discuss it afterwards. Written materials can augment lecture and demonstrations and are useful for the patient to keep for later reference.

There are also commercial materials that can be used, provided by various drug or equipment companies. **Teaching resources** are available online from the National Institutes of Health and other reputable sources. The nurse can use these prepared materials whenever possible to save time for actual teaching but must remember to customize them to the patient. They help provide pictures, colors, and interesting features that keep the patient's interest in learning alive. There are also many books, groups, and websites that the patient should be made aware of for resources after discharge.

READABILITY

Studies have indicated that learning is more effective if oral presentations and/or demonstrations are supplemented with reading materials, such as handouts. **Readability** (the grade level of the material) is a concern because many patients and families may have limited English skills or low literacy, and it can be difficult for the nurse to assess people's reading level. The average American reads effectively at the 6th to 8th grade level (regardless of education achieved), but many health education materials have a much higher readability level. Additionally, research indicates that even people with much higher reading skills learn medical and health information most effectively when the material is presented at the 6th to 8th grade readability level. Therefore, patient education materials (and consent forms) should not be written at higher than 6th to 8th grade level. Readability index calculators are available on the internet to give an approximation of grade level and difficulty for those preparing materials without expertise in teaching reading.

VIDEOS

Videos are a useful adjunct to teaching as they reduce the time needed for one-on-one instruction (increasing cost-effectiveness). Passive presentation of **videos**, such as in the waiting area, has little value, but focused viewing in which the nurse discusses the purpose of the video presentation prior to viewing and then is available for discussion after viewing can be very effective. Patients and/or families are often nervous about learning patient care and are unsure of their abilities, so they may not focus completely when the nurse is presenting information. Allowing the patients/families to watch a video demonstration or explanation first and allowing them to stop or review the video presentation can help them to grasp the fundamentals before they have to apply them, relieving some of the anxiety they may be experiencing. Videos are much more effective than written materials for those with low literacy or poor English skills. The nurse should always be available to answer questions and discuss the material after the patients/families finish viewing.

LEARNING CONTRACT

In order to be compliant with a therapeutic regimen, the patient needs information about the disease, the purpose of medications and treatments, and side effects and complications to watch for. A written **learning contract** organizes this information into specific learning goals, demonstrates the importance of the information, and ensures that all pertinent information is taught. Others on the healthcare team can note patient progress and easily determine what to teach next. The patient has a written plan to follow as well.

The learning contract should take into consideration the patient's age, sex, cultural and religious values, and educational level achieved. One must consider the patient's financial status, socio-economic status, living situation, and support network. The complex nature of a therapeutic regimen combined with distracters such as side effects, pain, denial, and fear can weaken the patient's resolve to maintain compliance. One must evaluate the patient's attitudes towards healthcare, coping mechanisms, and motivation and provide reinforcement as needed.

EDUCATIONAL GOALS, OBJECTIVES, AND PLANS

Once a topic for performance improvement education has been chosen, then goals, measurable objectives with strategies, and lesson plans must be developed. A class should stay focused on one topic rather than trying to cover many. For example:

Goal: Increase compliance with hand hygiene standards in ICU.

Objectives:

- Develop series of posters and fliers by June 1.
- Observe 100% compliance with hand hygiene standards at 2 weeks, 1-month, and 2-month intervals after training is completed.

Strategies: Conduct 4 classes at different times over a one-week period, May 25-31.

- Place posters in all nursing units, staff rooms, and utility rooms by January 3.
- Develop slide show presentation for class and provide online access to the presentation for all staff by May 25.
- Utilize handwashing kits.

Lesson plans: Discussion period: Why do we need 100% compliance?

- Slide show: The case for hand hygiene
- Discussion: What did you learn?
- Demonstration and activities to show effectiveness
- Handwashing technique

LEARNER OUTCOMES

When the quality professional plans an educational offering, whether it be a class, an online module, a workshop, or educational materials, the professional should identify **learner outcomes,** which should be conveyed to the learners from the very beginning so that they are aware of the expectations. The subject matter of the educational material and the learner outcomes should be directly related. For example, if the quality professional is giving a class on decontamination of the environment, then a learner outcome might be: "Identify the difference between disinfectants and antiseptics." There may be one or multiple learner outcomes, but part of the assessment at the end of the learning experience should be to determine if, in fact, the learner outcomes have been achieved. A survey of whether or not the learners felt that they had achieved the learner outcomes can give valuable feedback and guidance to the quality professional.

IMPLEMENTATION AND EVALUATION OF TEACHING PLAN

Implementation and evaluation of the teaching plan includes:

- Follow teaching plan but be flexible and alter plan to suit the patient's learning needs.
- Work with a healthcare team to follow the teaching plan and ensure consistency in teaching methods as well as coordinate efforts and take responsibility for altering the plan and evaluating learning to meet goals.
- Monitor patient's motivational level, encourage with positive feedback as needed, and record patient responses to teaching and changes in behaviors as a result of all teaching sessions.
- Use tools, such as checklists, rating scales, observed behavior, written tests, and the nature of the questions from the patient when evaluating the effectiveness of the teaching plan in reaching the patient's goals for learning.
- Evaluate the plan after each session and at the end.

Communicate information taught and patient learning to any home health or community nurses involved. They can then continue the patient's teaching by evaluating behavior in the home and continuing to address learning needs as they arise.

EVALUATING EFFECTIVENESS OF EDUCATION

Education, like all interventions, must be evaluated for **effectiveness**. Two determinants of effectiveness include:

- **Behavior modification** involves thorough observation and measurement, identifying behavior that needs to be changed and then planning and instituting interventions to modify that behavior. The nurse can use a variety of techniques, including demonstrations of appropriate behavior, reinforcement, and monitoring until new behavior is adopted consistently. This is especially important when longstanding procedures and habits of behavior are changed.
- **Compliance rates** are often determined by observation, which should be done at intervals and on multiple occasions, but with patients, this may depend on self-reports. Outcomes is another measure of compliance; that is, if education is intended to improve patient health and reduce risk factors and that occurs, it is a good indication that there is compliance. Compliance rates are calculated by determining the number of events/procedures and degree of compliance.

EDUCATIONAL NEEDS OF NEW MOTHERS

The educational needs of the new mother and family vary depending on age, background, education, experience, and expectations. The needs of the adolescent mother with no experience may be quite different from those of the multiparous mother. Assessing individual needs can be difficult in the short time women are usually hospitalized, so education should cover a wide range of topics. A checklist of topics may be a helpful starting point for the mother to indicate her needs. Because mothers are usually fatigued for the first 24-48 hours, teaching after that time is most effective, but many mothers leave the hospital on the second day. Demonstration with return demonstration is an effective method to ensure that a mother can carry out tasks, but education should anticipate other needs and concerns that may arise. Mothers often have concerns about a variety of issues, such as childcare, contraception, and resuming sexual relations. Pamphlets, website information, or videos that can be sent home with the mother are very helpful.

SAFE POSITIONING FOR INFANTS

Infants should be placed on their **backs** for sleeping. Sleeping on the stomach increases the risk of **sudden infant death syndrome (SIDS)**.

- Position the infant on the back when unattended or sleeping, but alternate the direction the head faces to prevent one side of the head from flattening (**positional molding**).
- Provide supervised time each day with the infant lying on the abdomen (only on firm surfaces) to strengthen head and neck muscles and to prevent positional molding.
- Hold the infant, rather than leaving them in a carrier.
- Position baby in side-lying position, alternating from one side to the other, using specially designed supports to maintain the position.

INFANT CAR SEAT

All infants, regardless of age, must be placed properly in an infant car seat during transit. Holding an infant while the car is in motion is not safe. Car seats should be new or in very good condition and fastened according to the manufacturer's guidelines to ensure safety.

- Place the car seat in the back seat and away from any side airbags.
- Always securely buckle the child into the seat.
- Face the infant seat toward the rear of the car.
- Recline the seat so the infant's head does not fall forward.
- Place padding around (not under) the infant if the infant slouches to one side.
- Place blankets over the straps and buckles, not under.

UMBILICAL CORD CARE

Education surrounding the umbilical cord should include the following information:

- Protect the cord from moisture, with top of diaper folded under the cord instead of covering it.
- If the cord becomes soiled, wash with mild soap and water, rinse, and dry. Swabbing with alcohol is no longer recommended and may increase skin irritation.
- Avoid covering the cord stump with clothing, which may cause irritation.
- Give the infant only sponge baths until the cord falls off in about 10-14 days.
- Report signs of infection, such as erythema, swelling, or purulent discharge.

Note: The umbilical cord changes color from grayish-brown to black as it dries and finally falls off.

FECAL ELIMINATION

The first stool (**meconium**) is usually passed within 24 hours and is black and tarry looking. The stool then transitions to greenish as the baby nurses or takes formula, and by the third day, the stool is usually yellow or yellow-green for breastfed babies and yellow or light brown for formula-fed babies. Typically, babies have 2-3 stools daily by day 3 and ≥4 daily by day 5, but this may vary.

- Report abnormalities, such as bloody stools, watery stools, very hard stools, clay-colored or whitish stools, black stools (after meconium has passed), and "currant jelly" stools.
- Cleanse skin thoroughly after defecation with mild soap and water, plain water, or unscented baby wipes.
- Examine skin carefully for irritation.

URINARY ELIMINATION

Urination is estimated according to the number of **wet diapers** in a 24-hour period. Typically, the infant has 1 wet diaper the first day, 2 the next, and so on until urination stabilizes at 6-8 wet diapers by about day 6.

- Check diaper frequently. Infants often urinate during or after feeding.
- Change diapers when wet, gently cleansing skin with mild soap and water, plain water, or unscented baby wipes.

CRADLE CAP

Cradle cap may appear as scaly, crusted, or flaky skin on the scalp and other parts of the face. It is not contagious and usually clears by 1 or 2 months. It is not usually a sign of poor hygiene.

- Cleanse scalp or affected areas thoroughly, gently rubbing the area with a terry cloth or brushing to loosen crust or flakes.
- If persistent, try softening the crusts with olive oil. Leave it in for 15 minutes, and then brush or gently comb to loosen crusts or flakes. Finally, wash with baby shampoo.

DIAPER RASH

Diaper rash usually results from leaving the infant in soiled/wet diapers and/or not adequately cleansing the skin, although breastfed infants sometimes react to foods the mother has eaten. A rash may also indicate an allergic response to baby wipes or other products, such as lotions or creams. Antibiotics may cause diaper rash. In some cases, a **fungal infection** may occur, usually characterized by red, weepy open areas. Purulent discharge may indicate infection.

- Change diapers as soon as possible when wet or soiled.
- Cleanse skin gently with water.
- Remove diaper and expose skin to air whenever possible.
- Apply barrier cream or ointment especially formulated for diaper rash to prevent or treat diaper rash.
- Contact physician if rash worsens and does not respond to treatment, as antifungals, cortisone, or topical antibiotics may be indicated.

CHOKING OR GAGGING IN INFANT

Education regarding chocking/gagging should include the following:

- Ensure small hazardous items, such as pins and cotton balls or materials, such as baby powder are out of reach.
- DO NOT prop bottle for feeding.
- Burp infant regularly during feedings, whether breast or bottle.
- Keep baby in upright position with head elevated during feedings.
- Check nipple of bottle to ensure it is dripping and not running freely.
- If the infant is choking, secure face down on forearm, tilted downward, and use the heel of the hand to thump on the mid-back. Repeat as necessary. If choking does not resolve with evidence of breathing immediately, call 911 and begin CPR.

Note: Prevention is important, as most **choking and gagging episodes** can be avoided.

BURPING THE INFANT

Both breastfed and bottle-fed babies require **burping** because they swallow air when feeding, although bottle-fed babies tend to require more burping. Infants often show indications (grimacing, squirming, spitting up, and crying) that they are uncomfortable and need to burp.

- Burp the infant routinely after 2 or 3 ounces of formula or after nursing on one breast.
- Position the infant on the shoulder with a burp cloth under the infant's head and gently pat or rub the infant's back.
- Change to a different position if the baby doesn't burp. Try on the opposite shoulder or with the infant sitting on the lap supported by one hand while the other hand pats or rubs the infant's back.

BATHING THE INFANT

The infant should receive **sponge baths** until the umbilical cord falls off at 10-14 days, and then a bath in an **infant tub** (NOT in an adult tub). Mild soap/shampoo intended for babies or water alone may be used for the bath.

- Make sure the environmental temperature is warm.
- Fill tub with 2-3 inches of water.
- ALWAYS check water temperature to make sure it is warm and NOT hot.
- Set water heaters ≤120 °F to prevent inadvertent scalding.
- Support the baby during the bath with one arm under upper back to support the neck and head while holding the infant under the axillae.
- Pour water over the child with the free hand and use that hand to wash the hair and the body.
- Lift the baby from the tub and wrap in a towel to dry.
- Dry thoroughly, making sure all skin folds and crevices are dry to prevent irritation and rashes.
- Avoid use of lotions or creams.

FONTANELS

The infant's fontanels (anterior and posterior) are covered by thick membranous tissue and should feel flat but firm.

- Do not be afraid to touch the fontanels or cleanse the scalp.
- Report **bulging** above the level of the skull, as this may indicate increased intracranial pressure.
- Report a **soft fontanel** that sinks below the level of the skull, as this may indicate dehydration.

CIRCUMCISION

Circumcision rates have dropped by 10% over the last 30 years, with about 58% of male infants now being **circumcised** in the United States. The American Academy of Pediatrics has confirmed that the benefits outweigh the risks, though they do not have a formal recommendation for circumcision and instead leave that decision up to the parents. Benefits including decreased risk of prostate cancer, urinary tract infections, and sexually transmitted infections such as HIV. Most parents make their decision based on cultural or religious beliefs or the factor of cost, as some insurance companies and many Medicaid programs do not cover the cost of circumcision. While at one time infants were not thought to experience pain, it is now clear that they do, so circumcision should be done using a local anesthesia or topical EMLA cream.

POST-CIRCUMCISION CARE

After circumcision, the end of the foreskin is typically swollen and red, and a small amount of bleeding may persist for 24 hours.

- Change the diaper immediately, because urine may cause pain to the open tissue.
- Cleanse the area gently with water and pat dry.
- Apply petroleum jelly gauze to the incision area as directed by the individual physician.
- Avoid using soap or commercial cleansing products, such as baby wipes, until the circumcision heals.
- Report any change, such as increased swelling, redness, temperature, or purulent discharge.

CARE OF THE UNCIRCUMCISED PENIS

The infant's foreskin is different from that of the adult male. It does not **separate and retract** until the child is around 5 years old.

- Do NOT attempt to retract the foreskin.
- Do NOT use cotton swabs to clean.
- Wash the penis with soap and water or just water during the routine bath.

SHAKEN BABY SYNDROME

Shaken baby syndrome is believed to be the result of vigorous shaking of a neonate, causing acute subdural hematoma with subarachnoid, and retinal hemorrhages. The shaking of the brain may damage vessels and nerves with resultant cerebral edema. Parents should be advised of the importance of always supporting and protecting the neonate's head and avoiding activities that may injure the child, such as throwing and catching a neonate or small child. Parents should be advised that sometimes children may not exhibit obvious neurological symptoms immediately after trauma but have learning disabilities and behavioral disorders that appear in school.

NEONATAL CPR

Most cardiac arrests in newborns are associated with respiratory arrest rather than cardiac arrest, so **cardiopulmonary resuscitation** of newborns follows the ABC protocol rather than the compressions only protocol used for adults. The parent should be advised to take a CPR course, especially if the neonate is at risk and if arrest occurs, immediately call 911 for help or ask someone else to call and begin CPR:

- **Airway:** Tilt the head slightly back and lift the chin to open the airway.
- **Breathing:** If the neonate does not begin breathing, administer 2 puffs to ventilate the lungs. For small neonates, place the mouth to cover the neonate's nose and mouth and ventilate each time for approximately one second, observing the chest to ensure it is rising. For the infant with a heart rate ≥ 60/minute without normal breathing, administer one breath every 2-3 seconds (20-30 breaths per minute).
- **Compressions:** Infants that require chest compressions should receive two breaths per 30 compressions (30:2) for a single rescuer, and two breaths per 15 compressions for two rescuers (15:2). The chest should be depressed approximately 1.5 inches, using two fingers or two thumbs while encircling the hands around the baby's body. The optimum rate of compressions is approximately 100-120 per minute.

Discharge Planning for Patients with Special Needs

DISCHARGE PLANNING FOR PATIENTS WITH SPECIAL NEEDS

DISCHARGE REQUIREMENTS FOR PRETERM INFANT

In the past, discharge requirements were based on factors such as weight and post-conceptual age. Current requirements are instead based on physiological and functional readiness. Hospitals vary, but requirements generally include:

- All medical or surgical problems that require hospitalization are resolved.
- The infant is feeding appropriately, as evidenced by:
  - Primary caregiver feeding the infant with the prescribed method (gavage, gastrostomy, or special positioning)
  - Weight gain of 15-30 grams per day over several days
  - Feeds accomplished without respiratory difficulty
- Temperature stability is maintained in an open crib.
- Parents are trained appropriately concerning the administration of medications, CPR, and the proper use of a car seat.
- The infant has passed all pre-discharge tests:
  - Hearing screening
  - Other tests as needed (anemia, ROP exams, sleep study, head ultrasound)
- Age-appropriate immunizations were administered.
- The discharge environment has been evaluated.
- Appropriate post-discharge follow-up appointments are scheduled with specialists and the primary care physician.

DISCHARGE EDUCATION FOR THE SPECIAL-NEEDS NEONATE

Family involvement and education are vital for the successful discharge of a **special-needs neonate** to ensure proper care. Bringing home a premature infant or one who has special needs is a daunting task for any parent, so preparation is essential.

- Educate the parents or guardians about appropriate care methods.
- Explain how to interpret the infant's cues concerning his or her needs and how to respond appropriately.
- Point out the different states of alertness during their infant's sleep and wake cycles. Identify the appropriate times and methods for infant interaction.
- Coach the parents to ensure that they perform each skill correctly and retain it. Observe interactions between the infant and parents in the nursery to help ensure continued wellness of the infant after discharge.
- Encourage kangaroo care immediately after birth for stable newborns as it is an excellent method to foster bonding between the neonate and the mother. For neonates who require resuscitation and medical intervention, delay kangaroo care until the neonate is stable.
- If the parents are not ready, contact a social worker for follow-up.

CEREBRAL PALSY AND COGNITIVE/LANGUAGE DELAYS

Important elements of discharge planning and parent teaching for patients with cerebral palsy and cognitive/language delays include:

- **Motor delays (especially with cerebral palsy)**: Parents need realistic information about what to expect and how to cope with motor delays and prevent further complications. The nurse should review the child's life care plan, including the need for follow-up therapy and the availability of resources. Instructions and education may vary according to the cause or type of CP. For example, sudden stimuli may increase spastic muscle contractions with spastic CP. Parents need information about specific feeding and positioning needs.
- **Cognitive/language delays**: Assessment of cognition and language delays often occurs over a period of time and cannot always be accurately predicted at birth. Parents should be educated about the levels of cognitive ability common to infants and methods to stimulate cognition. Additionally, parents should understand normal language development, including milestones, and interactions that promote language development.

FOLLOW UP SCREENING FROM NEONATE TO CHILDHOOD

Many screening procedures are available, including extensive laboratory testing that may be indicated if there is cause for concern that an infant may have a disorder. However, some basic screening should be done for all infants and children:

- **Genetic disorders**: Screening is usually done at birth according to state guidelines, and then may be indicated if there is concern that a child has a disorder that requires treatment.
- **Hearing**: Testing is usually done with newborns and then every 2-3 years until age 18.
- **Height and weight**: These are monitored monthly during the first year and then at least yearly until age 18 to determine if the child's development is within the normal range.
- **Vision**: This is screened at birth, at 3-4 years, and periodically between 5-18. Vision problems may become obvious when the child enters school and can't see the board or has trouble reading.
- **Fasting blood sugar**: Done every 2 years for those at risk.
- **Head circumference**: Measurement is done at birth, 1 year, and 2 years.
- **Blood pressure**: This is usually checked during infancy (6-12 months) and then periodically throughout childhood.
- **Dental screening**: Bottle-fed babies may require earlier screening as they often fall asleep with the bottle in their mouths, leading to infant caries. Dental screening is done periodically throughout childhood, especially after the new teeth come in, to evaluate for malocclusion or other problems.
- **Alcohol/drug use**: Neonates are screened for parental abuse. Screening of use may be done periodically for children between 11-18 years, especially if they are at risk.
- **Developmental screening**: There are a number of screening tests that are available and can be used if a child appears to have a developmental delay or abnormality. Screening tests must be age-appropriate. The tests are not diagnostic but can help to confirm developmental abnormalities. Tests may assess motor skills, language, and cognitive ability.

Maternal and Family Grief

TYPES OF GRIEF

Anticipatory grief occurs when a child is diagnosed with a terminal illness. The parent begins to mourn over the loss of the child before he or she expires.

Delayed grief occurs when the grieving process is postponed months to years after the loss of a child. Initially, the parent may not be able to grieve appropriately because of an inability to cope, or the pressing need to care for other family members.

Incongruent grief occurs when the mother and the father are out of sync in their grieving process, creating a source of stress and conflict in the marriage. It may be due to the differences in how men and women grieve:

- **Women** are often more expressive about their loss and more emotional. They are more likely to look for support from others.
- **Men** often grieve in a more solitary and cognitive manner. They are generally more oriented to fact-gathering or problem-solving.

Incongruent grief may also exist because the **bond** that develops between a pregnant woman and the developing fetus is unique and generally very intense. The mother's bond begins before the birth of the child, while the father often forms a strong bond after the birth of the child.

FACTORS THAT INFLUENCE GRIEVING FAMILIES

The emotions that individuals and families experience with the loss or severe illness/disability of an infant are varied and dependent on many **factors that influence grief**:

- **Cultural influences**: Different cultures have their own practices and beliefs concerning sickness, death, and dying, and varying rituals and ceremonies for processing loss.
- **Family system**: The family's composition, the roles of its various members, and its economic circumstances affect its expression of grief. A large family with extended community support processes grief differently from a single mother living far from home.
- **Siblings**: The impact on other children in the family must be considered, in addition to the impact on the parents.
- **History of loss**: Many diseases have a genetic component, and this may not be the first child to be affected.

MINIMIZING DILEMMAS SURROUNDING SEVERE ILLNESS OF AN INFANT

Dealing with neonates who are severely ill and not likely to survive is distressing to the staff responsible for their care. Caregivers can have dilemmas concerning adequate pain control, do not resuscitate (DNR) status, the family's cultural norms and religious beliefs that differ from their own, or grieving parents. Studies have shown that formal palliative care teams can help with issues that families face and with staff concerns. Specific procedures that may help staff deal with dying neonates include:

- Formal training in palliative care
- Assigning nurses who are comfortable with administering palliative care to dying neonates whenever possible
- Debriefing meetings shortly after a traumatic death or event to allow staff concerns to be discussed
- Consistent procedures established concerning organ donation

INTERVENTIONS FOR SPECIFIC CIRCUMSTANCES

Parents may need extra support in circumstances that lead to grief:

- **Chronic sorrow**: If grief is prolonged and the individual does not seem to be able to move forward, the individual should be encouraged to talk about feelings and express grief openly and to seek outside support, such as a therapist or support group.
- **Death of a twin or other multiple**: The parents should be allowed to hold the child if possible and encouraged to name the child, talk about the child, and express feelings of loss. Some parents may want to keep a tangible memory, such as a clipping of hair or a handprint or footprint of the child. Some may benefit from a support group.
- **Repeated obstetric loss** (recurrent abortion, still birth, preterm delivery): The losses should be acknowledged by those caring for the parents ("I'm so sorry...") and the parents encouraged to express feelings about their loss.

HELPING FAMILIES DEAL WITH THEIR DYING INFANT

The loss of an infant is an incredibly difficult time for families. In order to provide **compassionate care for the grieving family**, follow these steps:

- Recognize and acknowledge their emotions.
- Provide a private area for family members to gather.
- Allow the family members to take pictures or gather other mementos of the infant (identification bracelets, etc.).
- Discuss possible end-of-life care.
- Acknowledge that the grieving process can be a lifelong process and that each individual experiences grief in a different manner.
- Ensure the family is aware of counseling services provided by the hospital.
- Give the family contact information for local grief support groups.

> **Review Video: The Five Stages of Grief**
> Visit mometrix.com/academy and enter code: 648794

PATHOLOGIC/COMPLICATED GRIEF RESPONSES

Pathologic/Complicated grief occurs when the grieving process does not become resolved over time. The person continues to have intrusive thoughts and severe emotions for a period of greater than 6 to 12 months and typically has sleep disturbances, shows lack of interest in activities, withdraws from others, and feels severely lonely. With complicated grief, the person is at risk of comorbidities, such as depression and PTSD. **Types of complicated grief** includes:

- **Absent**: The person shows little emotion or response to grief but may experience a delayed grief reaction months or years later.
- **Chronic**: Prolonged grief that persists for years with little resolution, often associated with a codependent relationship.
- **Conflicted**: The person has ambivalent feelings about the deceased and may have little emotion initially but may feel delayed and increased grief associated with feelings of guilt.
- **Traumatic**: Associated with traumatic loss that did not allow any time to prepare. Some may react with anger or guilt.

PALLIATIVE CARE FOR CHILDREN

Palliative care is providing pain relief and comfort to the neonate who is not responding to current methods of treatment and has a poor prognosis. The goal of palliative care is to achieve the best possible quality of life for the patient and his or her family. Consider the cultural and spiritual beliefs of the family during this difficult time. In its *Policy Statement of Palliative Care for Children*, the American Academy of Pediatrics recommends the following guidelines:

- Respect for the dignity of patients and family
- Access to compassionate and competent care
- Support for the caregivers
- Improved professional and social support
- Continuing improvement through research and education
- The availability of an interdisciplinary pediatric palliative care team 24 hours a day

Family Dynamics and Psychosocial Support

FAMILY TYPES

Some of the different types of families are described below:

- **Nuclear**: This **husband-wife-children** model was once the most common family type but is no longer the norm. In this model, the husband is the provider, and the mother stays home to care for the children. This makes up only about **7%** of current American families.
- **Dual career/dual earner**: This model, where **both parents work**, is the most common in American society, including about **66%** of two-parent families. One parent may work more than another, or both may work fulltime. Income disparities may affect family dynamics.
- **Childless**: **10-15%** of families have no children because of **infertility** or **choice**.
- **Extended**: These may include **multigenerational families** or **shared households** with friends, parents, or other relatives. Childcare responsibilities may be shared or primarily assumed by an extended family member, such as a grandparent.
- **Extended kin network**: Two or more nuclear families live close together, share goods and services, and support each other, including sharing childcare. This model is common in the Hispanic community.
- **Single-parent**: This is one of the fastest-growing family models. Typically, the mother is the single parent, but in some cases, it is the father. The single parent may be widowed, divorced, or separated, but more commonly, has never married. In cases of divorce or abandonment, the child may have minimal or no contact with one parent, often the father. Single parents often face difficulties in trying to **support and care for a child** and may suffer **economic hardship.**
- **Stepparent**: Because of the high rate of divorce, stepparent families are common. This can result in **stress** and **conflict** when a new child enters the picture. There may be jealousy and resentment on the part of siblings and estranged family members. In some cases, families work together to achieve harmony and provide added support to children.
- **Binuclear/co-parenting**: In this model, children share time between two primarily nuclear families because of **joint custody agreements**. While this may at times result in conflict, the child benefits from having a continued relationship with both parents.
- **Cohabiting**: **Unmarried heterosexual couples** live together. The relationships within this model may vary, with some similar to the nuclear family. In some cases, people are in committed relationships and may avoid marriage because of economic or personal reasons. A planned child may strengthen the relationship, but an unplanned child may cause conflict.
- **Gay/lesbian**: Whether gay and lesbian couples marry or cohabit, they create families in non-traditional ways. For example, lesbian couples may use sperm donors. Gay couples often adopt. Children in these families may face social pressures because of their parents' lifestyles.

MATERNAL ATTACHMENT PROCESS

By the time of birth, most mothers have developed an emotional connection with their infants and demonstrate a number of typical steps in the **maternal attachment process**.

- **Touching**: The mother usually begins by lightly touching the infant's extremities with her fingertips and running her palm over the baby's trunk. This exploration of the infant can proceed very quickly in minutes, or be more tentative and take days. Early skin-to-skin contact with the infant tends to accelerate this process.
- **En face positioning**: The mother increases the amount of face-to-face eye contact with the infant, typically holding the infant close to her face and responding to eye contact by speaking in a sing-song, high-pitched tone (baby talk).
- **Responding**: The mother tends to respond verbally to sounds the infant makes.

Initially, the mother may feel separate and distant from the child, especially if she doesn't feel an immediate bond, and she should be reassured that these feelings are normal.

ACQUAINTANCE

During the acquaintance period, the first few days, responding helps the mother to recognize **clues** the child is giving about needs, such as hunger. The mother's ability to respond to those needs strengthens the bond and helps her gain confidence in her parenting ability. During this time, the infant is also learning to recognize **routines**, such as nursing when held toward the breast.

MUTUAL REGULATION

During this phase, which may vary in duration, the mother is learning to **balance** the needs of the infant against her own needs, and she may have some negative feelings, such as resenting her lack of sleep or feeling frustrated by the infant's crying. The mother may be afraid to express any negative feelings, fearful that people will think she is a "bad" mother, but these feelings are normal and are likely to continue until the mother and infant reach a mutual balance. The ability of the mother and infant to recognize each other's cues and respond to them is termed **reciprocity**.

MATERNAL ATTACHMENT/BONDING ASSESSMENT

Assessment of maternal attachment/bonding should be done prior to discharge so that any issues and needed interventions can be discussed. In doing the assessment, the nurse evaluates the mother's:

- Progression in touching and face-to-face eye contact with extended times and indications of attraction, such as verbally responding to the infant and cuddling the infant. If there has been no progression, the nurse should assess contributing environmental, cultural, and social factors that may be interfering.
- Consistency in caring for the infant and seeking knowledge about and validation of her infant care; adjusting care to the needs of the infant. Sensitivity to infant's needs, such as recognizing discomfort or hunger quickly and exhibiting pleasure at infant's response to her efforts.
- Pleasure in the infant, expressed by calling the infant by name, noting family traits/characteristics, showing overt happiness. If the mother shows displeasure or apathy, this may indicate poor attachment, but might also indicate that the mother is experiencing pain or weakness.

PATERNAL ATTACHMENT

Paternal attachment, referred to as engrossment, occurs in many ways similar to maternal attachment. The father may feel pride and wonderment at the child and develop a strong sense of nurturing. Early and frequent contact with the infant promotes engrossment, so the nurse should ensure that the father is not overlooked after delivery but is able to hold, touch, and respond to the child as soon as possible.

SIBLING AND FAMILY ATTACHMENT

Siblings should be allowed to visit the mother and infant as early as possible and be encouraged to hold or care for the infant as appropriate for their ages. Siblings sometimes feel left out or overshadowed by the new infant, so it's important that the parents take time to talk to the siblings and give them attention as well. Grandparents and other family members also form attachments to the infant and should be included.

SIBLING RESPONSES/INTERVENTIONS

If there are abnormalities or complications with the neonate, this may cause stress to the **siblings**. Younger children may be hostile and older children ashamed. They may feel guilty about their responses, and they may feel neglected as parents go through the stages of grief and are unable to provide the support that the siblings need. In some cases, parents may express their concern by focusing their anxiety on one of the siblings, becoming hypercritical. In these cases, staff may need to intervene by discussing observations with the parents and encouraging other family members to provide support to the siblings. Parents' groups that involve the entire family can be very helpful. Whenever possible, children should be included in education and demonstrations and encouraged to ask questions. Age-appropriate books and other materials that explain medical conditions and treatments should be available for siblings.

PREPARATION OF SIBLINGS FOR BIRTH OF INFANT

Preparation of siblings prior to the birth of an infant can decrease anxiety and sibling rivalry by helping the children feel that they are participants in the process and are valued. Children should be prepared for physical changes in the mother, changing family dynamics, and infant care. Formal classes may be available for children ages 3-12 to help them identify and express their concerns, and to teach them about pregnancy and childcare. Booklets, books, and videos are also available. The parent or teacher may use dolls to demonstrate childcare and allow the children to practice holding and caring for the baby. When possible, children should have contact with an infant, such as that of a friend or family member. Children may help to decorate the infant's room or prepare a welcome gift, such as a drawing or toy. Children should be told who will care for them during labor and delivery and should visit the mother and infant as soon after delivery as possible.

BARRIERS TO PARENT-INFANT INTERACTION

There are many **barriers to parent-infant interaction**, especially with preterm infants or those with genetic disabilities or birth defects that require prolonged hospitalization or treatment. Barriers include:

- **Physical separation**: When the infant cannot be held or fed, when the child is transported to a different facility outside of the area, or when the mother is discharged and the infant remains hospitalized, attachment can be difficult to form.
- **Lack of clear understanding of handicaps or developmental problems**: Lack of infant response is sometimes interpreted as rejection, and parents may be frightened by abnormalities.
- **Attitude of medical staff**: Negative attitudes may cause the parent to grieve rather than attach to the child. Staff members need to encourage the parents to become involved in the child's care and to provide stimulation. Staff often needs to demonstrate care to parents, who may be intimidated by the infant's condition and medical needs.
- **Environmental overload**: The equipment (alarms, ventilators, monitors) and environmental constraints (no chairs) may overwhelm parents.

CULTURAL/LIFESTYLE FACTORS AFFECTING FAMILY INTEGRATION

VALUES

Values based on attitudes, ideas, and beliefs often connect family members to common **goals**. However, these values may be influenced by many **external factors**, such as education, social norms, and attitudes of peers, other family, and coworkers, so values may change and impact family integration.

ROLES

In some families, roles are clearly defined by **gender** and **task** (homemaker and breadwinner), but the roles blur or are **shared** in many families, and in some cases, the father becomes the primary caregiver while the mother works. Other common roles include peacemaker, nurturer, and social planner. How these roles are perceived and actualized affects the manner in which a child is integrated into the family.

DECISION-MAKING

Family power structures vary widely, but in many families, **power** rests with one person who makes ultimate decisions and whose opinions affect other family members. In cultures with a strong emphasis on tradition, power often lies with the father, a grandparent, or another family member. However, it should not be assumed that the families of a given cultural background will always have the same power structure. Instead, power may be **shared** or it may rest with either the mother or the father.

SOCIOECONOMIC

Employment trends, marriage rates, and economic trends all affect **family integration**. Many people have become unemployed and are unable to support their families, resulting in severe **stress**, which may be exacerbated by the arrival of a new child. The divorce rate is high, leaving many parents with inadequate funds to support a child. Even if both parents are employed, the cost of living continues to escalate, including the cost of caring for a child.

MOTHER RELINQUISHING CHILD FOR ADOPTION

A mother relinquishing her child for **adoption** may have feelings of ambivalence and sadness. Many who relinquish their infants for adoption are young and unmarried. Adoptions may be closed or open, so procedures will vary. In some open adoptions, the adoptive parent(s) may accompany the mother and participate in the birth, with the birth mother relinquishing the child immediately after birth. In this case, the adoptive parents should be treated as the actual parents of the child, while staff should recognize the needs of the birth mother and provide for her emotional and physical support. In other cases, the child is first relinquished to an agency, such as Social Services, which then places the child. If possible, prior to the birth, the birth mother should indicate how she wants to handle the birth. Some want to hold and spend time with the child; others do not. The birth mother should be in a single room, rather than with other mothers, to protect her privacy.

MOOD DISORDERS

POSTPARTUM DEPRESSION

Postpartum major mood disorder, commonly referred to as postpartum depression, occurs in about 10-15% of mothers. Onset may occur before or during pregnancy or any time within the first year postpartum, but is most common within the first few months postpartum. Duration varies but is usually 3-14 months. Risk factors include primiparity, history of depression, bipolar disease, or previous postpartum depression, lack of stable and supportive social and family relationships, family history of psychiatric illness, and ambivalence about pregnancy. Symptoms are typical of depression and include sadness, crying, insomnia or excess sleeping, difficulty concentrating or making decisions, phobias, anxiety, lack of interest in activities, and feeling out of control or helpless. The mother may be irritable and hostile, especially toward the child. She may also be suicidal. Treatment may include psychotherapy, antidepressants, antipsychotics, and/or lithium. In some cases, the child may need to be cared for by others until the mother's depression lessens.

> **Review Video: Peripartum Depression**
> Visit mometrix.com/academy and enter code: 975380

POSTPARTUM PSYCHOSIS

Postpartum psychosis may occur up to 3 months postpartum, but symptoms are usually evident within the first 3 weeks, with sudden onset of **psychotic Criterion A symptoms**, such as delusions, hallucinations, insomnia, anorexia, paranoia, and suicidal or homicidal ideation. In 4% of cases, mothers have committed infanticide, sometimes because of voices urging them to do so, so postpartum psychosis is a **medical emergency** that often requires hospitalization. Mothers should be carefully supervised when caring for their children until symptoms have abated, or children may need to be removed from the mother until the mother stabilizes. While postpartum psychosis is most common in mothers with a history of mental illness (such as schizophrenia or bipolar disease), it can occur in mothers with no such history. The cause is unclear but may be a combination of **hormonal imbalance** and **stress/anxiety**. Treatment includes psychotherapy, mood stabilizers, antipsychotics, and benzodiazepines. Antidepressants may cause mood cycling if psychosis is associated with bipolar disorder.

Professional Issues

Ethical Principles

ETHICAL PRINCIPLES

Autonomy is the ethical principle that the individual has the right to make decisions about his or her own care. In the case of children or patients with dementia who cannot make autonomous decisions, parents or family members may serve as the legal decision maker. The nurse must keep the patient and/or family fully informed so that they can exercise their autonomy in informed decision-making.

Justice is the ethical principle that relates to the distribution of the limited resources of healthcare benefits to the members of society. These resources must be distributed fairly. This issue may arise if there is only one bed left and two sick patients. Justice comes into play in deciding which patient should stay and which should be transported or otherwise cared for. The decision should be made according to what is best or most just for the patients and not colored by personal bias.

Beneficence is an ethical principle that involves performing actions that are for the purpose of benefitting another person. In the care of a patient, any procedure or treatment should be done with the ultimate goal of benefitting the patient, and any actions that are not beneficial should be reconsidered. As conditions change, procedures need to be continually reevaluated to determine if they are still of benefit.

Nonmaleficence is an ethical principle that means healthcare workers should provide care in a manner that does not cause direct intentional harm to the patient:

- The actual act must be good or morally neutral.
- The intent must be only for a good effect.
- A bad effect cannot serve as the means to get to a good effect.
- A good effect must have more benefit than a bad effect has harm.

NURSING CODE OF ETHICS

There is more interest in the **ethics** involved in healthcare due to technological advances that have made the prolongation of life, organ transplants, prenatal manipulation, and saving of premature infants possible, sometimes with poor outcomes. Couple these with healthcare's limited resources, and **ethical dilemmas** abound. Ethics is the study of **morality** as the value that controls actions. The American Nurses Association Code of Ethics contains nine statements defining **principles** the nurse can use when faced with moral and ethical problems. Nurses must be knowledgeable about the many ethical issues in healthcare and about the field of ethics in general. The nurse must help a patient to reveal their values and morals to the health care team so that the patient, family, and team can resolve moral issues pertaining to the patient's care. As part of the healthcare team, the nurse has a right to express personal values and moral concerns about medical issues.

BIOETHICS

Bioethics is a branch of ethics that involves making sure that the medical treatment given is the most morally correct choice given the different options that might be available and the differences inherent in the varied levels of treatment. In the health care unit, if the patients, family members, and the staff are in agreement when it comes to values and decision-making, then no ethical dilemma exists; however, when there is a difference in value beliefs between the patients/family members and the staff, there is a bioethical dilemma that must be resolved. Sometimes, discussion and explanation can resolve differences, but at times the institution's ethics committee must be brought in to resolve the conflict. The primary goal of bioethics is to determine the most morally correct action using the set of circumstances given.

ETHICAL DECISION-MAKING MODEL

There are many ethical decision-making models. Some general guidelines to apply in using ethical decision-making models could be the following:

- Gather information about the identified problem
- State reasonable alternatives and solutions to the problem
- Utilize ethical resources (for example, clergy or ethics committees) to help determine the ethically important elements of each solution or alternative
- Suggest and attempt possible solutions
- Choose a solution to the problem

It is important to always consider the **ethical principles** of autonomy, beneficence, nonmaleficence, justice, and fidelity when attempting to facilitate ethical decision-making with family members, caregivers, and the healthcare team.

ETHICAL ASSESSMENT

While the terms *ethics* and *morals* are sometimes used interchangeably, ethics is a study of morals and encompasses concepts of right and wrong. When making **ethical assessments,** one must consider not only what people should do but also what they actually do, as these two things are sometimes at odds. Ethical issues can be difficult to assess because of personal bias, which is one of the reasons that sharing concerns with other internal sources and reaching consensus is so valuable. Issues of concern might include options for care, refusal of care, rights to privacy, adequate relief of suffering, and the right to self-determination. Internal sources might include the ethics committee, whose role is to make decisions regarding ethical issues. Risk management can provide guidance related to personal and institutional liability. External agencies might include government agencies, such as the public health department.

ETHICAL ANALYSIS OF A SITUATION

Assessment of the situation is done to reveal the ethical, legal, and professional **conflicts** that are present. Those who are involved are identified, including the patient, family, and healthcare personnel. The decision maker is determined if it is not the patient. Information about the situation is collected to determine medical facts about the disease and condition of the patient, options for treatment, and nursing diagnoses. Any pertinent legal information is included. The patient and family's cultural, religious, and moral values are determined. Possible courses of action are listed and compared in terms of outcomes for the patient using the utilitarian or deontological theory of ethics. Professional codes of ethics are also applied. A decision is made and evaluated as to whether it is the most morally correct action. Ethical arguments for and against the decision are given and responded to by the decision maker.

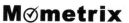

PROFESSIONAL BOUNDARIES

GIFTS

Over time, patients may develop a bond with nurses they trust and may feel grateful to the nurse for the care provided and want to express thanks, but the nurse must make sure to maintain professional boundaries. Patients often offer **gifts** to nurses to show their appreciation, but some adults, especially those who are weak and ill or have cognitive impairment, may be taken advantage of easily. Patients may offer valuables and may sometimes be easily manipulated into giving large sums of money. Small tokens of appreciation that can be shared with other staff, such as a box of chocolates, are usually acceptable (depending upon the policy of the institution), but almost any other gifts (jewelry, money, clothes) should be declined: "I'm sorry, that's so kind of you, but nurses are not allowed to accept gifts from patients." Declining may relieve the patient of the feeling of obligation.

SEXUAL RELATIONS

When the boundary between the role of the professional nurse and the vulnerability of the patient is breached, a boundary violation occurs. Because the nurse is in the position of authority, the responsibility to maintain the boundary rests with the nurse; however, the line separating them is a continuum and sometimes not easily defined. It is inappropriate for nurses to engage in **sexual relations** with patients, and if the sexual behavior is coerced or the patient is cognitively impaired, it is **illegal**. However, more common violations with adults, particularly elderly patients, include exposing a patient unnecessarily, using sexually demeaning gestures or language (including off-color jokes), harassment, or inappropriate touching. Touching should be used with care, such as touching a hand or shoulder. Hugging may be misconstrued.

ATTENTION

Nursing is a giving profession, but the nurse must temper giving with recognition of professional boundaries. Patients have many needs. As acts of kindness, nurses (especially those involved in home care) often give certain patients extra attention and may offer to do **favors**, such as cooking or shopping. They may become overly invested in the patients' lives. While this may benefit a patient in the short term, it can establish a relationship of increasing **dependency** and **obligation** that does not resolve the long-term needs of the patient. Making referrals to the appropriate agencies or collaborating with family to find ways to provide services is more effective. Becoming overly invested may be evident by the nurse showing favoritism or spending too much time with the patient while neglecting other duties. On the other end of the spectrum are nurses who are disinterested and fail to provide adequate attention to the patient's detriment. Lack of adequate attention may lead to outright neglect.

COERCION

Power issues are inherent in matters associated with professional boundaries. Physical abuse is both unprofessional and illegal, but behavior can easily border on abusive without the patient being physically injured. Nurses can easily **intimidate** older adults and sick patients into having procedures or treatments they do not want. Regardless of age, patients have the right to choose and the right to refuse treatment. Difficulties arise with cognitive impairment, and in that case, another responsible adult (often the patient's child or spouse) is designated to make decisions, but every effort should be made to gain patient cooperation. Forcing the patient to do something against his or her will borders on abuse and can sometimes degenerate into actual abuse if physical coercion is involved.

PERSONAL INFORMATION

When pre-existing personal or business relationships exist, other nurses should be assigned care of the patient whenever possible, but this may be difficult in small communities. However, the nurse should strive to maintain a professional role separate from the personal role and respect professional boundaries. The nurse must respect and maintain the confidentiality of the patient and family members, but the nurse must also be very careful about **disclosing personal information** about him or herself because this establishes a social relationship that interferes with the professional role of the nurse and the boundary between the patient and the nurse. The nurse and patient should never share secrets. When the nurse divulges personal information, he or she may become vulnerable to the patient, a reversal of roles.

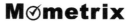

Professional/Legal Issues

INFORMED CONSENT FOR NEONATES

Parents/guardians of neonates must provide **informed consent** for all treatment the infant receives. This includes providing the parents/guardians with a thorough explanation of all procedures, treatments, and associated risks. Parents/guardians should be apprised of all options and allowed input on the type of treatments. Parents/guardians should also be apprised of all reasonable risks and any complications that might be life-threatening or might increase morbidity. The American Medical Association has established guidelines for informed consent:

- Explanation of diagnosis
- Nature of and reason for treatment or procedure
- Risks and benefits
- Alternative options (regardless of cost or insurance coverage)
- Risks and benefits of alternative options
- Risks and benefits of not having a treatment or procedure

Providing informed consent is a requirement of all states.

ADVANCE DIRECTIVES AND DO-NOT-RESUSCITATE ORDERS FOR INFANTS

In accordance with federal and state laws, individuals have the right to self-determination in health care, including making decisions about end-of-life care through **advance directives,** such as living wills and the right to assign a surrogate person to make decisions through a durable power of attorney. Parents/guardians have the right to make these decisions for minors. Parents/guardians should routinely be questioned about an advance directive, as they may present at a healthcare organization without the document.

If parents/guardians indicate the desire for a **do-not-resuscitate (DNR) order** for a seriously ill child, that child should not receive resuscitative treatments for terminal illness or conditions in which meaningful recovery cannot occur. For those with DNR requests or those withdrawing life support, staff should provide the child palliative rather than curative measures, such as pain control and/or oxygen, and emotional support to the child and family. Religious traditions and beliefs about death should be treated with respect.

NURSE-PATIENT RATIOS

Nurse-patient ratios refer to the number of patients assigned to a nurse. For example, if one nurse is assigned responsibility for 4 patients, the ratio is 1:4. Ratios are an area of concern because studies have consistently shown better outcomes for patients with lower nurse-patient ratios. However, the lower the ratio, the higher the costs. Only California currently has mandated nurse-patient ratios. The California law, often cited as a model, requires a 1:1 ratio in the operating room and for trauma patients in the ER, and a 1:2 ratio for patients in ICU, NICU, post-anesthesia recovery, and labor and delivery, as well as ICU patients in the ER. Ratios in other areas range from 1:3 to 1:6 (the maximum). Massachusetts has a mandate for ICU only: 1:1 or 1:2. A number of other states require staffing committees to establish staffing policies, and some states require public reporting of nurse-patient ratios even though they do not mandate the ratios.

MEDICAL RECORD DOCUMENTATION

Proper **documentation** is a cornerstone in nursing care. It is a way to communicate patient status to other caregivers. It provides a snapshot of the patient's condition during that moment in time. It documents care given, responses to that care, and further interventions taken. Documentation should be streamlined as much as possible to make efficient use of nursing time. Documentation should be thorough and provide enough information for a subsequent reviewer to reach the same conclusions as the nurse did when giving care. Proper documentation is also the best defense against litigation. Information charted in real time may need to be reviewed by the one who charted it several years later, so it is imperative that the nurse document all of the information required to defend their actions.

SENTINEL EVENTS IN PERINATAL SERVICES

A sentinel event is one that requires specific actions by a Joint Commission–accredited institution. These events are so serious that they require immediate investigation and response. The **criteria** for these events in perinatal services are any event that results in:

- Unexpected death or loss of function
- Harm due to a medication error or suicide
- Maternal death during the intrapartum period
- Death of a full-term infant
- Infant abduction
- Release of the infant to the wrong family
- Blood group incompatibility causing a hemolytic transfusion reaction
- Wrong surgery
- Retention of the foreign body after surgery
- Hyperbilirubinemia above 30 mg/dL

AREAS OF OBSTETRICAL NURSING PRONE TO LITIGATION

Certain areas of care are more highly scrutinized during litigation. The policies and procedures guiding care in these areas should be reviewed continually to be sure they are in line with national standards. **Litigation** is common in the areas of FHR interpretation, documentation, and communication; telephone triage; labor induction; the use of misoprostol or oxytocin; hyperstimulation interventions; response to pain; nursing role during regional anesthesia; use of fundal pressure; interventions for shoulder dystocia; management of the second stage of labor; use of forceps and vacuum extraction; expedited cesarean births; vaginal birth after cesarean birth (VBAC); care of multiple gestations; unintended prematurity; neonatal resuscitation; and prevention of Group B streptococcal infection in the newborn.

MALPRACTICE AND NEGLIGENCE RISKS FOR THE NEONATAL NURSE PRACTITIONER

Neonatal nurse practitioners, as all advance practice nurses, are usually insured for **malpractice** at a higher rate than registered nurses because their scope of practice is much wider. An NNP may be sued individually or as part of a medical group to which the NNP is associated. Because a suit is a civil matter, loss of judgment may not be reported to the state board of nursing. If a charge of negligence is brought to the attention of the board, the board may initiate an investigation and disciplinary action. Negligence may involve a number of failures, such as not referring a patient when needed, incorrect diagnosis, incorrect treatment, and not providing the patient/family with adequate or essential information. Once an NNP has established a duty to a patient—by direct examination or even a casual in-person or over-the-phone conversation that involves professional advice—the NNP may be liable for malpractice if he or she does not follow up with adequate care.

TYPES OF NEGLIGENCE

Risk management must attempt to determine the burden of proof for acts of **negligence**, including compliance with duty, breaches in procedures, degree of harm, and cause. Negligence indicates that *proper care* has not been provided, based on established standards. *Reasonable care* uses rationales for decision-making in relation to providing care. State regulations regarding negligence may vary, but all have some statutes of limitations. There are a number of different types of negligence:

- **Negligent conduct**, meaning that an individual failed to provide reasonable care or to protect/assist another, based on standards and expertise.
- **Gross negligence**, or willfully providing inadequate care while disregarding the safety and security of another.
- **Contributory negligence**, in which the injured party has contributed to his/her own harm.
- **Comparative negligence**, which attributes a percentage of negligence to each individual involved.

ETHICAL PRINCIPLES ENDORSED BY NANN AND ANA

Both the National Association of Neonatal Nurses (NANN) and the American Nurses Association (ANA) have **codes of ethics** that outline the responsibilities of the neonatal nurse. General concepts emphasized include:

- Respect the human rights of patients and families regardless of race, gender, etc.
- Use nursing skills for the advancement of human welfare.
- Remember, the nurse's primary responsibility is to the patient.
- Respect family autonomy and provide accurate information.
- Ensure that patient's and family's rights and privacy are maintained in accordance with HIPAA regulations.
- Ensure that colleagues are competent; report incompetents, impaired colleagues, or those with questionable behavior.
- Maintain competence through accountability, responsibility, and continuing education.
- Enhance the nursing environment through participation in policy development and participation in professional organizations.

PROFESSIONAL ORGANIZATIONS

Many **professional neonatal and pediatric nursing organizations** are available for neonatal nurses to join. A professional organization is a group of practitioners who share a common interest. They are able to form a collective voice that can influence standards of practice, institutional policies, and governing regulations and laws. They may have admission standards for those wishing to join and provide ethical guidelines for members. Other benefits often include educational opportunities in a chosen area of specialty, newsletters concerning healthcare trends and issues that affect their specialty area, and gatherings where peers meet for discussions. Some organizations available for neonatal nurses include:

- The Academy of Neonatal Nurses (ANN)
- The Association of Women's Health, Obstetric, and Neonatal Nurses (AWHONN)
- The National Association of Neonatal Nurses (NANN)
- The National Association of Pediatric Nurse Practitioners (NAPNP)

BOARD OF NURSING

Each state has its own Nurse Practice Act, which is governed by the state **Board of Nursing**. The Nurse Practice Act outlines requirements for licensure and certification and delineates the scope of practice of nurses, including duties and delegation. Typically, licensure is granted to those who complete an accredited LVN/LPN or RN program and pass the nursing exam (NCLEX) or receive endorsement because of licensure in another state. The neonatal nurse practitioner (NNP) must practice within the standards of advanced practice under the Nurse Practice Act in the state in which the person works and the individual's scope of practice, which is directly related to the individual's educational preparation and certification. In some cases, NNP certification in one state is automatically recognized in other states through the Compact agreement. Educational experience and scope of practice must relate to patient population in terms of age, disease, diagnosis, and treatment.

ORGANIZATIONS REGULATING THE PHILOSOPHY OF CARE IN BIRTHING FACILITY

The philosophy of care in a birthing unit must be an agreement that all care given be based on evidence and national standards and guidelines. All policies and procedures should be written with the guidance of these materials. They should be reviewed as needed in the light of additional evidence and changes in guidelines by major professional organizations. These organizations include the Association of Women's Health, Obstetric and Neonatal Nurses (AWHONN), the American College of Obstetricians and Gynecologists (ACOG), the American College of Nurse Midwives (ACNM), the American Academy of Pediatrics (AAP), the American Society of Anesthesiologists (ASA), the Joint Commission (TJC), the Centers for Disease Control (CDC), the American Heart Association (AHA), and the Food and Drug Administration (FDA).

NEONATAL NURSE PRACTITIONER

A neonatal nurse practitioner (NNP) is a registered nurse who also has a graduate degree in nursing with a concentration in advanced care of the neonate. The NNP manages daily care of several neonates in the Intensive Care Unit. The NNP assesses physical signs, evaluates laboratory results and clinical data, consults with specialists, writes orders, and interacts with parents to provide support and updates on the clinical status of their neonate. The NNP is responsible for delivery room management of the high risk neonate, intubation, placement of umbilical lines, lumbar punctures, percutaneous placement of arterial and central lines, and insertion of chest tubes. These activities are performed under the direction and supervision of an attending neonatologist.

PREREQUISITES FOR RN TO BECOME NNP AND EXPANSION IN SCOPE FROM RN TO NNP

Prerequisites for an RN to become a Neonatal Nurse Practitioner include a current state nursing license demonstrating successful completion of a nursing program and completion of a post-baccalaureate accredited graduate program at the doctorate or master's level in neonatal nursing. In order to receive NNP certification from the National Certification Corporation (NCC), the graduate program must have been at least one academic year in duration with at least 200 hours didactic and 600 clinical. The certification exam must be taken within 8 years of graduation. While both the RN and NNP monitor patients and provide direct nursing care, the NNP has a broader **scope of practice** and prescriptive authority and can order medications and treatments while the RN cannot. Additionally, the NNP can establish an independent practice (supervisory requirements may vary from state to state) and work directly with patients and family to establish plans of care. The NNP may bill Medicare, Medicaid, and insurance companies directly for services provided while the RN may not.

Evidence-Based Practice

CLASSES OF EVIDENCE-BASED PRACTICE

Evidence-based practice is treatment based on the best possible evidence, including a study of current research. Literature is searched to find evidence of the most effective treatments for specific diseases or injuries, and those treatments are then utilized to create clinical pathways that outline specific multi-departmental treatment protocols, including medications, treatments, and timelines. Evidence-based guidelines are often produced by specialty organizations that undertake the task of searching and analyzing literature to produce policies, procedures, and guidelines that become the standard of care for the disease. These guidelines are then used when a patient fits the disease criteria for that guideline.

Evidence-based nursing aims to improve the quality of nursing care by examining the reasons for all nursing practices and determining those that have the most positive outcomes. Evidence-based nursing focuses on the individual nurse utilizing evidence-based observations to influence decision-making.

EVIDENCE-BASED PRACTICE GUIDELINES

The creation of evidence-based practice guidelines includes the following components:

- **Focus on the topic/methodology:** This includes outlining possible interventions and treatments for review, choosing patient populations and settings, and determining significant outcomes. Search boundaries (such as types of journals, types of studies, dates of studies) should be determined.
- **Evidence review:** This includes review of literature, critical analysis of studies, and summarizing of results, including pooled meta-analysis.
- **Expert judgment:** Recommendations based on personal experience from a number of experts may be utilized, especially if there is inadequate evidence based on review, but this subjective evidence should be explicitly acknowledged.
- **Policy considerations:** This includes cost-effectiveness, access to care, insurance coverage, availability of qualified staff, and legal implications.
- **Policy:** A written policy must be completed with recommendations. Common practice is to utilize letter guidelines, with "A" being the most highly recommended, usually based on the quality of supporting evidence.
- **Review:** The completed policy should be submitted to peers for review and comments before instituting the policy.

CRITICAL PATHWAYS

Clinical/critical pathway development is done by those involved in direct patient care. The pathway should require no additional staffing and cover the entire scope of an illness. Steps include:

1. Selection of patient group and diagnosis, procedures, or conditions, based on analysis of data and observations of wide variance in approach to treatment and prioritizing organization and patient needs
2. Creation of interdisciplinary team of those involved in the process of care, including physicians to develop pathway
3. Analysis of data including literature review and study of best practices to identify opportunities for quality improvement
4. Identification of all categories of care, such as nutrition, medications, and nursing
5. Discussion and reaching consensus

6. Identifying the levels of care and number of days to be covered by the pathway
7. Pilot testing and redesigning steps as indicated
8. Educating staff about standards
9. Monitoring and tracking variances in order to improve pathways

LEVELS OF EVIDENCE IN EVIDENCE-BASED PRACTICE

Levels of evidence are categorized according to the scientific evidence available to support the recommendations, as well as existing state and federal laws. While recommendations are voluntary, they are often used as a basis for state and federal regulations.

- **Category IA** is well supported by evidence from experimental, clinical, or epidemiologic studies and is strongly recommended for implementation.
- **Category IB** has supporting evidence from some studies, has a good theoretical basis, and is strongly recommended for implementation.
- **Category IC** is required by state or federal regulations or is an industry standard.
- **Category II** is supported by suggestive clinical or epidemiologic studies, has a theoretical basis, and is suggested for implementation.
- **Category III** is supported by descriptive studies, such as comparisons, correlations, and case studies, and may be useful.
- **Category IV** is obtained from expert opinion or authorities only.
- **Unresolved** means there is no recommendation because of a lack of consensus or evidence.

OUTCOME EVALUATION

Outcome evaluation is an important component of evidence-based practice, which involves both internal and external research. All treatments are subjected to review to determine if they produce positive outcomes, and policies and protocols for outcome evaluation should be in place. **Outcome evaluation** includes the following:

- **Monitoring** over the course of treatment involves careful observation and record-keeping that notes progress, with supporting laboratory and radiographic evidence as indicated by condition and treatment.
- **Evaluating** results includes reviewing records as well as current research to determine if outcomes are within acceptable parameters.
- **Sustaining** involves discontinuing treatment but continuing to monitor and evaluate.
- **Improving** means to continue the treatment but with additions or modifications in order to improve outcomes.
- **Replacing** the treatment with a different treatment must be done if outcome evaluation indicates that current treatment is ineffective.

EVIDENCE-BASED NURSING INTERVENTIONS

Evidence-based nursing interventions enable nurses to provide high-quality patient care that is based upon research and knowledge, as opposed to giving care that is based upon tradition or information that is out of date. An evidence-based nursing approach is based on the integration of practical clinical experience with medical and clinical research; it utilizes proven clinical guidelines and assessment practices. Evidence-based nursing interventions allow nurses to make patient care decisions based on cutting-edge research that has been scientifically validated. Studies show that evidence-based nursing practice yields improved patient outcomes, enables nurses to practice up-to-date methods, improves nurse confidence and decision-making skills, and enhances Joint Commission standards.

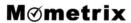

RESOURCES

There are numerous information resources for evidence-based nursing interventions. These resources include evidence-based textbooks; databases such as CINAHL Plus, COCHRANE library, Mosby's Nursing Index, NursingConsult, and Nursing@Ovid; evidence-based nursing metasites such as the Academic Center for EBN, Joanna Briggs Institute, McGill University, ONS-EBN section, and EBN-University of Minnesota; online evidence-based nursing journals such as Clinical Nurse Specialist, Clinical Nursing Research, Evidence-Based Nursing, Journal of Nursing Care Quality, Journal of Advanced Nursing, Journal of Nursing Scholarship, Nurse Researcher, Nursing Research, Western Journal of Nursing Research, and Worldviews on Evidence-Based Nursing; and various online tutorials.

OBTAINING RESULTS OF RESEARCH TO USE IN EVIDENCE-BASED PRACTICE

When searching for **current evidence** in print and online literature, the nurse should look for **systematic reviews, analyses, and reports**. PUBMED lists all literature and can be searched for all published articles on a particular subject. These articles can be analyzed to determine treatments that have the best evidence of efficacy. Subject and methodological terms and clinical filters can be used to find necessary information, including a specific medical subject heading (MH), subheading (SH), publication type (PT), and text word (TW). The nurse should also search the National Guideline Clearinghouse, Cochrane Databases, Agency for Healthcare Research and Quality, and US Preventive Services Task Force Recommendations for evidence and guidelines. When trials of a treatment provide evidence of effectiveness, the evidence is weighed for strength and confidence. Those that provide the strongest evidence of efficacy become recommendations and guidelines for use in the field. Research is also done on a smaller scale by specialists who publish in peer-reviewed journals their research results related to the use of a particular intervention.

ELEMENTS OF RESEARCH

The following are elements of research:

- **Variable**: An entity that can be different within a population
- **Independent variable**: The variable that the researchers change to evaluate its effect
- **Dependent variable**: The variable that may be changed by alterations in the independent variable
- **Hypothesis**: The proposed explanation to describe an expected outcome in a study
- **Sample**: The selected population to be studied
- **Experimental group**: The population within the sample that undergoes the treatment or intervention
- **Control group**: The population within the sample that is not exposed to the treatment of intervention being evaluated

The nurse must be taught and must understand the process of critical analysis and know how to conduct a survey of the literature. **Basic research concepts** include:

- **Survey of valid sources**: Information from a juried journal and an anonymous website or personal website are very different sources, and evaluating what constitutes a valid source of data is critical.
- **Evaluation of internal and external validity**: Internal validity shows a cause-and-effect relationship between two variables, with the cause occurring before the effect and no intervening variable. External validity occurs when results hold true in different environments and circumstances with different populations.

- **Sample selection and sample size**: Selection and size can have a huge impact on the results, but a sample that is too small may lack both internal and external validity. Selection may be so narrowly focused that the results can't be generalized to other groups.

VALIDITY, GENERALIZABILITY, AND REPLICABILITY

Many research studies are most concerned with **internal validity** (adequate unbiased data properly collected and analyzed within the population studied), but studies that determine the efficacy of procedures or treatments, for example, should have **external validity** as well; that is, the results should be **generalizable** (true) for similar populations. **Replication** of the study under different circumstances and with different subjects and researchers should produce similar results. For various reasons, some people may be excluded from a study so that instead of randomized subjects, the subjects may be highly selected so when data is compared with another population in which there is less or more selection, results may be different. The selection of subjects, in this case, would interfere with external validity. Part of the design of a study should include considerations of whether or not it should have external validity or whether there is value for the institution based solely on internal validation.

HYPOTHESIS

A hypothesis should be generated about the probable cause of the disease/infection based on the information available in laboratory and medical records, epidemiologic study, literature review, and expert opinion. For example, a hypothesis should include the infective agent, the likely source, and the mode of transmission: "Wound infections with *Staphylococcus aureus* were caused by reuse and inadequate sterilization of single-use irrigation syringes used during wound care in the ICU."

Hypothesis testing includes data analysis, laboratory findings, and outcomes of environmental testing. It usually includes case-control studies, with 2-4 controls picked for each case of infection. They may be matched according to age, sex, or other characteristics, but they are not infected at the time they are picked for the study. Cohort studies, whose controls are picked based on having or lacking exposure, may also be instituted. If the hypothesis cannot be supported, then a new hypothesis or different testing methods may be necessary.

CRITICAL READING

There are several steps to critical reading to evaluate research:

- **Consider the source** of the material. If it is in the popular press, it may have little validity compared to something published in a peer-reviewed journal.
- **Review the author's credentials** to determine if a person is an expert in the field of study.
- **Determine the thesis**, or the central claim of the research. It should be clearly stated.
- **Examine the organization** of the article, whether it is based on a particular theory, and the type of methodology used.
- **Review the evidence** to determine how it is used to support the main points. Look for statistical evidence and sample size to determine if the findings have wide applicability.
- **Evaluate** the overall article to determine if the information seems credible and useful and should be communicated to administration and/or staff.

Major Study Types Utilized in Statistical Analysis

When conducting research, the nurse should be aware of the **types of studies** available and when each type of study is appropriate and most reliable:

- **Case-control studies** are simple. They use pre-existing cases with and without the disorder of interest. For example, case-control studies may be done with mesothelioma and exposure to possible pleural irritants. These are good for rare diseases to determine cause and effect.
- **Cross-sectional studies** utilize a cross-section of data from the population and analyze variables at one time point. They are not good for determining cause and effect, but they are useful for correlating characteristics with disorders.
- **Cohort studies** follow a cohort of a population for a period of time and attempt to make a link with diseases. As in the previous example, researchers could follow a group exposed to asbestos and study the incidence of mesothelioma.
- **Randomized controlled trial** is the gold standard, with patients assigned to the control or experimental group. This is a difficult type of test to design and implement but very useful, as the data is often well-controlled. It is the most expensive type of study.

Bias in Research

Selection bias occurs when the method of selecting subjects results in a cohort that is not representative of the target population because of inherent error in design. For example, if all patients who develop urinary infections are evaluated per urine culture and sensitivities for microbial resistance, but only those patients with clinically-evident infections are included, a number of patients with sub-clinical infections may be missed, skewing the results. Selection bias is only a concern when participants in studies are specifically chosen. Many surveillance studies do not involve the selection of subjects.

Information bias occurs when there are errors in classification, so an estimate of association is incorrect. Non-differential misclassification occurs when there is similar misclassification of disease or exposure among both those who are diseased/exposed and those who are not. Differential misclassification occurs when there is a differing misclassification of disease or exposure among both those who are diseased/exposed and those who are not.

Qualitative and Quantitative Data

Both qualitative and quantitative data are used for analysis, but the focus is quite different:

- **Qualitative data**: Data are described verbally or graphically, and the results are subjective, depending upon observers to provide information. Interviews may be used as a tool to gather information, and the researcher's interpretation of data is important. Gathering this type of data can be time-intensive, and it can usually not be generalized to a larger population. This type of information gathering is often useful at the beginning of the design process for data collection.
- **Quantitative data**: Data are described in terms of numbers within a statistical format. This type of information gathering is done after the design of data collection is outlined, usually in later stages. Tools may include surveys, questionnaires, or other methods of obtaining numerical data. The researcher's role is objective.

CONTINUOUS QUALITY IMPROVEMENT

Continuous quality improvement is a multidisciplinary management philosophy that can be applied to all aspects of an organization, whether related to such varied areas as the cardiac unit, purchasing, or human resources. The skills used for epidemiologic research (data collection, analysis, outcomes, action plans) are all applicable to the analysis of multiple types of events, because they are based on solid scientific methods. Multi-disciplinary planning can bring valuable insights from various perspectives, and strategies used in one context can often be applied to another. All staff, from housekeeping to supervising, must be alert to not only problems but also opportunities for improvement. Increasingly, departments must be concerned with cost-effectiveness as the costs of medical care continue to rise, so the quality professional in the cardiovascular unit is not in an isolated position in an institution but is just one part of the whole, facing similar concerns as those in other disciplines. Disciplines are often interrelated in their functions.

JURAN'S QUALITY IMPROVEMENT PROCESS

Joseph Juran's quality improvement process (QIP) is a 4-step method of change (focusing on quality control) which is based on a trilogy of concepts that includes quality planning, control, and improvement. The steps to the QIP process include the following:

1. **Defining** the project and organizing includes listing and prioritizing problems and identifying a team.
2. **Diagnosing** includes analyzing problems and then formulating theories related to cause by root cause analysis and test theories.
3. **Remediating** includes considering various alternative solutions and then designing and implementing specific solutions and controls while addressing institutional resistance to change. As causes of problems are identified and remediation instituted to remove the problems, the processes should improve.
4. **Holding** involves evaluating performance and monitoring the control system in order to maintain gains.

FOCUS PERFORMANCE IMPROVEMENT MODEL

Find, organize, clarify, uncover, start (FOCUS) is a performance improvement model used to facilitate change:

1. **Find**: Identifying a problem by looking at the organization and attempting to determine what isn't working well or what is wrong.
2. **Organize**: Identifying those people who have an understanding of the problem or process and creating a team to work on improving performance.
3. **Clarify**: Determining what is involved in solving the problem by utilizing brainstorming techniques, such as the Ishikawa diagram.
4. **Uncover**: Analyzing the situation to determine the reason the problem has arisen or that a process is unsuccessful.
5. **Start**: Determining where to begin in the change process.

FOCUS, by itself, is an incomplete process and is primarily used as a means to identify a problem rather than a means to find the solution. FOCUS is usually combined with PDCA (FOCUS-PDCA), so it becomes a 9-step process; however, beginning with FOCUS helps to narrow the focus, resulting in better outcomes.

Nurse's Involvement in Quality Improvement

The following are ways in which nurses can be involved in quality improvement in their facility:

- **Identify situations** in the nursing unit that require improvement and might benefit patient outcomes (cost containment, incident reporting, etc.) if changed.
- **Identify potential items** that can be measured to be able to test the problem or to be able to monitor patient outcomes.
- **Collect data** on those measurements and determine current patient outcomes.
- **Analyze the data** and identify procedures, methods, etc., that can be utilized to potentially make positive changes in patient outcomes, doing research if necessary.
- **Make recommendations for changes** to be implemented to determine the effect on patient outcomes.
- **Implement recommendations** after approval from administrative personnel.
- **Collect data** using the same measurements and determine if the changes improved patient outcomes or not.

Risk Management

Risk management attempts to prevent harm and legal liability by being proactive and by identifying a patient's **risk factors**. The patient is educated about these factors and ways that they can modify their behavior to decrease their risk. Treatments and interventions must be considered in terms of risk to the patient, and the patient must always know these risks in order to make healthcare decisions. Much can be done to avoid mistakes that put patients at risk. Patients should note medications and other aspects of their care so that they can help prevent mistakes. They should feel free to question care and to have their concerns heard and addressed. When mistakes are made, the actions taken to remedy the situation are very important. The physician should be made aware of the error immediately, and the patient notified according to hospital policy. Errors must be evaluated to determine how the process failed. Honesty and caring can help mitigate many errors.

Nursing Malpractice, Negligence, Unintentional Torts, and Intentional Torts

- **Malpractice** is unethical or improper actions or lack of proper action by the nurse that may or may not be related to a lack of skills that nurses should possess.
- **Negligence** is the failure to act as any other diligent nurse would have acted in the same situation.
- Negligence can lead to an **unintentional tort**. In this case, the patient must prove that the nurse had a duty to act, a duty proven via standards of care, and that the nurse failed in this duty and harm occurred to the patient as a result of this failure.
- **Intentional torts** differ in that the duty is assumed and the nurse breached this duty via assault and battery, invasion of privacy, slander, or false imprisonment of the patient.

> **Review Video: Medical Negligence**
> Visit mometrix.com/academy and enter code: 928405

Patient Safety

IMPORTANCE OF COMMUNICATION TO PATIENT SAFETY

Many adverse incidents related to **patient safety** result from errors or failures in **communication**. In fact, over 30% of malpractice claims result from communication failures. Communication is especially a concern during hand-off procedures. Critical information about the patient may be undocumented, forgotten, overlooked, or misplaced. For this reason, standardized hand-off procedures, such as SBAR (**s**ituation, **b**ackground, **a**ssessment, **r**ecommendation) or I-PASS (**i**llness severity, **p**atient summary, **a**ction list, **s**ituation awareness/contingency planning, **s**ynthesis by receiver) should be utilized. While an initial error in communication may not directly harm a patient, the decisions made by subsequent healthcare providers may cause harm because the healthcare providers lacked essential information. Additionally, communication failures may occur because healthcare providers don't take the time to talk with patients or family or to listen attentively and gather their input. Problems may arise if healthcare providers fail to document medications, treatments, or observations in a timely manner. Many electronic health records utilize limited narration in favor of checklists, and checking all the boxes may become a rote activity, leading to errors.

INTERPROFESSIONAL PRACTICE AND PATIENT SAFETY

Interprofessional practice often begins with interprofessional education in which members of two or more professions study and learn together in order to build relationships and to have a better understanding of the contributions of each profession and the role of the profession in ensuring **patient safety**. For example, in obstetrics, an interprofessional group may include a nurse, midwife, ultrasonographer, and breastfeeding specialist. Each has a different but equally important role in patient care. A better understanding of roles and responsibilities leads to better collaboration and fewer patient safety issues. Additionally, collaboration promotes cross training and awareness of patient needs. Key elements in interprofessional practice include leadership (definitions, who leads and how leadership is determined), monitoring (continually assessing processes and outcomes), communication (methods and styles of effective communication), and support (mutual and organizational). Studies indicate that interprofessional education and practice especially improves communication among participants, a critical element in patient safety.

PERINATAL PATIENT SAFETY NURSE

Large birthing facilities may designate a nurse as a **perinatal patient safety nurse**. This is usually an advanced practice nurse who focuses on mother/baby safety during care. This nurse monitors nursing care for adherence to safety procedures and provides education as needed. The overall coordination of efforts to evaluate and improve care to result in a safe, optimal outcome for both mother and baby is a major part of this role. This complies with the Joint Commission's recommendations and with the goals of Healthy People 2030 that seek to improve the nursing and medical care that is given to all persons. The unit manager and staff of smaller birthing units must take this responsibility on themselves to ensure the safety of care given in their unit.

THE JOINT COMMISSION'S PERINATAL CARE CORE MEASURE

The Joint Commission's Perinatal Care Core Measures are those measures that require data collection for accredited hospitals that have at least 300 live births each year and any hospital that wants Perinatal Care certification. From January 2021 onward, there are 4 core measures:

- **PC-01 Elective delivery**: Elective vaginal or cesarean delivery at ≥37 weeks and <39 weeks of gestation
- **PC-02 Cesarean birth**: Nulliparous patient with term singleton in vertex position
- **PC-05 Exclusive Breast Milk Feeding**: Only breast milk feeding during entire hospital stay
- **PC-06 Unexpected Complications in Term Newborns**: Percentage with unexpected complications among full-term neonates with no pre-existing conditions (such as prematurity, congenital malformations, genetic disorders, exposure to maternal drug use, poor fetal growth, and genetic disorders)

MATERNAL SAFETY BUNDLES PRESENTED BY THE AIM

The **Alliance for Innovation on Maternal Health** (AIM), a maternal safety and quality improvement initiative, has developed a series of **Patient Safety Bundles and Tools** to improve maternal outcomes and prevent complications:

- **Maternal Mental Health, Depression and Anxiety**: Identify tools, establish screening, provide education, support, and follow-up.
- **Maternal Venous Thromboembolism**: Use risk assessment tools and appropriate prophylaxis.
- **Obstetric Care for Women with Opioid Use Disorder**: Assess and provide education (patient, staff), utilize community resources, emphasize available therapies, and establish clinical pathways.
- **Obstetric Hemorrhage**: Maintain hemorrhage cart, establish protocols, response team and massive transfusion protocols.
- **Postpartum Care Basics for Maternal Safety** (from birth to the comprehensive PP visit and transition from maternity to well-woman care): Develop personalized PP care plan, provide counseling and anticipatory guidance, screen for common morbidities, implement protocols. Provide discharge planning, information about community resources, and education.
- **Prevention of Retained Vaginal Sponges after Birth**: Educate staff, utilize sponge detection system.
- **Reduction of Peripartum Racial/Ethnic Disparities**: Provide staff education, obtain demographic information, and practice shared decision making.
- **Safe Reduction of Primary Cesarean Birth**: Educate and train providers, offer standardized pain management and fetal assessment, and develop protocols for problems.
- **Severe Hypertension in Pregnancy**: Use standardized screening and assessment and provide triage and rapid access to medications.
- **Support After a Severe Maternal Event**: Creation of unit-based procedures to provide support after severe events, assessment of maternal mental status, provision of timely and effective interventions, and monitoring patient outcomes for report generation.

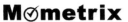

DECREASING FAMILY STRESS IF NEONATE REQUIRES INTENSIVE CARE

Having a neonate admitted to the neonatal intensive care unit is a very stressful event for a family. It interrupts family interactions and the bonding process that occurs when a neonate goes home to spend time with family members. Interventions to decrease **family stress** and encourage bonding between the neonate, mother, and family include:

- Have facilities available for families to stay close to their infant to encourage bonding.
- Maintain a play area for siblings so they are not isolated from parents.
- Permit liberal visiting times for family members.
- If it is known before birth that the infant will require critical care, let the family visit the unit and ask questions.
- Give the family contact information for support groups comprised of other parents who have children with similar illnesses.
- Encourage hands-on parental care, including kangaroo care, by both parents.

COUNSELING TECHNIQUES FOR FAMILIES WITH NEONATES IN NICU

Counseling techniques for families and extended families with a neonate in the NICU include:

- **Talk with families and listen:** Assess the family members' understanding of the neonate's condition and the situation to determine if it is realistic or distorted. If distorted, try to ascertain the reason and provide useful information in a non-threatening manner to help them more fully understand. Avoid overwhelming family members with too much information, especially initially. Listen attentively and show respect at all times. Acknowledge family members feeling of guilt and explain that these feelings are normal. Pay attention to body language when delivering information.
- **Assess coping strategies/grief:** Determine how the family members cope with stress and handle grief. Provide support and information about resources and support groups that are available and may be appropriate.
- **Encourage expression of feelings:** Remain supportive of family members' feelings and responses, even if negative, and encourage them to interact and share feelings with others. Suggest keeping a journal, diary, or blog to write about their feelings and experiences.

SHARED DECISION-MAKING AND PARENT-STAFF DISAGREEMENTS

Shared decision making requires that staff members treat the parents with respect, listen to their opinions and feelings, provide full information about treatments and the neonate's condition, encourage the parents to participate in care, and encourage parents to collaborate and share in decision-making at every step in the NICU provision of care.

When **disagreements occur between parents and staff members**, it is important to respond with patience and empathy. The nurse should try to determine why the parents disagree or are angry. For example, are they afraid a treatment is harmful? Do they not understand what the treatment consists of? Have they been reading advice on the internet or getting advice from others? Have they developed a dislike or distrust for staff members? Do they feel left out of decision-making process? Do they resent lack of control? Is a treatment at odds with their cultural or religious beliefs? The staff members should ask parents what they want and why, and provide as complete information as possible, including pros and cons.

NICU Nurse Practice Test #1

1. Which of the following is NOT a physical sign of cold stress in a neonate?

    a. Bradycardia

    b. Hypertonia

    c. Lethargy

2. Hyperthermia is defined as a core body temperature above what temperature?

    a. 37.5 °C

    b. 38 °C

    c. 39 °C

3. A 29-week neonate presents with the following arterial blood gas values:

- pH – 7.36
- pCO_2 – 52
- HCO_3^- – 30

These values would indicate which of the following?

    a. Compensated metabolic acidosis

    b. Compensated respiratory acidosis

    c. Uncompensated respiratory acidosis

4. What is the most common complication of ECMO (extra corporeal membrane oxygenation)?

    a. Bleeding

    b. Infection

    c. Thrombosis

5. With regard to oxygen delivery, which of the following scenarios would be an appropriate indication for using a nasal cannula in an infant?

    a. A 32-week-old, gavage-fed infant who requires 2 lpm O_2 to maintain a SpO_2 greater than 90%

    b. A 33-week-old infant who requires FiO_2 of 0.5 (50%) to maintain SpO_2 greater than 90%

    c. A 34-week-old infant who is bottle-feeding and requires 0.5 lpm O_2 to maintain a SpO_2 greater than 90%

6. Maternal HELLP syndrome is characterized by which set of symptoms?

    a. Hemolysis, elevated liver enzymes, low platelet count

    b. Hemorrhage, episodic liver lesions, pulmonary insufficiency

    c. Hypertension, electrolyte loss, low protein

7. What diseases comprise TORCH syndrome?

    a. Toxoplasmosis, Ollier disease, rheumatic fever, chlamydia, hepatitis

    b. Toxoplasmosis, other diseases, rubella, cytomegalovirus, herpes simplex

    c. Toxoplasmosis, ochronosis, Rh disease, cholera, histoplasmosis

8. Which of the following patient scenarios is NOT a candidate for mechanical ventilation?

a. 27-week infant weighing 980 g, respiratory rate 80/min, mild retractions
b. 34-week infant weighing 2400 g, respiratory rate 42/min, in oxyhood at FiO_2 30%
c. 38-week infant weighing 3200 g, respiratory rate 60/min, grunting, marked retractions, in oxyhood at FiO_2 45%, SpO_2 falling

9. Which of the following infants are at LOW risk for insensible water loss?

I. 28-week-old infant in an open-bed warmer
II. 30-week-old infant in closed Isolette incubator
III. Term infant, born on way to hospital
IV. 36-week-old infant in open bassinet with respiratory rate 64/min

a. I
b. IV
c. II

10. Which of the following is an indication for total parenteral nutrition?

a. Short-gut syndrome
b. Transient diarrhea
c. Vomiting

11. Which of the following provides the appropriate daily caloric intake for the associated infant?

a. Healthy 2500 g infant receiving 55 cc expressed human milk by gavage every 3 hours
b. Healthy 3400 g infant receiving 3.5 oz fortified preterm formula by bottle every 4 hours
c. Post-surgical 2800 g infant receiving 60cc half-strength formula by bottle every 3 hours

12. Which of the following findings are associated with fetal alcohol syndrome?

I. Large head
II. Cardiac defects
III. SGA (small for gestational age)
IV. Delayed development

a. I, III, IV
b. I, II, III, IV
c. II, III, IV

13. What is a serious sequela regarding meconium aspiration in the infant?

a. Cardiac anomalies
b. Gastroschisis
c. PPHN (persistent pulmonary hypertension of the newborn)

14. What is the function of pulmonary surfactant in the neonate?

a. Prevents bronchoconstriction of the smooth bronchial muscles
b. Prevents alveolar collapse
c. Increases surface tension in lungs to provide more structure

15. What is the most common cause of pneumothorax in a neonate?

a. Atrial/septal defects
b. RDS (respiratory distress syndrome)
c. Shock

16. A neonate presents with cyanotic legs and toes but upper extremities and head are pink. Respiratory rate is 55/min and heart rate is 120/min with a loud murmur. What is the likely type of cyanosis that is exhibited?

a. Central cardiac cyanosis
b. Central pulmonary cyanosis
c. Differential cyanosis

17. What conditions exist in Tetralogy of Fallot?

I. Left ventricular hypertrophy
II. Pulmonary stenosis
III. Atrial septal defect
IV. Overriding aorta

a. I, III
b. I, III, IV
c. II, IV

18. Being an ethical and responsible nurse requires which of the following?

a. Keeping knowledge and skills current
b. Making decisions independently
c. Subjective charting

19. Which of the following could be considered possible signs and symptoms of grief in the parents of an ill neonate?

I. Palpitations, syncope, and vertigo
II. Guilt and shame
III. Nightmares, insomnia, and other sleep disturbances
IV. Withdrawal from interpersonal relationships
V. Hostility and agitation

a. I, III, IV
b. I, II, III, IV, V
c. II, IV, V

20. A baby was a born at 30 weeks' gestation. She is going home on room air. She does well with bottle feedings and has successfully nursed twice in the NICU. The mother wants to continue breastfeeding at home. Which of the following topics would be important to include in the discharge planning/teaching at this time?

a. Lactation consult
b. Physical therapy
c. Special equipment needs

21. Which of the following statements regarding anticipatory grieving is FALSE?

a. It is common for parents to have feelings of guilt, shame, and remorse toward their malformed infant.
b. It is normal for parents to display emotional withdrawal from a critically ill infant.
c. It is normal for parents to exhibit persistent emotional detachment from their infant for long after the infant begins to show signs of improvement or survival.

22. Which of the following does NOT usually present a barrier to parent/infant interaction?

    a. Adolescent parents

    b. Involved, large extended family

    c. Well-educated parents

23. Which of the following genetic diseases is the common name for trisomy 18?

    a. Down syndrome

    b. Edwards syndrome

    c. Patau syndrome

24. What is the leading cause of hearing loss in infants?

    a. Congenital cytomegalovirus infection

    b. Intraventricular hemorrhage

    c. Side effect from maternal medication ingestion

25. A boy was born at 35 weeks' gestation an hour ago. His mother was in labor for 26 hours and was running a fever of 38.5 °C during labor. During labor the mother had an intrauterine fetal monitoring device in place. The baby now has respiratory distress, cyanosis, a core body temperature of 36 °C, and is very lethargic. Which of the following is the most likely cause of his condition?

    a. Candidiasis

    b. Group B streptococcus

    c. MRSA (methicillin-resistant *Staphylococcus aureus*)

26. Which of the following statements is usually associated with neonatal abstinence syndrome (NAS)?

    a. NAS can be caused by iatrogenic exposure of opiates to the neonate for the purpose of sedation and/or analgesia.

    b. Lethargy, hypotonia, and decreased reflexes are hallmark signs of NAS.

    c. Symptoms of withdrawal always appear immediately after birth and last 1-3 days.

27. Which of the following are true regarding physiologic signs of pain in the neonate?

    I. Increased heart rate

    II. Increased oxygenation

    III. Changes in muscle tone

    IV. Different from those of adults

    V. Feeding difficulties

    a. I, II, IV

    b. I, II, III

    c. I, III, V

28. What nonpharmacologic methods can be effective in reducing pain in the neonate?

I. Swaddling
II. Placing neonate in tucked, flexed, side lying position for procedures
III. Subdued lighting
IV. Music
V. Use of white noise

a. I, III
b. I, II, V
c. I, II, III, IV, V

29. What is the proper placement position of the neonate in kangaroo care?

a. Swaddled tightly, cradled on caregiver's chest
b. Unclothed (diaper is acceptable), placed vertically on caregiver's bare chest
c. Unclothed, cradled on caregiver's lap

30. A 6-day-old boy was born at 36 weeks' gestation. He weighs 6 lbs. He just underwent circumcision. What is the most appropriate dose of acetaminophen for pain control?

a. 1 cc pediatric acetaminophen liquid, orally every 6 hours
b. ½ of a 120 mg acetaminophen suppository, per rectum every 8 hours
c. 0.3 cc concentrated infant acetaminophen drops, orally every 6 hours

31. Which of the following characteristics are most common in the average infant abductor?

I. Female
II. Criminal record
III. Visits the nursery prior to the abduction
IV. Appears suspicious and paranoid
V. Desires to replace a lost infant or is unable to conceive

a. I, II, V
b. I, III, IV
c. I, III, V

32. What is one of the purposes of HIPAA regulations?

a. Ensure patient confidentiality
b. Provide a safe working environment for hospital employees
c. Regulate hospital policies and procedures

33. Which of the following factors have been linked to SIDS?

I. Prematurity
II. Sleeping in prone position
III. Being born to an older (over 35 years) mother
IV. Exposure to cigarette smoke while in the womb and after birth
V. Hard mattresses

a. I, II, IV
b. I, II, III, V
c. II, III, V

34. A couple expecting their first child seeks genetic counseling for a maternal family history of cystic fibrosis. The woman is a carrier of the cystic fibrosis gene but the man is not. What are the chances that their child will have cystic fibrosis disease?

    a. 1:2
    b. 25%
    c. 0%

35. Which of the following symptoms are associated with an infant of a diabetic mother (IDM)?

    I. LGA
    II. Hyperglycemia
    III. Hypoglycemia
    IV. SGA
    V. Jaundice

    a. I, II, III
    b. I, III, V
    c. I, IV, V

36. An infant girl was born at 38 weeks by NSVD. Shortly after birth she presents with retractions and cyanosis at rest, but these symptoms resolve when she cries vigorously. She is also unable to nurse. What is a likely cause of this?

    a. Aspiration pneumonia
    b. Choanal atresia
    c. Respiratory distress syndrome

37. What are common risks associated with post-term infants?

    I. Meconium aspiration
    II. Cord compression
    III. Shoulder dystocia
    IV. Transient hypoglycemia
    V. Seizures

    a. I, III, IV
    b. I, II
    c. I, II, III, IV, V

38. What is the recommended dose of naloxone in neonates who are exhibiting moderate respiratory depression?

    a. 0.01 mg/kg
    b. 0.1 mg/kg
    c. 1 mg/kg

39. With regard to resuscitation, chest compressions (cardiac massage) should be initiated in a neonate when heart rate dips below what value (assuming adequate and effective ventilation is in place)?

    a. 60 bpm
    b. 90 bpm
    c. 120 bpm

40. What is the Kleihauer-Betke test used to determine?

a. Apnea of prematurity
b. Fetal blood loss
c. Respiratory insufficiency

41. Which pathogen is responsible for most nosocomial infections in the NICU?

a. Group B *Streptococci*
b. Rotavirus
c. *Staphylococcus aureus*

42. Which of the following is NOT an effective method in preventing nosocomial infections in the NICU?

a. Frequent handwashing
b. Keeping infants on ventilators as long as possible to maintain a closed sterile system of ventilation
c. Starting enteral feedings as soon as possible

43. Which of the following factors would interfere with the measurement of oxygen saturation (SpO_2)?

I. Bright ambient lights
II. Shivering
III. Cold extremities
IV. Vasodilation
V. Placing probe on lower extremities

a. I, II, III
b. I, II, IV
c. I, II, V

44. Which of the following initial stabilization measures should be instituted during the delivery of an infant with a known omphalocele in the NICU?

I. Place infant in supine position.
II. Cover exposed organs with saline-soaked gauze.
III. Insert orogastric tube.
IV. Insert UAC/UVC lines.
V. Closely monitor temperature and urine output.

a. I, II, III, V
b. II, III, V
c. II, IV, V

45. What is the normal rate of urinary output for a neonate?

a. 0.25-0.75 cc/kg/hr
b. 1-3 cc/kg/hr
c. 3-6 cc/kg/hr

46. What is the L:S ratio test used to determine?

a. Cardiac function
b. Estimated gestational age
c. Fetal lung maturity

47. Which of the following symptoms can be associated with amniotic band syndrome?

    I. Limb deformity
    II. Cleft deformity of face
    III. Chest deformity
    IV. Congenital limb amputation

    a. I, II, III
    b. I, III, IV
    c. I, II, III, IV

48. Transient tachypnea of the newborn (TTN) is more likely to occur in babies born under which of the following circumstances?

    a. Babies born before 33 weeks' gestation
    b. Babies delivered by C-section
    c. SGA babies

49. Which of the following is an appropriate intervention for an infant with GE reflux?

    a. Elevating the head of the bed
    b. Larger, less frequent feedings
    c. Placing infant in prone position after feeding

50. Which of the following statements is FALSE regarding neonatal hyperbilirubinemia?

    a. It can be associated with breastfeeding.
    b. It is usually a benign finding.
    c. It is a serious condition that often leads to kernicterus.

51. A pregnant mother that is 30 weeks pregnant presents with right upper quadrant pain, nausea, vomiting and hypertension. She is most likely suffering from which of the following?

    a. Cholestasis
    b. HELLP syndrome
    c. Influenza

52. A woman who is known to have hepatitis B, is delivering her first baby. What should the treatment of the infant include?

    a. Waiting until the infant is at least 5 years of age to administer hepatitis B immunoglobin
    b. Hepatitis B vaccine given within the first year of life
    c. Hepatitis B vaccine and hepatitis B immunoglobulin given within 12 hours of birth

53. The nurse is talking to new parents whose child was born with a cleft lip and palate due to Amniotic Band Syndrome. They are concerned that this may happen to any more children they have in the future. What is the best response to this?

    a. There is no known genetic cause of Amniotic Band Syndrome and it is very rare this will happen again in future pregnancies.
    b. This is an autosomal dominant genetic trait and there is a 50% chance this could happen in future pregnancies.
    c. Once one child is born with this condition, all future children will also inherit it.

54. What is a major risk factor for chorioamnionitis?

    a. Premature rupture of the membranes

    b. Maternal tobacco use during pregnancy

    c. There are no known risk factors for chorioamnionitis

55. What is measured with the quad screen test?

    a. Amniotic fluid levels, maternal fasting blood sugar, inhibin-A, and maternal HIV status

    b. Fetal DNA testing, fetal glucose level, estriol, and alpha-fetoprotein levels

    c. Alpha-fetoprotein, human chorionic gonadotropin, estriol, and inhibin-A

56. When monitoring the fetal heart rate during labor, which of the following is most likely to be most dangerous to the fetus?

    a. Early decelerations during the late stages of labor

    b. Late decelerations without accelerations

    c. Occasional, brief variable decelerations followed by accelerations

57. Which of the following medications may be given to slow down preterm labor contractions that initiated at 30 weeks gestation?

    a. Cytotec

    b. Terbutaline

    c. Pitocin

58. Which breech presentation at birth presents with the buttocks only passing through the birth canal first?

    a. Frank breech

    b. Footling breech

    c. Complete breech

59. In which of the below conditions does the placenta detach from the wall of the uterus prematurely, depriving the fetus of oxygen and nutrients?

    a. Abruptio placentae

    b. Cord prolapse

    c. Placenta previa

60. Which of the following potential side effects can occur as a result of forceps being used during delivery?

    a. Sudden infant death

    b. Facial palsy

    c. Cerebral palsy

61. Small for gestational age is defined as which of the following?

    a. An infant born after 37 weeks gestation and weighing 2500 grams or less

    b. An infant born before 37 weeks gestation and weighing 2500 grams or less

    c. An infant born after 37 weeks gestation and weighing less than 2000 grams

62. A new mother is visiting her infant in the NICU. She expresses concern over the tiny white bumps on her child's nose and chin. What should the nurse explain to her?

    a. The bumps can usually be removed by applying some pressure and pinching the bumps.

    b. A referral to dermatologist can be ordered for further evaluation of this.

    c. This is due to plugged pores in the skin and it will go away on its own.

63. While assessing a newborn in the NICU, the nurse notices that he has pitting edema on the right side of his scalp. What should the next step be?

    a. Immediately contact the neonatologist on call and let him know of your findings.

    b. Continue to monitor for any change in the symptoms.

    c. Stop all IV fluids and monitor closely to see if the swelling decreases.

64. The parents of a newborn ask the nurse about the white bumps they have noticed along their baby's upper gum line. Of the following, which would be the best response?

    a. He is starting to develop teeth at a very young age.

    b. These are small cysts that will go away on their own within 1-2 weeks.

    c. These are skin lesions on his gums that need to be evaluated as soon as possible by a dentist.

65. What are the four heart defects seen with Tetralogy of Fallot?

    a. A large ventricular septal defect, pulmonary stenosis, right ventricular hypertrophy, and an overriding aorta

    b. A patent ductus arteriosus, pulmonary hypertension, cor pulmonale, and aortic stenosis

    c. A thoracic aortic aneurysm, aortic stenosis, pulmonary stenosis, and a ventricular septal defect

66. When the nurse is assessing a newborn's respiratory status, which would indicate the newborn is developing respiratory distress?

    a. Nasal flaring

    b. Pink skin color

    c. Respiratory rate of 40 breaths per minute

67. The nurse is caring for a child with end stage renal disease. What is a sign that he may be in fluid overload?

    a. A decrease in blood pressure

    b. An increase in blood pressure

    c. A red, burning rash on the legs

68. What is a contraindication to performing daily chlorhexidine baths on infants in the NICU?

    a. The common infant allergy to chlorhexidine

    b. Poor skin integrity in premature infants

    c. Increased risk of respiratory compromise from noxious fumes from the chlorhexidine

69. When the nurse is assessing a newborn, what is the reflex that results in abduction and extension of the infant's arms as the hands open?

    a. Grasp reflex

    b. Moro reflex

    c. Asymmetrical tonic reflex

70. According to the American Heart Association, when should chest compressions be started in the pediatric patient?

    a. If there is no detectable pulse

    b. If the pulse is less than 60 beats per minute or there are signs of poor perfusion

    c. If there is a normal pulse but signs of respiratory distress

71. A 4-week-old infant in the NICU is taking formula orally. The baby is crying very often and acts hungry, however, she projectile vomits after she eats even a small amount of formula. The nurse notices a small lump in the infant's upper abdomen. What is another symptom that would most likely be present?

    a. A hard, rigid abdomen

    b. Waves from peristalsis across the baby's abdomen

    c. A high fever, usually >102 degrees

72. A premature infant is in distress and has not responded to resuscitative measures. A volume expander is indicated at this time. What is the risk of giving this type of medication too quickly?

    a. Hypercoagulability resulting in pulmonary emboli

    b. Supraventricular tachycardia

    c. Intraventricular hemorrhage

73. In what order should resuscitative efforts in the premature infant with hydrops fetalis and bilateral pleural effusions be performed?

    a. Cutting of the umbilical cord, resuscitative measures, then emergency thoracentesis

    b. Cutting of the umbilical cord, emergency thoracentesis, then resuscitative measures

    c. Emergency thoracentesis, cutting of the umbilical cord, then resuscitative measures

74. How many calories does a preterm infant require per day?

    a. 50-100 kcal/kg/day

    b. 100-150 kcal/kg/day

    c. 150-200 kcal/kg/day

75. An infant with a known congenital diaphragmatic hernia is born at 38 weeks gestation. He requires resuscitation shortly after delivery due to the weakening of the diaphragm from the hernia. Generally speaking, how does the survival rate for this infant compare to another infant requiring resuscitation without a diaphragmatic hernia?

    a. Lower

    b. Higher

    c. Equal

76. The nurse is assessing an infant with renal disease. Over the past 4 hours, he has had 100 mL of urine output. He weighs 6 lbs., or 2.73 kg. What would the initial interpretation of this be?

    a. Severe polyuria

    b. Severe oliguria

    c. Normal urine output for weight of the infant

77. Which of the following will have the greatest amount of insensible water loss?

    a. Normal size and full-term
    b. Small size and earlier gestational age
    c. Small size and full-term

78. At what point after birth is gut priming performed?

    a. Within 12 hours of birth
    b. 2nd day of life
    c. 3rd day of life

79. What method should be used to feed the preterm infant with a weak sucking reflex?

    a. Gavage feeding
    b. PEG tube
    c. Thickened liquids given orally

80. All of the following are early feeding cues EXCEPT

    a. Sucking on fingers
    b. Persistent crying
    c. Opening mouth wide when touched on the chin

81. Oral sucrose is given to infants for what reason?

    a. Prevent dehydration
    b. Pain relief
    c. An increase in heart rate and blood pressure

82. A premature infant in the NICU has a nasogastric drain. The results of her arterial blood gases are as follows: pH 7.5, HCO_3^- 29, pCO_2 37. Based on these values, which acid-base disorder has this infant developed?

    a. Respiratory alkalosis
    b. Respiratory acidosis
    c. Metabolic alkalosis

83. How does the protein content in colostrum compare to the protein content in mature human milk?

    a. The protein content is lower in colostrum than mature milk.
    b. The protein content is equal in both.
    c. The protein content is higher in colostrum than mature milk.

84. Which of the following is an indication for parenteral nutrition in the premature infant?

    a. Oxygen saturation less than 90%
    b. Very low birth weight infants (less than 1500 g)
    c. Difficulty latching on for breastfeeding

85. Which vitamin should be given to infants at risk for bronchopulmonary dysplasia?

    a. Vitamin C
    b. Vitamin B
    c. Vitamin A

86. Which of the following conditions may require total parenteral nutrition indefinitely?

a. Short bowel syndrome
b. Low birth weight infants
c. Pyloric stenosis

87. Which of the following is NOT a potential risk when using an extracorporeal membrane oxygenation (ECMO) device?

a. Blood clots
b. Bleeding
c. Electrolyte imbalance

88. What is an elevated serum lactate level in an infant in the NICU associated with?

a. Rapid lung maturation
b. Increased risk of death
c. Poor GI absorption of nutrients

89. What change in arterial blood gas values would be expected in a patient with compensated respiratory acidosis?

a. $PaCO_2$ is elevated, and blood pH is decreased.
b. $PaCO_2$ is decreased, and blood pH is normal.
c. $PaCO_2$ is elevated, blood pH is normal, and serum bicarbonate (HCO_3^-) is elevated.

90. What is the difference between hypoxia and hypoxemia?

a. Hypoxia is increased oxygen at the tissue level, while hypoxemia is an increase in the oxygen level within arterial blood.
b. Hypoxia is decreased oxygen available at the tissue level, while hypoxemia is a decrease in the oxygen level within arterial blood.
c. Hypoxia is the patient's subjective sensation of not breathing in enough air, while hypoxemia is an increase in the oxygen level within arterial blood.

91. The nurse has an order to give dobutamine intravenously. She knows that

a. This can only be given in oral form.
b. This can only be given through a peripheral IV site.
c. This should be given through a central line.

92. A newborn in the NICU has been receiving gentamicin and ampicillin for the treatment of gram-negative sepsis. He is on a fairly high dose of gentamicin and has been for the past 3 days. In addition to the risk of developing renal impairment from the medication, he is also at risk for which of the following?

a. Permanent discoloration of his teeth later in life
b. Cataract development
c. Hearing loss

93. What is the mineral concentration that is often very low after the administration of intravenous Lasix?

a. Calcium
b. Magnesium
c. Iron

94. **Which of the following is the most immediate concern for fetuses of mothers who have used cocaine during their pregnancy?**

    a. Cleft lip or palette
    b. Patent ductus arteriosus
    c. Premature delivery

95. **Signs and symptoms of acute alcohol withdrawal in the newborn with neonatal abstinence syndrome should appear within what timeframe?**

    a. Minutes to 4 hours after birth
    b. 3-12 hours after birth
    c. 24-36 hours after birth

96. **Proven benefits from the kangaroo method include all of the following EXCEPT**

    a. Stabilizing blood pressure and heart rate
    b. More rapid PDA closure
    c. Pain relief

97. **The newborn with hypothermia has an increased risk of developing which of the following?**

    a. Hypoglycemia
    b. Metabolic alkalosis
    c. Respiratory acidosis

98. **An infant in the NICU is receiving carbamazepine (Tegretol) for seizure control. When would be the best time to obtain a blood sample to check a drug level?**

    a. Just before giving a regular scheduled dose
    b. Two hours after giving a dose
    c. Mid-way between doses

99. **Which combination of drugs is compatible when given together intravenously?**

    a. Sodium bicarbonate and furosemide (Lasix)
    b. Phenytoin (Dilantin) with D5W
    c. Amiodarone and atropine

100. **What are the most common symptoms of sudden withdrawal of a beta-blocker medication?**

    a. Hypertension, increased heart rate, cardiac dysrhythmias, tremors, and sweating
    b. Hypotension, decreased heart rate, fatigue, and lethargy
    c. Hallucinations, seizures, and irritability

101. **An infant in the NICU is being treated for meningitis with ampicillin. The dosage is 400 mg/kg/day divided over every 8 hours. The infant being cared for weighs 6 pounds 8 ounces. How many milligrams should be given with each dose?**

    a. 300 mg
    b. 325 mg
    c. 393 mg

102. A newborn with congenital cytomegalovirus infection is being treated with IV ganciclovir. When giving this intravenously, over what time period should it be infused?

   a. 30 minutes
   b. 60 minutes
   c. 90 minutes

103. Which of the following medications is NOT indicated for use in the infant in respiratory distress?

   a. Formoterol (Perforomist)
   b. Albuterol
   c. Dexamethasone

104. A pediatric patient in the NICU is receiving an infusion of dopamine. Once it is completed, when should the effects from the medication be gone?

   a. Within 10 minutes
   b. Within 1 hour
   c. Within 4 hours

105. Which of the following routes is NOT recommended when administering naloxone (Narcan) to infants?

   a. Intravenous
   b. Intramuscular
   c. Endotracheal

106. A newborn in the NICU turns his head towards the sound of a monitor alarm sounding. This sound is heard multiple times during the day, and after a while, he no longer responds to it. What is this lack of reaction called?

   a. Habituation
   b. Nature vs. nurture
   c. Deconditioning

107. Which of the following is an autonomic response to stress?

   a. Stable vital signs
   b. Appropriate response to reflex testing
   c. Flushing

108. Studies have shown that having cycled light in the NICU (bright during the day and dim at night), can result in which of the following?

   a. An increased amount of time requiring mechanical ventilation
   b. Infants being able to feed sooner
   c. A disruption in the normal circadian rhythm

109. A preterm infant in the NICU is receiving tube feedings until he is able to attempt oral feedings. What activity can help him with the transition from tube to oral feedings?

   a. Playing soft music during tube feedings
   b. Give him a pacifier to suck on during the tube feedings
   c. Gently rub his stomach during tube feedings

110. Which activity has been found to decrease apneic episodes in newborns?

    a. Rocking movement

    b. Softly singing

    c. Large feedings

111. The nurse is assessing a newborn and notices some faint perioral cyanosis. What should the first response be?

    a. Initiate oxygen via a mask.

    b. Activate the facility's Code Blue protocol.

    c. Assess the rest of their body to see if there is any cyanosis present in the extremities or if the infant is exhibiting any retractions or other signs of respiratory distress.

112. What is a patent ductus arteriosus?

    a. A widening of the mitral valve resulting in mitral regurgitation

    b. An opening in the septal wall between the left and right ventricles

    c. An opening between the pulmonary and aortic arteries

113. When should surfactant be administered?

    a. As a first line therapy for respiratory distress in infants

    b. To infants in severe respiratory distress that did not respond to CPAP

    c. If the infant is requiring FiO_2 of 30% to maintain an oxygen saturation above 90% while on CPAP

114. What is a common cause of a cardiac tamponade in the newborn?

    a. Incorrect location of a central venous catheter tip

    b. Chest wall trauma during passage through the birth canal

    c. Chest compressions in the event of cardiac arrest

115. If left untreated, coarctation of the aorta can lead to which of the following?

    a. Congestive heart failure

    b. Patent ductus arteriosus

    c. Tetralogy of Fallot

116. Which of the following heart conditions will cause weak peripheral pulses and cool extremities?

    a. Patent ductus arteriosus

    b. Hypoplastic left heart syndrome

    c. Pulmonary stenosis

117. Transposition of the great vessels can involve the superior and inferior vena cavas, the pulmonary artery and pulmonary veins, or which of the following?

    a. Femoral artery

    b. Tricuspid valve

    c. Aorta

118. With which genetic condition is the NICU nurse likely to see an atrioventricular septal defect, or a ventricular septal defect in less severe cases?

    a. Cerebral palsy
    b. Down syndrome
    c. Cystic fibrosis

119. Which of the following congenital heart defects is considered a cyanotic condition?

    a. Tetralogy of Fallot
    b. Aortic stenosis
    c. Atrial septal defect

120. The nurse is checking the blood pressure of a newborn. It is 64/40. What should the next step be?

    a. Begin monitoring it very closely, at least once every 10 minutes, to assess for changes
    b. Activate the Code Blue protocol for the facility
    c. Record the blood pressure as a normal reading and continue the assessment of the newborn

121. A premature infant in the NICU has a G-tube and the nurse is starting his scheduled feeding. The formula is backing up in the tube and not flowing smoothly. What would the next intervention be?

    a. Contact the neonatologist on call for further instructions.
    b. Flush the tube with 20 cc of a carbonated soft drink.
    c. Flush the tube with 5-10 cc warm water and try aspirating and flushing if there is resistance.

122. The nurse is evaluating a newborn. The infant is having retractions with respirations and a low, grunting sound can be heard with his rapid breathing. Which of the following is the most likely diagnosis?

    a. Neonatal sepsis
    b. Meconium aspiration syndrome
    c. Cystic fibrosis

123. What is the most common cause of respiratory distress in the newborn?

    a. Forceps-assisted delivery
    b. Transient tachypnea of the newborn
    c. High birth weight

124. What is the ideal timeframe in which surfactant should be given to the newborn with respiratory distress?

    a. Within 1 hour of birth
    b. At 12 hours of birth
    c. At least 24 hours after birth

125. During the first few months of life, the newborn is only able to digest those proteins found in which of the following?

    a. Formula or human milk
    b. Formula, human milk, or cow's milk
    c. There are no limitations to which proteins the newborn is able to digest

126. The nurse is caring for an infant in the NICU. The newborn has not had a bowel movement in the first 48 hours of his life and has vomited whenever oral feedings are attempted. What is one of the problems that may be present?

    a. Short gut syndrome
    b. Colitis
    c. Hirschsprung's disease

127. A newborn has an NG tube in place due to an intestinal obstruction. In order to prevent aspiration of saliva, which of the following is essential?

    a. Perform continuous oral suction.
    b. The aspirate should drain into a drainage bag and the stomach contents should be aspirated at least every 30 minutes.
    c. Administer feeds at a trickle pace until the obstruction has resolved.

128. What intestinal disorder can occur as a result of malrotation?

    a. Ulcerative colitis
    b. Meconium ileus
    c. Volvulus

129. Which of the following infants is most likely to develop necrotizing enterocolitis?

    a. A premature infant being fed human milk pumped by his mother
    b. A premature infant being formula fed
    c. A full-term infant being formula fed

130. What is the difference between an omphalocele and a gastroschisis?

    a. An omphalocele is a fluid collection in the abdomen, while a gastroschisis is a decrease in fluid in the abdomen.
    b. An omphalocele occurs when the abdominal contents protrude through the umbilicus, but a gastroschisis occurs when there is no membrane covering the abdominal organs.
    c. An omphalocele occurs when the brain ventricles are dilated, while a gastroschisis occurs when loops of bowel are dilated.

131. Parents of a newborn have opted to not have their son circumcised. Which of the following should be included in the care instructions?

    a. The child should receive an annual exam by a urologist to evaluate the uncircumcised penis.
    b. The foreskin should be retracted as much as it allows without force, and cleaned with soap and water, then should be dried well.
    c. Though the circumcision was not done in the hospital, they will need to follow-up with their pediatrician so it can be done before age 2.

132. When administering blood or blood products, which of the following statements is true?

    a. A patient with A- blood can receive blood from a donor who is O- or O+.
    b. A patient with A+ blood can receive blood from a donor who is AB+.
    c. A patient with AB+ blood can receive blood from a donor of any blood type.

133. The nurse is administering blood to a premature infant who is anemic. A possible transfusion reaction may be occurring if the patient develops which of the following?

    a. Dysuria
    b. The hiccups
    c. Tenderness at the IV site

134. What is the most common cause of ambiguous genitalia in a genetic female newborn?

    a. Maternal use of prednisone during the first trimester
    b. Congenital adrenal hyperplasia
    c. Developmental anomaly of having only one ovary

135. A newborn has been diagnosed with neonatal testicular torsion that has left one testicle unsalvageable. The other testicle is not affected. The parents are asking if their son will have fertility problems when he is older because of this. What is the most appropriate response?

    a. There is a very low chance of this causing any fertility issues long-term.
    b. He will need to see an endocrinologist for hormone testing to determine the long-term effects on fertility.
    c. There is usually an approximately 50% chance that he will be infertile.

136. Clinical symptoms of neonatal renal vein thrombosis include which of the following?

    a. Leukocytosis
    b. Bence-Jones protein in the urine
    c. Thrombocytopenia

137. What is the difference between measuring a total bilirubin and a direct bilirubin?

    a. Total bilirubin is the amount of direct and indirect bilirubin, while direct bilirubin is the unbound amount of bilirubin that normally passes from the liver to the small intestine.
    b. Total bilirubin is the amount of bilirubin bound to albumin, while direct bilirubin is the total amount of bound and unbound bilirubin.
    c. Total bilirubin is a measure of the bilirubin excreted through the urine, while direct bilirubin is the amount of protein-bound bilirubin stored in the liver.

138. In which of the following scenarios would the Kleihauer Betke test be useful?

    a. A 36-year-old pregnant female at 38 weeks gestation, contractions 2 minutes apart
    b. An 18-year-old pregnant female at 37 weeks gestation, having Braxton-Hicks contractions
    c. A 29-year-old pregnant female at 26 weeks gestation having abdominal pain following a fall down a steep flight of stairs

139. What is the most common cause of direct hyperbilirubinemia in the newborn?

    a. Trauma during passage through the birth canal
    b. Liver immaturity
    c. Congenital kidney disease

140. What condition can occur in the newborn as a result of Rh incompatibility?

    a. Hydrops fetalis
    b. Sick sinus syndrome
    c. Sickle cell anemia

141. In which group is hypoxic ischemic encephalopathy more common?

    a. All infants, regardless of age, are at equal risk

    b. Premature infants

    c. Full-term infants

142. The nurse is caring for a newborn with spina bifida. The mother expresses concern that a fall she had 2 weeks before delivery could have caused the birth defect. Which of the following is the best response?

    a. Spina bifida is due to trauma during labor and delivery, not due to her fall.

    b. There is a chance that trauma during pregnancy may have caused the abnormality.

    c. Spina bifida develops during the first month of pregnancy and her fall did not cause this.

143. What is the mildest form of an intraventricular hemorrhage of the brain in a newborn also called?

    a. Normal pressure hydrocephalus

    b. A germinal matrix hemorrhage

    c. Elevated pressure hydrocephalus

144. Periventricular leukomalacia is often the cause of which chronic condition?

    a. Acute lymphocytic leukemia

    b. Cerebral palsy

    c. Systolic ejection murmurs

145. The nurse has received a lab report on the CSF of a newborn who underwent a lumbar puncture. The lab report shows the glucose level in the sample is 100 mg/dL. What does this value mean?

    a. The newborn is most likely diabetic.

    b. The newborn likely has meningitis.

    c. The newborn has a normal CSF glucose level.

146. Which of the following is used to test for congenital cytomegalovirus infection?

    a. Saliva

    b. Feces

    c. Nasal swab

147. The feces of house cats can cause which parasitic infection?

    a. Toxoplasmosis

    b. Shigella

    c. Giardia

148. What is early onset group B strep infection in the newborn most likely to cause?

    a. Meningitis

    b. Malabsorption syndromes

    c. Sepsis

149. When will a child with late congenital syphilis generally show symptoms?

    a. Within the first month life

    b. Within the first year of life

    c. After the second year of life

150. Which of the following infections is the most common in the newborn?

  a. Polio virus
  b. Varicella virus
  c. Enterovirus

151. The parents of a newborn are asking the nurse what PKU is and if it is really necessary to have this tested as part of the newborn screening process. What is the best response?

  a. The PKU screen is not a necessary test and can be eliminated from the tests to be performed.
  b. PKU can be a fatal illness and it is highly recommended that this be performed.
  c. The test can be postponed until the newborn is a few months old.

152. The new parents of a child with Down syndrome tell the nurse that they want to have more children in the future, but they are concerned about the risk of having another child with this condition. Which of the following is the most appropriate response?

  a. There is no chance to have this happen again because it is not hereditary.
  b. The chance of that happening is very low, about 1 out of 100 pregnancies.
  c. There is a 50% chance they will have another child with Down syndrome.

153. Due to a family history of sickle cell anemia, a newborn has been screened for and diagnosed with sickle cell disease. His mother is concerned about him participating in normal sports activities when he gets older. What is the most appropriate response to this?

  a. He can participate, but needs to be careful to avoid dehydration or overly strenuous exercise.
  b. He will not be able to participate in any organized sports.
  c. There are no limitations to physical activity with sickle cell disease.

154. Which of the following electrolytes can help to reduce the incidence of neurological deficits in premature infants?

  a. Magnesium
  b. Calcium
  c. Phosphorous

155. An infant has been identified as having galactosemia. The mother wants to know if she can still breastfeed him. Which of the following would be the best response?

  a. She should pump until the infant is well enough to begin breastfeeding again.
  b. He will not be able to breastfeed because of the risk of ingesting galactose in the milk.
  c. He will not be able to breastfeed, but he can drink regular cow's milk without difficulty.

156. Which syndrome affects almost half of the infants of diabetic mothers?

  a. Cleft lip and palate
  b. Hydrocephalus
  c. Fetal macrosomia

157. Of the following, which is an example of an autosomal recessive disease?

  a. Down syndrome
  b. Edward's syndrome
  c. Cystic fibrosis

158. What does it mean if a disease is autosomal dominant?

    a. Both parents need to pass on the gene for the disease to occur.

    b. One parent needs to pass on the gene for the disease to occur.

    c. Neither parent passes on the gene for the disease to occur; it is a genetic mutation that occurs during fetal development.

159. Which of the following is a defect in chromosome 22?

    a. DiGeorge syndrome

    b. Trisomy 13

    c. Trisomy 18

160. Is Turner's syndrome more commonly seen in male or female newborns?

    a. It affects both genders equally.

    b. It affects males only.

    c. It affects females only.

161. Which of the following is a condition that prevents a newborn from being able to breathe after birth?

    a. Polycythemia

    b. Candidiasis

    c. Bilateral choanal atresia

162. In the 1940s and 1950s, what was the leading cause of blindness in children in the United States?

    a. Amblyopia

    b. Myopia

    c. Retinopathy of prematurity

163. The nurse is assessing a newborn diagnosed with tracheomalacia. Which of the following is an exam finding that may be seen?

    a. Expiratory stridor

    b. A webbed neck

    c. Polydactyly

164. What is a medical emergency that can lead to hypovolemic shock in the newborn?

    a. Cephalohematoma

    b. Subgaleal hemorrhage

    c. Micrognathia

165. During pregnancy, what is a suspicious finding on ultrasound that may indicate an esophageal atresia?

    a. A fetus that is large for gestational age

    b. Polyhydramnios

    c. Oligohydramnios

166. What is the purpose for CCHD screening in newborns?

    a. To identify infants with severe congenital heart disease

    b. To identify infants born with a cleft lip or palate

    c. To identify infants born with fetal alcohol syndrome

167. When the nurse is teaching tracheostomy care at home, which of the following is important for the caregivers to understand?

a. Cleaning and changing the trach tube must be done under sterile conditions.
b. The trach tube can be reused after it has been cleaned properly.
c. The trach tube can only be changed by a Respiratory Therapist who will come to the home.

168. Parents of a newborn in the NICU are concerned about their baby having an IV placed in their scalp. To reassure them, what should the nurse explain?

a. There are no mature nerve endings in the scalp and it is not painful for the infant to have the IV in that location.
b. The peripheral veins are not yet mature enough to handle IV therapy.
c. The IV needs to be in an area with less fat so the vein can be clearly visualized.

169. Which of the following is one of the main advantages to using the Teach-Back system for educating patients and their families?

a. Improving education documentation in the patient's medical record
b. To ensure that information that is taught is fully understood
c. To limit the number of people involved in the patient's care

170. Which of the following is best when communicating with a non-English speaking patient and her family?

a. Have another family member interpret if possible
b. Improvise by using pictures and video to teach
c. Arrange to have an interpreter familiar with medical terminology present

171. Of the following, which is an example of beneficence in nursing?

a. Helping patients with their ADLs when they are not able to do them on their own
b. Confirming that medical interventions will not harm the patient
c. Ensuring all patients are treated fairly regardless of their background

172. Of the following, which is an example of nonmaleficence in nursing?

a. Letting the CNA help a patient with her ADLs rather than doing it yourself
b. Waiting until a patient has had pain medication before performing wound care
c. Being truthful and honest regarding patient condition and care options

173. The nurse accidentally administers the wrong dosage of medication to an infant in the NICU, resulting in a poor outcome. What is this an example of?

a. Medical negligence
b. Medical malpractice
c. Slander

174. What is the purpose of quality improvement?

a. To improve employee satisfaction
b. To monitor the leadership skills of the administration of a healthcare facility
c. To implement specific changes, which have a measurable improvement for a group of patients

175. The nurse receives a phone call from the grandmother of a patient. She has not been able to reach the child's parents because they have been staying at his bedside, but she is asking for a status update about his condition. What is the best response?

   a.   Tell her how he has been doing.
   b.   Explain that, in order to speak with her, she will need to submit a release of information form signed by the parents.
   c.   Tell her you are not able to give her any information, but that you will let the parents know she called and ask them to contact her.

Answer Key and Explanations for Test #1

1. B: Hypertonia is not present in an infant experiencing cold stress. An infant can actually become hypotonic with lax muscle tone during cold stress situations—especially premature infants who may already exhibit some degree of hypotonia due to their immaturity. Hypotonia can also be seen in hypoxia, so it is important to determine the cause and correct it if possible. If an infant exhibits symptoms of hypertonia, investigation as to its cause and subsequent management is warranted.

2. A: Normal body temperature range for a neonate is 36.5-37.5 °C (97.7-99.5 °F). According to the World Health Organization, hyperthermia is stated as being a core body temperature greater than 37.5°C. The other answers do indicate a hyperthermic state, but they are not the reference point for determining hyperthermia.

3. B: In this scenario, a pH that is WNL (within normal limits) does not mean this is a normal blood gas. All measurements must be taken into consideration for proper interpretation. Acidosis or alkalosis has one of three causes: respiratory, metabolic, or mixed. Usually, in an otherwise healthy premature neonate, an abnormal blood gas is due to underdeveloped lungs which leads to a buildup of CO_2 in the bloodstream. The indicator for a respiratory imbalance is pCO_2. High pCO_2 usually indicates a case of respiratory acidosis. When coupled with a high level of HCO_3^- (bicarbonate—which is base), it is an indication of the body trying to compensate for the high CO_2 in the bloodstream. Whether an imbalance is compensated or uncompensated is determined solely by the pH. If the pH is within normal range, the state is compensated.

4. A: Bleeding is the most common complication of ECMO, probably due to the large amounts of heparin that are used to prevent the blood from clotting in the mechanical process. Bleeding can be seen in any internal organ, but is most concerning when it occurs in the brain. For this reason, infants on ECMO are frequently and regularly evaluated for intracranial hemorrhages.

5. C: Nasal cannulas are appropriate for infants that require less than 1 lpm (liter per minute) O_2. Cannulas will also allow for uninterrupted bottle feeding. Infant nasal cannulas will only provide an O_2 flow of less than 1 lpm. Infants that require higher flow rates or concentrations of FiO_2 greater than 0.4 (40%) will require alternate delivery methods.

6. A: HELLP syndrome is a triad of specific maternal hematologic findings, characterized by hemolysis, elevated liver enzymes, and low platelet count. It is believed that HELLP syndrome occurs in about 1:1500 normal pregnancies and is seen in as much as 20% of women who are exhibiting preeclampsia or eclampsia. The cause is unknown, and it is often misdiagnosed as other illnesses and/or conditions. The only effective treatment of HELLP syndrome is delivery of the baby; therefore, the chance for premature delivery of the infant is high.

7. B: TORCH syndrome includes toxoplasmosis, other diseases, rubella, cytomegalovirus, and herpes simplex. The "other" category of diseases in TORCH syndrome includes syphilis, coxsackievirus, varicella-zoster, parvovirus, and HIV. TORCH syndrome can cause multiple, devastating effects on the fetus/neonate including jaundice, microcephaly, intellectual disability, deafness, eye problems, autism, and death. Prognosis varies depending of type of infection and the stage of pregnancy when contracted. If the cause is bacterial and the mother is treated early with antibiotics, the prognosis for the infant is good. However, no effective treatment is available if the cause is viral. In the case of viral TORCH syndrome, prevention by way of maternal vaccination is key.

8. B: Many factors contribute to the need for mechanical ventilation in a neonate. One must take into consideration all aspects of respiratory function to determine if mechanical ventilation is necessary. General guidelines include signs of impending respiratory failure (respiratory rate greater than 60/min, retractions, grunting, nasal flaring), apnea, and presence of existing respiratory failure. Other factors may also be indications for mechanical ventilation, including certain congenital anomalies that may interfere with respiration, septic infants, and infants weighing less than 1000 g.

9. C: Insensible water loss is defined as evaporative water loss through the skin and respiratory tract. Open-air warmers and bassinets can pose a risk for increased insensible water loss through the skin via exposure to environmental air currents. This is especially true with open warmers, as infants are either nude or just wearing a diaper, thus exposing a majority of skin to the surrounding air. This is why it's important to position warmers and bassinets out of drafts. Tachypnea (respiratory rate greater than 60/min) increases insensible water loss through rapid respiration. Babies born in uncontrolled environments are subject to greater insensible water loss due to improper drying and swaddling in the field.

10. A: Total parenteral nutrition (TPN) is a means of providing essential nutrients to the patient while bypassing the GI tract. Since this often requires long-term IV access, it is considered appropriate only when complete bowel rest is called for. In the neonate, this might include short-gut syndrome, gastroschisis, bowel obstruction, or prolonged diarrhea. TPN administration carries many risks, and must therefore be used only when medically necessary.

11. A: The total daily calorie requirement for a normal, growing preterm infant is between 105-120 kcal/kg/day for enteral feedings. Human milk and regular formula contain 20 kcal/oz. Fortified preterm formulas contain 22-24 kcal/oz. Half-strength human milk or formula contains 10 kcal/oz. Parenteral nutritional requirements are about 20% less at 85-100 kcal/kg/day. Many factors come into play when determining appropriate caloric intake for an infant, including activity, body temperature, and stress level of the infant. Infants under more stress (like those who have just had surgery) will require more calories/day.

12. C: Fetal alcohol syndrome (FAS) is characterized by cardiac defects (atrial or ventricular septal defects), small head, growth restriction, developmental delays, and facial abnormalities (small upper jaw, thin upper lip, small eyes with epicanthal folds). Most infants with FAS do not have normal brain development and will require work with many varied health care providers over the course of their life.

13. C: The presence of meconium in the amniotic fluid can have dire consequences in the neonate if the neonate inhaled the meconium-stained fluid while in utero or during delivery. Meconium aspiration can negatively impact an infant's lung function severely, and can cause a pneumothorax or PPHN. The symptoms of meconium aspiration may include cyanosis, respiratory distress with labored/rapid breathing, slow heartbeat, and a barrel-shaped chest.

14. B: Pulmonary surfactant is composed of proteins and phospholipids. It is a substance that is produced and secreted by the lungs. It reduces surface tension and acts as a lubrication of the alveolar surfaces. This prevents the walls of alveoli from sticking together during exhalation, preventing alveolar collapse. Preterm infants less than 32 weeks' gestation are at greater risk for having surfactant deficiencies, since adequate surfactant production usually occurs later in gestation. The leading cause of respiratory distress syndrome in neonates is pulmonary surfactant insufficiency.

15. B: Respiratory distress syndrome is a serious and fairly common problem for preterm neonates due to the lack of pulmonary surfactant needed to maintain alveolar integrity. When RDS is severe, the infant may require mechanical ventilation which significantly increases the air pressure in the neonatal lungs. It is trauma from this increased air pressure on already-compromised and noncompliant alveoli that can cause them to rupture, thus causing pneumothoraxes in the neonate.

16. C: There are three main types of cyanosis: central, peripheral, and differential. In differential cyanosis, the infant's lower extremities are usually cyanotic while the upper extremities and head remain pink. The main cause of differential cyanosis (DC) is the presence of a PDA (patent ductus arteriosus). DC occurs when unoxygenated blood is shunted through the PDA opening in the heart and is pumped out into the descending aorta to the lower extremities causing cyanosis in only the lower extremities. Large PDAs can cause very loud, mechanical-sounding murmurs.

17. C: Tetralogy of Fallot (ToF) is a congenital cardiac defect that occurs in approximately 1:2000 live births. It is characterized by the presence of four structural defects within and surrounding the heart. The four components are right ventricular hypertrophy, pulmonary stenosis, ventricular septal defect, and overriding aorta. ToF is the major cause of the so-called "blue baby syndrome."

18. A: In an ever-evolving field such as neonatology, it is vitally important to keep current on one's skills and knowledge base as new technologies and treatment modalities are continually being improved upon. It is also crucial to base charting on objective data that can be measured and quantified. Feelings are an important part of nursing, but they do not belong in the charting. Although it is beneficial that a nurse be able to work independently without requiring constant supervision, a nurse should always consult other colleagues in the decision-making process.

19. B: Grief can manifest itself in many diverse ways. It is important to understand that grief can be expressed directly, come out "sideways," or be suppressed or turned inwardly. When grief is turned inward, it can have profound psycho-physiological effects that can manifest themselves in cardiac, respiratory, neuromuscular, or other somatic symptoms. When grief is expressed outwardly, significant changes in behavior and personality can be observed. It's important to help parents identify and acknowledge their grief so that they might work through it in more positive ways.

20. A: When discharging any infant whose mother plans on breastfeeding at home, it is always good practice to coordinate a lactation consult. This will ensure the best chance for successful home breastfeeding by providing a professional/competent source of evaluation, encouragement, training, and troubleshooting. Since this child is not going home with any special equipment, and is not exhibiting any physical problems that require therapy, it is not necessary to plan for physical/occupational therapy or additional durable medical equipment at this time. It is, however, important to teach the parents/caregivers about the potential developmental challenges associated with prematurity. Encourage the parents to call their healthcare provider if they develop any questions or concerns.

21. C: After delivery of a critically ill or malformed infant, parents often exhibit emotional withdrawal or detachment from the infant. This is a normal coping mechanism in which the parents are attempting (subconsciously) to shield themselves from feelings of sadness, guilt, disappointment, or shame. This behavior becomes pathologic and dysfunctional when it persists despite improvement in the infant's condition and subsequent imminent survival of the infant.

22. C: Being well educated does not seem to negatively affect the parent/child interaction. In fact, it is the opposite that is the case. In parents who are of low-education levels (especially if the parents are also of a low intelligence level), a general lack of knowledge or decreased capacity for learning can cause significant problems with healthy parent/child interaction. The same holds true for young parents or parents with very large, overly involved families. The intentions of these families may be good, but often times can hinder appropriate parent/child interactions.

23. B: Edwards syndrome is a fairly common genetic condition that occurs in about 1:5000 live births. It is not an inherited disease. The chance of having a child with Edwards syndrome increases as the mother's age increases. Most children with Edwards syndrome are female (at a ratio of about 3:1). Trisomy 18 is a devastating condition in which about 50% of all infants die in utero. Of those who survive, 95% die within the first year. It causes significant and devastating malformations and failures in multiple organ systems.

24. A: Congenital cytomegalovirus (CMV) occurs when an infected mother transmits the disease to her fetus. It is estimated that the transmission rate from primarily infected mothers to their fetus is between 30-50%. Of those infants born with congenital CMV, the vast majority will be asymptomatic and will not suffer any problems related to CMV later in their life. However, 10-15% of infants will exhibit symptoms that may include seizures, hepatosplenomegaly, hearing loss, and microcephaly.

25. B: Many factors put an infant at risk for developing group B Strep infections including a maternal fever greater than 38 °C, prolonged labor lasting over 18 hours, use of internal fetal monitoring devices, prematurity, and a mother who is positive for group B Strep. Mothers are now routinely screened for group B Strep between 37+0 to 37+6 weeks gestation. Treatment for group B Strep includes antibiotics, respiratory/ventilatory support, IV fluids, and oxygen therapy.

26. A: There are two causes of NAS: passive exposure to opioids and non-opioids in utero from a "using" mother through the placenta and iatrogenic exposure by the direct administration of opiates to the neonate. When the umbilical cord is cut, passive exposure immediately ends. Withdrawal symptoms can occur within hours after birth to up to 2 weeks of age. The majority of symptoms occur within 72 hours. NAS causes a host of symptoms including CNS hyperirritability, GI dysfunction, respiratory distress, increased and exaggerated reflexes, marked sleep disturbance, tremors, and restlessness.

27. C: Physiologic signs of pain in the neonate are the same as they are in adults. Pain causes an increase in many metabolic processes including heart rate, blood pressure, ICP, and respiratory rate. It causes a decrease in oxygenation. It can manifest as hyper- or hypotonicity and can cause disturbances in sleeping and feeding patterns.

28. C: There are many nonpharmacologic interventions that can lessen the severity of pain in the neonate. Comfort measures play an important role in pain management and may prevent the intensification of pain in the neonate. Comfort measures are effective in the alleviation of mild pain but, alone, they may be inadequate in cases of moderate to severe pain. Controlling the neonate's environment to decrease sensory stimulation is a major component in providing effective comfort measures.

29. B: Kangaroo care is a method of providing noninvasive, non-painful touch that is not associated with caregiving activities. Its purpose is to promote social contact between caregiver and neonate by providing a positive touch experience. This can help prevent the neonate from developing touch aversion. In kangaroo care, the infant is naked (with or without diaper) and is placed vertically on the bare chest of the caregiver between his/her breasts. This provides skin-to-skin full body contact which can have marked calming effects of the neonate. It may also promote parent/child bonding.

30. A: FDA guidelines recommend a dose of 10-15mg/kg of acetaminophen every 6 hours for neonates. For the infant in the given scenario, the dose range would be 27-41 mg. Using partial suppositories is not recommended because the exact dosing cannot be accurately determined. Though answer C used to be correct, the FDA has pulled the concentrated infant drops (80 mg/0.8 cc) off the market as of 2011. It is no longer available and has been replaced by pediatric-strength (160 mg/5 cc) liquid.

31. C: Infant abductors are usually women around 30 years of age. They are often overweight with low self-esteem. Most have no prior criminal records. The majority of them exhibit normal behavior and will often visit the nursery prior to the abduction in order to learn about the security measures that are in place and to choose their target/targets. The motive for many of these abductors stems from wanting to either replace a child they've lost or because they are not able to conceive.

32. A: HIPAA is an acronym that stands for Health Insurance Portability and Accountability Act. It was established in 1996. Part 1 of the act protects the health care insurance coverage of workers and their families when they change job statuses. Part 2 of the act addresses many areas regarding the security and privacy of health information and data.

33. A: According to the American Academy of Pediatrics, there are several known precipitating or contributing factors which have been linked with sudden infant death syndrome (SIDS). In addition to the factors listed, others include being born to a teenage mother, living in poverty conditions, soft bedding/mattresses, multiple birth babies (twins, triplets, etc.), the absence of prenatal care, and sleeping in the same bed as parents. It is important for the neonatal nurse to not only know these factors, but also to teach these to new parents.

34. C: Cystic fibrosis (CF) is an autosomal recessive disease. This means that both parents must have the CF gene in order to possibly pass it on to their children. If only one parent possesses the CF gene, the chance that their child will have the disease is 0. The chance that their child will be a carrier of the CF gene is 1:2. The chance that their child will be completely normal is also 1:2.

35. B: The hallmark sign of an infant of a diabetic mother is that they are usually large for gestational age (LGA). They are also at great risk for developing hypoglycemia so it is important to monitor all IDM for hypoglycemia regardless of whether they are exhibiting symptoms or not. Newborn jaundice is also a common complication of IDM.

36. B: Choanal atresia is a congenital condition in which the nasal passages are extremely narrowed or completely blocked by tissue. Since babies are obligate nose-breathers, they will attempt breathing through their nose. When this is not possible, retractions and cyanosis will ensue as the baby attempts nose-breathing. Because of the size/configuration of the infant tongue and soft palate, the oral airway is easily obstructed when the infant is at rest. When the infant cries, the palate raises and the tongue moves enough to temporarily open the airway. Bilateral choanal atresia can be life-threatening. It can be corrected surgically through the insertion of nasal stints.

37. C: Post-term infants (born at greater than 41 weeks' gestation) are at risk for developing a host of problems. First and foremost, they are at risk for meconium aspiration since a large number of post-term infants pass meconium in utero. Umbilical cord compression is a potentially serious problem as a result of oligohydramnios, which can occur post-term. Since most post-term babies are large, there is the possibility for macrosomia-related problems and subsequent birth injuries. Other potential problems include hypoglycemia, seizures, and respiratory insufficiency.

38. A: The usual dose of naloxone in an infant who is showing moderate respiratory depression from exposure to narcotic analgesics is 0.01 mg/kg given IM, IV, or SC. If the infant is in severe respiratory distress and requires mechanical ventilation from a narcotic overdose, a high dose of naloxone (0.1 mg/kg) is indicated.

39. A: Per the American Heart Association, the current recommendation is that external chest compressions be given if the heart rate is sustained below 60 bpm if adequate assisted ventilation with oxygen is in place. The rate of compressions should be about 90/min with 30 coordinated breaths per minute.

40. B: The Kleihauer-Betke test is a blood test that determines the presence and quantity of fetal hemoglobin in the mother's bloodstream. Fetal hemoglobin retains its red staining while adult hemoglobin becomes very pale after fixing. The presence of 10 fetal hemoglobin cells per microscope field is equivalent to approximately 1 cc of fetal blood. This is an effective method in determining the extent of fetal blood loss.

41. C: Methicillin-resistant *Staphylococcus aureus* (MRSA) is the primary strain of bacteria that is responsible for most cases of hospital-acquired infection/illness. MRSA has become the most prevalent and potentially dangerous pathogen found in hospitals today. It has evolved to the point where it has become resistant to many, if not most, antibiotics.

42. B: Hospital-acquired pneumonia is a common nosocomial infection in the NICU. By rapidly weaning infants off mechanical ventilators as quickly as is medically safe, the risk for developing nosocomial pneumonia is greatly reduced because the pathogen's method of entry into the host is eliminated at the time of extubation.

43. A: SpO_2 is the percent of hemoglobin that is saturated with oxygen. The pulse oximeter is a device used to measure SpO_2. The pulse oximeter uses a noninvasive probe that is attached to a finger or toe. It works by emitting light and calculating the absorption of specific wavelengths of light to determine how much of the hemoglobin is saturated. Because the machine utilizes a light source, any bright external light could potentially interfere with its functioning. Factors like vasoconstriction or shivering can interfere with the probe's ability to accurately measure the hemoglobin. This is why it's important to make certain the patient's peripheral perfusion is adequate and that the patient is kept calm and still if possible.

44. B: Initial stabilization practices for the infant with an abdominal wall defect (either gastroschisis, or omphalocele) involve measures aimed at protecting the exposed organs and minimizing their trauma. This can be obtained by covering the exposed organs with warm saline-soaked gauze with some form of evaporative barrier (even plastic wrap would work) to keep them from drying out. It is recommended to place the infant in a side-lying position with support of the exposed organs. Although IV access should immediately be established, UAC/UVC lines are absolutely contraindicated with abdominal wall defects. An orogastric tube should be inserted and placed on low-intermittent suction to aid in decompression of the stomach. Extreme vigilance should be given to monitoring the infant's temperature and urine output since the infant is at great risk for temperature instability and possible damage to the internal urinary system.

45. B: Expected urinary output rate for a neonate less than 2 days old is 1-3 cc/kg/hr. It takes a day or so for newborn kidneys to reach their optimal functioning level, so a slightly lower rate of 1 cc/kg/hr is acceptable (albeit on the low side). After the infant is about 48 hours old, kidney function should increase to about 2-4 cc/kg/hr. Any deviation from this range should be investigated to determine the underlying cause.

46. C: The L:S ratio test (lecithin-sphingomyelin ratio) is a marker of fetal lung maturity. Lecithin and sphingomyelin are excreted in equal proportions until about 32 weeks' gestation, at which time lecithin concentration increases dramatically while sphingomyelin levels remain the same. The L:S ratio is measured in the amniotic fluid. Lecithin and sphingomyelin are both surfactants, but lecithin is the substance responsible for making them work more effectively thus preventing collapse of the neonate lung. A ratio of 2:1 indicates that the fetal lungs are mature, thereby decreasing the chance of the infant developing respiratory distress syndrome.

47. C: Amniotic band syndrome (also known as ADAM complex, pseudoainhum, Streeter's dysplasia, amniotic band sequence) is a rare condition in which the amnion (inner layer of placenta) has been damaged and fiber-like bands of the amnion have broken off (been torn away) and become entangled and/or wrapped around the developing fetus. The bands usually get tangled around the limbs of the fetus. This reduces blood supply to the entrapped areas and cause them to develop abnormally or (in extreme cases) amputate the limb altogether. Amniotic bands can also entrap the face or chest. When this occurs, clefts of the affected area can develop.

48. B: TTN is a respiratory disorder that occurs shortly after delivery. It is seen in babies who are born at or near full term. In TTN, the respiratory rate is greater than 60 breaths/minute, which usually lasts less than 24 hours. Babies born by C-section are at risk due to retention of amniotic fluid in the lungs which can temporarily interfere with respiration. In an NSVD, the lungs are better drained of the amniotic fluid via the squeezing of the chest wall during vaginal delivery. The amniotic fluid is eventually reabsorbed and the condition resolves.

49. A: GE reflux is common in healthy infants. It is estimated that over half of all newborns exhibit signs of GE reflux within the first 3 months of life. Most cases of GE reflux resolve within the first 12 months. Since it is such a common finding in neonates, it is important to institute measures that help reduce the risk/frequency of reflux episodes. These interventions include small, frequent feedings with frequent burping, elevating the head of the bed, placing infant in supine position, thickening feedings, and keeping the infant upright for 30 minutes after feeding.

50. C: Neonatal hyperbilirubinemia (aka newborn jaundice or physiological jaundice) is a common condition in a newborn. It is usually a benign finding that is self-limiting. It can be associated with breastfeeding for one of three reasons: (a) decreased oral intake due to mother's decreased milk production, (b) infants who do not breastfeed well, or (c) due to substances in the human milk that affect bilirubin breakdown in the infant. It usually resolves on its own within the first 2-3 weeks of life. Occasionally hyperbilirubinemia requires phototherapy treatment to aid in the breakdown of bilirubin in the skin. In extremely rare cases, hyperbilirubinemia can lead to kernicterus, but this is usually associated with hyperbilirubinemia that has some other underlying cause.

51. B: HELLP syndrome is a serious liver disorder that can occur in the last trimester in pregnancy. It is characterized by hemolysis, elevated liver enzymes, and low platelets. Most women who develop HELLP syndrome also have preeclampsia, which is the greatest risk factor for developing this condition. The mother will have very high blood pressure, nausea, abdominal pain, and swelling. Treatment begins with delivery of the baby, even if it is premature. Symptomatic treatment with IV fluids, anti-hypertensives, and vasodilators are given to the mother. It can be fatal if it is not treated.

52. C: Hepatitis B is transmitted from the mother to the fetus during pregnancy. Approximately 40% of infants of hepatitis B positive women will develop the disease, and up to 25% of those will die from chronic liver disease. It is imperative to administer the hepatitis B vaccine and hepatitis B immunoglobulin to these infants within 12 hours of birth. Routine vaccination of all infants is usually given within 24 hours of birth.

53. A: There is no known genetic risk for developing Amniotic Band Syndrome. There are also no known behaviors during pregnancy that increase the risk for this condition. It occurs when thick, fibrous bands within the amniotic fluid wrap around the limb or face of the fetus in utero. It can cut off the blood supply to the affected area and result in amputation or deformity of the affected limb. If the bands wrap around the face, it can result in cleft lip and palate. There is a greater than 30% chance that Amniotic Band Syndrome will cause a club foot deformity.

54. A: Chorioamnionitis is an acute infection and inflammation of the membranes and is commonly caused by a premature rupture of the membranes. This eliminates the protective barrier surrounding the fetus and increases the risk for pathogens to ascend into the uterus. Less commonly, chorioamnionitis can occur in the absence of membrane rupture. Long-term effects of this condition to the neonate include stillbirth, premature birth, sepsis, chronic lung disease, and brain injury or cerebral palsy. The mother can develop postpartum infections and sepsis.

55. C: The quad screen is performed at 15-20 weeks of pregnancy via a blood test. It measures alpha-fetoprotein, human chorionic gonadotropin, estriol, and inhibin-A. Alpha-fetoprotein is made in the liver of the fetus and elevated levels may indicate a neural tube defect such as spina bifida. Human chorionic gonadotropin is made by the placenta and levels vary during pregnancy. Estriol is a form of estrogen made by the placenta and levels increase during pregnancy. Inhibin-A is a hormone produced by the fetus and the placenta and abnormal levels may indicate the presence of Down syndrome.

56. B: Late decelerations present as smooth decreases in the heart rate that begin at the peak of a contraction. When late decelerations occur along with tachycardia and without an acceleration, or return to normal heart rate range, it can be a sign that the fetus is not getting enough oxygen. Early decelerations begin before the contraction peaks and usually occur as the fetus passes through the birth canal and the skull is compressed. They are generally not harmful. Variable decelerations occur when the umbilical cord is temporarily compressed and are very common during labor. They are usually not harmful when they occur later in labor and are followed by an acceleration. When variable decelerations occur early in labor and are severe, emergent delivery of the baby may be necessary.

57. B: Tocolytics are drugs that are given to slow down or stop preterm labor. They are generally not used before 23-24 weeks of pregnancy and may be used as late as 36 weeks of pregnancy. Terbutaline is in a class of drugs called beta-mimetics. It is used to decrease uterine contractions by relaxing the uterine musculature. It can cause nervousness, tremors, headache, and tachycardia. Cytotec is given as a pill or vaginal suppository to help soften the cervix to induce labor. Pitocin is used to increase uterine contractions and cervical dilation to induce labor.

58. A: A frank breech presentation is one in which the legs of the fetus are extended upward so that the feet are near the head. This results in the buttocks passing through the birth canal first. A complete breech occurs when the knees of the fetus are bent so that the feet are near the buttocks. A footling breech occurs when the fetus is foot down and one or both feet present first through the birth canal.

59. A: Abruptio placentae results in early detachment of the placenta from the wall of the uterus. The most common cause of this condition is hypertension in the mother, but trauma can also be a cause. The effects on the fetus can be critical because of the disruption of the oxygen and nutrient supply. A cord prolapse occurs when the umbilical passes through the birth canal before the fetus. Placenta previa occurs when the uterus attaches to the lower portion of the uterus and covers the cervix.

60. B: Forceps may be used during delivery to assist the neonate's passage through the birth canal, especially if the mother or infant is in distress. There is a risk of facial palsy (usually temporary) and minor facial or external eye injury. Rarely, a skull fracture or bleeding within the brain can occur.

61. A: An infant born at 37 weeks or later who weighs 2500 grams or less is considered small for gestational age. This differs from the premature infant who is born earlier than 37 weeks gestation, though they often weigh less than 2500 grams as well.

62. C: Milia are very common and occur when flakes of skin become trapped within pores. It is most common in newborns and occurs most often on the nose and chin. It is important to not pick or pinch these lesions because this could damage the tissue or lead to a skin infection. The lesions usually resolve on their own within a few weeks.

63. B: Pitting edema in the soft tissues of the scalp is not uncommon after birth, due to trauma on the baby's scalp while moving through the birth canal. This condition is called caput succedaneum and is most evident immediately after birth. It usually resolves rather quickly over the first 24-48 hours following birth and just needs to be monitored for any changes.

64. B: Whitish bumps, or cysts, along the gum or roof of the mouth are called Epstein's pearls. They are very common and occur in about 80% of newborns. These will resolve on their own within the first couple of weeks of life and do not require any treatment.

65. A: Tetralogy of Fallot is a very serious congenital heart defect that includes a large ventricular septal defect, pulmonary stenosis, right ventricular hypertrophy, and an overriding aorta. Though this is a serious condition, it is treated surgically during infancy and most children with this condition will go on to live into adulthood.

66. A: Nasal flaring is seen in newborns as an attempt to widen the nares and take in more oxygen. Other signs of respiratory distress include retractions, tachypnea, grunting, and abnormal breath sounds. Pink skin color and a respiratory rate of 40 breaths per minute are expected findings in the neonate.

67. B: Some of the signs of fluid overload include increased blood pressure, swelling in the extremities and face, abdominal bloating, shortness of breath, and tachycardia. The nurse will monitor the patient regularly for any of these symptoms. If the patient will be discharged home, the parents and/or caregivers will also need to be educated on these symptoms.

68. B: Daily chlorhexidine baths performed on infants in the NICU have been proven to reduce the incidence of many nosocomial infections. The primary concern with some infants is that the skin does not fully mature until the last quarter of gestation, so skin integrity may be a concern. The U.S. Food and Drug Administration has not approved the use of chlorhexidine in infants less than 2 months of age, but it is still used in most hospital settings as off-label usage.

69. B: The Moro reflex is checked by quickly lowering the infant's head relative to the trunk and when present, results in the abduction and extension of the infant's arms as the hands open. This reflex is present as early as 32 weeks gestation. It is no longer present by the time the infant is 6-months-old. The grasp reflex is the reflexive action of bending the fingers around an object placed in the palm. The asymmetrical tonic reflex is also called the "fencing" reflex. When the infant's head is turned to one side, the arm and leg of the side at which the face is turned extend and the arm and leg on the opposite side flex.

70. B: According to the American Heart Association, chest compressions should be started on the pediatric patient if the pulse is less than 60 beats per minute or if there are signs of poor perfusion. If one person is performing CPR, the rate is 30 compressions followed by 2 breaths. If 2-person CPR is being performed, the cycle should be 15 compressions followed by 2 breaths.

71. B: Pyloric stenosis is a condition in which the muscle tissue in the lower stomach, at the pylorus, becomes thickened and prevents food from passing into the small intestine. This is usually evident around 3-5 weeks of age and will cause an olive-shaped mass in the upper abdomen, peristaltic waves across the abdomen, projectile vomiting, and persistent crying because the infant is hungry. It is repairable with surgery, though the infant's fluid and electrolyte balance needs to be corrected.

72. C: Acute volume expansion in the neonate can be accomplished with an isotonic crystalloid solution, such as lactated Ringer's solution. This increases the pressure in the intravascular space, which causes water to move from the interstitial to intravascular spaces, increasing the circulating blood volume. Crystalloids have a half-life between 30 and 60 minutes and must be given in amounts three times the volume lost. If too much is given too quickly, however, fluid overload with intraventricular hemorrhage and pulmonary edema can result.

73. C: Hydrops fetalis is a potentially life-threatening condition in which accumulating fluid is present in at least two body cavities (abdomen, pleura, or pericardium). Traditionally, this has been treated through removal of the fluid after the umbilical cord has been cut and resuscitative measures started. It has recently been found that the prognosis is improved if the neonate remains attached to the placenta via the umbilical cord so they continue to receive oxygenated blood from the mother. The fluid can be drawn off and then the cord can be clamped before resuscitative measures are started.

74. B: The preterm infant needs 100-150 kcal/kg/day in order to complete development and gain weight. A term infant generally needs 100-120 kcal/kg/day for normal growth and development. Adequate nutrition to meet the nutritional needs of the preterm infant can help to prevent poor outcomes and help to improve adequate nervous system development.

75. A: The survival rate for this infant is lower than another infant requiring resuscitation without a diaphragmatic hernia. With a diaphragmatic hernia, the diaphragm becomes weakened and this can result in the stomach and other abdominal contents expending into the chest cavity. This, along with the weakened diaphragm, can result in a decreased ability to breathe. If detected in the prenatal period, assistance can standby during delivery to begin resuscitative measures promptly and improve the chances for survival.

76. A: A urine output >8 mL/kg/hr is categorized as severe polyuria. If not already present, a urinary catheter is usually inserted at this point to obtain a more accurate reading of urinary output. If this is a new change in urine output for the infant, the neonatologist on call should be contacted.

77. B: Insensible water loss is that water that passes through the skin and evaporates and the water that evaporates through the respiratory tract. Newborns have a relatively large surface area through which there can be increased amounts of insensible water loss. This loss will be at its greatest in the small early gestational age infant.

78. C: Gut priming is the practice of giving enteral nutrition in sub-nutritional quantities in order to stimulate the GI tract to function better. It is usually done at the 3rd day of life and is only indicated in babies weighing less than 1000 g. It is usually done for 2-3 days to stimulate hormone production, enzymes, peristalsis, and to boost the immune system. Gut priming can also help to increase the excretion of bilirubin.

79. A: Gavage feeding is used to provide nutrition to the infant with a poor sucking reflex, tachypnea, respiratory distress, impaired swallowing, or apneic spells. A nasogastric tube is placed and formula or human milk is slowly fed through the tube with a syringe. Often, the baby will be soothed or gently touched during the feeding to promote positive reinforcement with sucking. The feeding should be stopped if the baby exhibits signs of gasping or choking.

80. B: Early feeding cues, the signs that an infant is hungry, include opening the mouth when the chin is touched, sucking on fingers, smacking or licking the lips, or fussiness. Hard crying can be a late feeding cue, but the infant is usually easily consoled when held and then fed, and the crying does not tend to be persistent. Persistent crying is more likely to be a sign that there is pain or another discomfort that is not being relieved.

81. B: Oral sucrose has been used in infants as a mild analgesic. It is given before minor procedures to help relax the infant and provide pain relief. The sucrose solution activates the body's mechanism to produce natural opioid-like substances, such as endorphins.

82. C: Metabolic alkalosis will cause the arterial blood pH and bicarbonate levels to increase. Conversely, metabolic acidosis will cause arterial pH and bicarbonate levels to decrease. Respiratory acidosis will increase the arterial carbon dioxide level while decreasing the pH, and respiratory alkalosis will have the opposite results with a decrease in carbon dioxide level and an increased pH.

83. C: The first form of human milk that can be expressed is called colostrum. This is produced for the first few days, up to a week, following delivery. It has a higher protein content than mature human milk. Colostrum can contain up to 17% protein, while mature human milk contains only about 1% protein.

84. B: Parenteral nutrition is given via intravenous route. It is used when enteral feeding via a tube directly in the GI tract is not possible. This is most often due to a very low birth weight, less than 1500 g. Enteral feedings are delayed in these infants due to immature lung function requiring intubation, hypotension, hypothermia, and infection risk. Also, the GI tract in these infants may not tolerate feedings that require digestion by normal means.

85. C: Very low birth weight infants are at risk for developing bronchopulmonary dysplasia. Nutritional support can possibly help to decrease the development of this condition. Vitamin A helps with lung maturity, and supplementation with this vitamin may help to prevent this condition. Parenteral nutrition also helps with lung development to ensure the infant is receiving the proteins and lipids needed to help with lung maturity.

86. A: Short bowel syndrome in infants is a condition in which there are absorption problems due to a short bowel length. The short bowel may occur as a result of a birth defect affecting maturation of the bowel, an abdominal wall defect, enterocolitis, atresia, or volvulus. The goal with this condition is to eventually have the patient not rely on TPN for their nutritional needs, but sometimes it is necessary indefinitely. Low birth weight infants almost always go on to feeding regularly after the initial acute phase following delivery. Pyloric stenosis is surgically repairable and does not normally lead to permanent absorption issues that require long-term TPN.

87. C: An extracorporeal membrane oxygenation (ECMO) device is used in infants who are not able to breath or pump blood on their own. It is a type of heart-lung bypass machine that circulates blood from the infant, through an artificial lung to oxygenate the blood, and then back into the infant to circulate through the body. Some of the potential risks include the formation of blood clots, bleeding, or infection.

88. B: Lactic acid is increased in situations of tissue hypoxia, which can lead to severe metabolic acidosis. This can occur with sepsis, heart failure, shock, and multisystem organ failure. Studies have shown that elevations in serum lactate in the first week of life correlate with an increase in mortality rates. This risk is higher in infants born less than 1000 g.

89. C: Respiratory acidosis occurs when a person is not being adequately oxygenated. This results in an elevated $PaCO_2$ level and a decreased blood pH level. When the body attempts to compensate for this abnormality, the serum bicarbonate (HCO_3^-) level is elevated to offset the acidic level of the blood pH. This results in a continued $PaCO_2$, a normal blood pH level, and an elevated HCO_3^- level.

90. B: Hypoxia is a decrease in oxygen concentration at the tissue level. This is measured using a pulse oximeter and not by a lab test. On the other hand, hypoxemia is a true decrease in oxygen concentration within the blood. This is measured with a sample of arterial blood and should be 80-100 mmHg. It is labeled as a PaO_2 measurement.

91. C: Whenever possible, dobutamine should be given through a central line because it is caustic to the body's tissues. This medication is primarily used to improve the effectiveness of the heart to work as a pump and, to a lesser degree, can help with hypotension.

92. C: When gentamicin is given for more than 2 days, there is an increased risk of hearing loss. In order to decrease this risk, drug levels are measured at the point at which the drug level is highest and again when it is at its lowest (a peak and trough). This is to ensure the antibiotic remains at a therapeutic level rather than a toxic level.

93. A: Calcium excretion is increased when a person receives Lasix. In the newborn, this can affect bone formation and maturation. Calcium levels should be monitored and supplementation administered if necessary.

94. C: The most immediate concern for babies born to mothers who use cocaine is premature delivery with associated low birth weight. Most of the problems these children develop are evident later with cognitive development, behavior problems, and learning disabilities.

95. B: Symptoms of alcohol withdrawal in a newborn who was exposed to alcohol regularly during pregnancy generally occur 3-12 hours after birth. Withdrawal symptoms from opiates generally occur 24-36 hours after birth, but may be longer depending on the medication. For example, newborns that were exposed to methadone regularly while in utero may not show withdrawal symptoms until a week or longer after birth due to the long half-life of the drug.

96. B: The kangaroo hold involves having the baby in skin-to-skin contact with another person. This gained popularity in the 1970s in Colombia where there was a high infant mortality rate. It was found that infants who were held against their mother's chest in skin-to-skin contact tended to thrive when compared to those who did not receive that close contact. Vital signs stabilize, crying is decreased, pain is reduced, sleep is increased, and the infant feeds better. PDA closure has not been proven to correlate with kangaroo care.

97. A: Persistent hypothermia can lead to hypoglycemia. There may be a period of transient hyperglycemia when glycogen stores are used to increase glucose levels, but this is followed by hypoglycemia as energy demands exceed glucose supply. This can lead to metabolic acidosis.

98. A: There are some medications that require drug levels to be drawn to ensure the drug concentration is at a therapeutic level and not too high or too low. For carbamazepine (Tegretol), the best time to check the drug level is just prior to giving a dose. The therapeutic drug level for this medication is 4-12 mg/L.

99. B: Some medications are incompatible with each other when given intravenously. This can be a chemical incompatibility, a physical incompatibility, a therapeutic incompatibility, or a drug IV container incompatibility. Of the choices listed, phenytoin (Dilantin) is safe to mix with D5W. The other two choices are not compatible with each other. It is advised that an IV drug compatibility chart be available for reference at all nursing stations.

100. A: Therapeutic drugs can cause withdrawal symptoms when they are stopped suddenly, especially if the patient has been taking them for a long period of time. The primary mechanism of action of beta-blockers is to decrease heart rate, thereby decreasing blood pressure, and decreasing the risk of developing a cardiac dysrhythmia. When the medication is stopped suddenly, the opposite effect is seen with a significant response. This includes high blood pressure, elevated heart rate, increased risk of cardiac dysrhythmia, tremors, and sweating.

101. C: To calculate the correct dosage, the first step will be to convert the weight to kilograms. 6 pounds 8 ounces, or 6.5 pounds, is divided by 2.2 to convert the weight to 2.95 kg. The dosage is 400 mg/kg/day so in a full day, the infant should receive 1,180 mg in a full day (400 x 2.95 = 1,180). The dosage is spaced three times a day, every 8 hours, so each dosage should be 393 mg (1,180/3 = 393).

102. B: Ganciclovir should be given over a 60-minute time period when given intravenously. It is used primarily for immunodeficient patients with CMV retinitis. It is a very cytotoxic drug and its cytotoxic effects are increased if given over a shorter period of time than 60 minutes. These adverse effects include thrombocytopenia, granulocytopenia, and anemia. In male patients, it may cause aspermatogenesis.

103. A: Perforomist, a formoterol inhalation treatment, is not indicated for use in children. It is indicated for treatment of COPD symptoms in adults. Albuterol is a beta-2 agonist that works to relieve respiratory symptoms by dilating the airway. Dexamethasone is a steroid that can decrease inflammation within the airway.

104. A: The half-life of dopamine is less than 2 minutes, so the total time in which the effects from the medication are seen is around 10 minutes. Dopamine is used to improve heart function, increase blood pressure, and increase renal perfusion.

105. C: When given, the preferred route for administering Narcan in the infant is IV or IM. It should not be given via endotracheal administration. Narcan is not used as a first line drug in the infant with respiratory depression. Normal color and pulse must first be present before it is considered. It may cause seizures if given to the infant of an opioid-addicted mother.

106. A: Habituation is the process by which repeated exposure to some type of stimuli eventually fails to elicit a response. In this example, the newborn becomes accustomed to hearing the monitor alarms several times daily, so he no longer turns his head toward it. This has also been called the "Get Used To It" concept.

107. C: Autonomic responses to stressful stimuli occur involuntarily. These can include flushing, pallor, or cyanosis. The vital signs can change in response to stress, resulting in an elevated heart rate, elevated blood pressure, increase in respiratory rate, or a decrease in oxygen saturation. Visceral responses can also occur, resulting in nausea, vomiting, diarrhea, or constipation.

108. B: Positive effects have been seen in the NICU when the lighting is in a cyclical pattern. Bright lights during the day and dim at night has been shown to contribute to infants feeding sooner, establishing "normal" sleep patterns, increasing the rate of weight gain while in the NICU, and decreasing the amount of time on a ventilator. The cyclical lighting helps to promote a regular circadian rhythm within the body to establish a regular sleep and wake cycle, which promotes improved overall health.

109. B: Non-nutritive sucking is having an infant suck on something that does not give them milk. For infants who are tube fed, it can trigger an association with them between having a full stomach and sucking, which can help when transitioning to oral feedings. The sucking activity is also helpful in strengthening the oral muscles needed to suck, as well as being soothing and calming for the infant.

110. A: Studies have shown that a rhythmic rocking motion can decrease apneic episodes in the newborn. Rocking also helps to stimulate the vestibular sense, which maintains a sense of balance and equilibrium. It can assist with further developing visual and auditory tracking. It is thought that rocking helps infants to shift their focus on external stimuli.

111. C: The first step should be to assess the rest of the infant to see if this is truly cyanosis. It is not uncommon for the face to undergo some trauma while passing through the birth canal, which can cause some areas of bruising. It can be differentiated from cyanosis by assessing whether it is present in the distal extremities or if the infant is showing any signs of respiratory distress. Facial bruising may take several days to gradually fade.

112. C: Before a baby is born, its blood is oxygenated by the mother through the placenta. A vessel is formed connecting the pulmonary and aortic arteries, the ductus arteriosus. Shortly after birth, this vessel closes off so that the infant's blood can then receive oxygen from its own lungs. A PDA results when the ductus arteriosus remains open and oxygen-rich blood from the aorta mixes with the blood lacking oxygen from the pulmonary artery. If the rest of the heart is functioning normal, the baby is monitored and the PDA is allowed to repair itself. If this does not happen, the defect can be surgically corrected.

113. B: According to the American Academy of Pediatrics and the European Consensus Guidelines recommendations, CPAP should initially be applied to all respiratory distressed infants. Infants in severe respiratory distress that, with CPAP, are still requiring FiO_2 of greater that 40% in order to maintain an oxygen saturation greater than 90%, or infants that are apneic, should then be intubated and administered surfactant. Infants requiring a FiO_2 of less than 40% to maintain appropriate oxygen saturation should remain on CPAP and have an ABG drawn to determine next intervention steps.

114. A: Cardiac tamponade occurs when fluid accumulates with the pericardial sac, causing pressure on the outside of the heart. It is treated by inserting a needle through the chest wall, into the pericardium, and withdrawing the fluid. While cardiac tamponade is rare in neonates, it can occur in the newborn when a central venous catheter is in an incorrect position, applying pressure at the juncture of the inferior vena cava and the right atrium. Ensuring correct placement of the catheter is imperative to prevent this life-threatening complication.

115. A: Coarctation of the aorta occurs when there is narrowing in the aorta. It is a congenital condition that may not cause any symptoms in the newborn and may not be known to be present until adulthood. If symptomatic, the common symptoms are pallor, difficulty breathing, and poor feeding due to difficulty breathing. If it is left untreated, it can lead to congestive heart failure or even death.

116. B: Hypoplastic left heart syndrome is a congenital heart defect that results in the left side of the heart being smaller than normal. This decreases the amount of oxygenated blood that can be delivered through the body. It will result in decreased peripheral pulses due to the left ventricular dysfunction. Peripheral cyanosis will also occur due to the decrease in oxygen being sent to the extremities. Patent ductus arteriosus and pulmonary stenosis do not result in peripheral cyanosis.

117. C: Transposition of the great vessels can involve any of the great vessels of the body: the superior or inferior vena cava, the pulmonary artery or pulmonary veins, or the aorta. It usually involves a "swap" between the locations of the vessels and can result in poorly oxygenated blood or poor delivery of blood to the body. If the pulmonary artery and aorta are involved, the condition is called a transposition of the great arteries.

118. B: Approximately one-half of all children born with Down syndrome have a heart defect. The most common type of heart defect in these children is an atrioventricular septal defect, or a ventricular septal defect in less severe cases. This occurs when the septum between either the atria and ventricles, or just the ventricles, is not fully formed. This allows oxygenated blood and deoxygenated blood to mix, which can cause the heart to work harder to transport oxygenated blood throughout the body.

119. A: There are two congenital heart defects that are considered cyanotic conditions: Tetralogy of Fallot and transposition of the great vessels. They both interfere with the delivery of oxygenated blood through the peripheral circulation, resulting in peripheral cyanosis. Other congenital heart defects are considered acyanotic because they are not likely to result in peripheral cyanosis.

120. C: A normal newborn blood pressure is 64/40. This usually rises to 95/58 around the first month of age. Premature infants will have even lower blood pressures unless their medical condition results in an elevation in blood pressure. In this situation, the nurse should record the reading and continue with the newborn assessment.

121. C: A G-tube should be flushed with warm water before and after all feedings to ensure patency and remove any build-up of formula within the tube itself. Air should not be flushed into the tube and nothing should ever be forcibly pushed through the tube.

122. B: Meconium aspiration syndrome occurs when the infant inhales meconium during the labor and delivery process. It presents as labored or rapid breathing with retractions and grunting sounds with each breath. The infant may begin to appear cyanotic as this condition progresses. To treat this condition, surfactant may be given which has proven to be helpful. A laryngoscope may be inserted to perform suction below the level of the vocal cords. Mortality rates are higher for these infants than others and there may be some residual respiratory problems for the first 5-10 years of life.

123. B: Transient tachypnea of the newborn is the most common cause of respiratory distress in the newborn. It is triggered by excessive fluid in the lungs and usually resolves on its own. It occurs shortly after delivery. Supportive care with oxygen or CPAP may be necessary until the symptoms resolve. It is most common in babies born via Cesarean section.

124. A: Surfactant should be given as soon as the diagnosis of respiratory distress syndrome is made, preferably within 1 hour of birth. A repeat dose is then given 4-12 hours after birth as long as the infant is still intubated and requiring 30-40% oxygen. Surfactant is administered through the endotracheal tube over the course of a few minutes.

125. A: The digestive system of the newborn begins maturing soon after birth. For the first few months, however, the only proteins it is able to digest are those found in formula or human milk. That is why it is advised that cow's milk not be given to babies within the first year of life. The GI tract has also not fully matured with the necessary microorganisms that aide in digestion. Development and maturation of the GI tract continues for the first 2 years of life.

126. C: Hirschsprung's disease is a congenital condition in which nerve cells are absent from the lower part of the GI tract. This prevents the normal peristaltic movement to occur in the intestines, which pushes waste material through, resulting in a BM. The infant will usually have a distended abdomen and vomiting with this disease. It is treated with surgery to remove the affected part of the colon.

127. B: There is an increased risk of death by aspiration in newborns that have an NG tube. This is due to aspiration of saliva. Because of this, a drainage bag should be attached to collect the aspirate. The stomach contents should also be aspirated at least every 30 minutes to decrease this risk. Feedings are contraindicated in this patient due to the intestinal obstruction and only increase aspiration risks.

128. C: Around the 10th week of gestation, the intestines are forming and settle within the abdominal cavity. As the large intestine begins to further develops, it repositions itself above and on either side of the small intestine, which is centrally located in the abdomen. With malrotation, the large intestine remains positioned on the left side of the abdomen and the small intestine remains on the right. This can result in a twisting of the intestine, or a volvulus, which can cause ischemia of the area affected and even result in death if not treated. Surgical intervention is often necessary to correct this condition.

129. B: Necrotizing enterocolitis is most common in premature infants who are being formula fed rather than breastfed. With lung prematurity in the premature infant, there is an increased risk of decreased oxygenation to the lining of the intestines. Formula fed infants are not receiving any of the immune mediators that are helpful in fighting infection and which help to build up the normal protective microorganisms in the intestines. This can result in a necrotizing infection in the intestines that can lead to intestinal rupture and even death. This condition affects 10% of premature infants, but is rare in full-term infants.

130. B: Omphalocele is a condition in which there is an opening at the umbilicus through which the abdominal organs can protrude. A gastroschisis occurs when all of the abdominal organs are exposed because the outer membrane does not form over the abdomen to cover them. Both of these are congenital defects that occur early in development. The abdominal organs usually form outside the abdomen, but then return to the abdomen during development. There is no definitive known cause for either condition.

131. B: It is recommended that the newborn's foreskin be retracted as much as it will naturally allow, then cleaned with soap and water and dried fully in order to prevent infections. Forceful retraction should be avoided as it may cause irritation, bleeding, or fibrosis, and should be avoided for that reason. Bacteria, fungus, and moisture can be trapped within the foreskin, which can lead to a painful infection. Infections can become severe enough to cause significant swelling of the foreskin, which can prevent it from being able to be retracted down over the penis.

132. C: A person with AB+ blood is considered a universal recipient because they can receive blood or blood products of any type. A universal donor would be a person with type O- blood. The most restricted recipient blood type is O- because those patients can only receive O- blood or blood products.

133. C: One of the first signs that an acute intravascular hemolytic reaction is occurring is pain at the IV site. Other early signs include fever, chills, elevated heart rate, nausea, and dyspnea. This potentially life-threatening reaction usually occurs within 10 minutes of the beginning of the infusion of blood or blood products.

134. B: In newborns that are genetically female, the most common cause of ambiguous genitalia is congenital adrenal hyperplasia. Ambiguous genitalia result in genital characteristics that are not wholly female or wholly male. There can be features of both, externally and internally. Congenital adrenal hyperplasia results in the overproduction of male hormones, which causes the genitalia to take on both male and female features during development. This condition can result in a great deal of stress for the parents. Genetic testing is usually done to determine if the infant is genetically a male or female.

135. A: Unilateral neonatal testicular torsion generally has little, if any, effect on future futility. Bilateral torsion can result in bilateral testicular dysfunction, which can involve deficiencies in sex steroid hormones. Those patients should be seen by an endocrinologist to determine what sex steroid hormone replacement therapy will be necessary for normal development.

136. C: Clinical symptoms of renal vein thrombosis in the newborn include thrombocytopenia, hypertension, hematuria, proteinuria, and renal insufficiency. This condition is rare, but can occur in infants born to mothers with a history of diabetes mellitus. This is not an infectious condition, so you would not expect to see leukocytosis. Bence-Jones proteins in the urine are specific to multiple myeloma.

137. A: Bilirubin is measured as direct, indirect, or total. Direct bilirubin is the amount of bilirubin that is not bound to protein that passes from the liver to the small intestines. A small amount passes through the urine to give it a yellow color. The indirect bilirubin is bilirubin that is bound to albumin. The total bilirubin is the measure of both direct and indirect bilirubin combined.

138. C: The Kleihauer Betke test is a blood test used following maternal trauma, such as a bad fall down stairs or a car accident. It checks the maternal blood sample for fetal hemoglobin mixed with maternal blood. This occurs when there is trauma that results in a breach to the placental barrier, allowing fetal and maternal blood to mix in the mother's circulation. This can be fatal to the mother and the fetus if there is an Rh incompatibility between the two blood types.

139. B: Direct hyperbilirubinemia is also known as jaundice, yellow discoloration of the skin and sclera. The most common cause in newborns is due to the liver being immature and not being able to breakdown bilirubin. It is fairly common and most often responds to phototherapy for a few days.

140. A: Hydrops fetalis occurs as a result of Rh incompatibility between the newborn and the mother. The Rh incompatibility results in a large number of red blood cells in the infant to be destroyed. This causes severe edema. Approximately half of newborns with hydrops fetalis will not survive. This can be prevented if prenatal testing is done on the mother to determine her Rh status. If she is Rh negative, an injection can be given during the first trimester of her pregnancy to prevent this reaction from occurring.

141. C: Hypoxic ischemic encephalopathy is more common in full-term infants than premature infants. This condition results in damage or death to brain tissue due to lack of oxygen to the brain. It can occur when there is any condition, maternal or fetal, that results in a disruption in oxygenation of brain tissue. This can include a prolapsed cord, placental abruption, maternal hypotension, and others. This is the leading cause of impairment in newborns, though severity of the impairment may not be determined until 3 or 4 years of age.

142. C: Spina bifida is classified as a neural tube defect and it develops during the first month of pregnancy, when development of the spinal column occurs. Other neural tube defects include anencephaly and development of a Chiari malformation. With spina bifida, the spinal column does not completely close, resulting in at least some paralysis of the lower extremities. There is no cure for this condition, and any nerve damage present at birth is permanent.

143. B: An intraventricular hemorrhage in a newborn is classified into grades, depending upon the severity of the bleeding. Grade I, the mildest form, is also called a germinal matrix hemorrhage. Those infants most at risk for developing an intraventricular hemorrhage are those who are premature, at least 10 weeks preterm. This occurs because the blood vessels in the brain are very weak in the premature infant and can easily rupture, causing a brain bleed. Less than half of infants with a mild bleed will have long-term effects from it. Up to one-third of those with severe bleeds may die.

144. B: Periventricular leukomalacia often causes cerebral palsy in the affected child. It has also been associated with an increased chance of epilepsy. Periventricular leukomalacia occurs when there is necrosis of the white matter in the brain near the lateral ventricles. Premature infants are at greatest risk for developing this condition due to the risk of neonatal encephalopathy.

145. C: The normal glucose level in cerebrospinal fluid in a newborn is 35-120 mg/dL. A value of 100 would be normal for this infant. Diabetes mellitus may cause CSF glucose levels to be elevated. Meningitis can cause CSF glucose to be normal with viral meningitis, low with bacterial meningitis, and normal to low in fungal meningitis.

146. A: A congenital cytomegalovirus (CMV) infection can be diagnosed using saliva, urine, or blood specimens. Testing must be done within the first 2-3 weeks following birth. A mother who has CMV can pass this infection to the fetus through the placenta. Most infants will never develop any symptoms from the virus, but approximately 20% can develop hearing loss, vision loss, intellectual disabilities, seizures, or muscle weakness.

147. A: Cat feces can contain a parasite called toxoplasmosis. A pregnant woman may contract this parasite and then pass it onto the fetus through the placenta. For this reason, pregnant women should avoid contact with cat feces, such as when cleaning a litter box. Most pregnant women who become infected will not be aware of the infection. It can cause prematurity in about half of those infants who contract the parasite in utero. The infection can cause damage to the eyes, ears, nervous system, and skin in infants.

148. C: Early onset group B strep infection in the newborn is most likely to cause sepsis. It can also cause pneumonia. Meningitis can occur with early onset group B strep, but it is not as common as sepsis. Meningitis is more likely to occur with late onset of the infection. Group B strep infection is passed from the mother to the fetus. Screening pregnant women for group B strep is routine so that it can be treated with antibiotics to prevent transmission during pregnancy and birth.

149. C: Late congenital syphilis will reveal symptoms after a child is at least 2-years-old. This is transmitted to the newborn by a mother with syphilis. Early onset of the disease (less than 2 years of age) may cause a chronic runny nose, enlarged liver or spleen, skeletal abnormalities, or a bullous skin condition. Late onset can cause eye and ear problems, and skeletal abnormalities.

150. C: Enterovirus is a very common cause of infections. It often creates no symptoms in the infant, but can be very serious if it occurs in the first 2 weeks of life. Enterovirus infections are usually transmitted from the mother to the infant. They can cause cold symptoms, or be so severe that sepsis, meningitis, or respiratory failure develops. Enterovirus infections are most common in the summer and fall.

151. B: PKU, or phenylketonuria, is a metabolic disorder in which the body is not able to break down some of the amino acids in proteins. This leads to poor brain development and intellectual disabilities. It is highly recommended that this test be performed on all newborns so that treatment can be started and the devastating effects of this illness can be avoided.

152. B: The risk of having a child with Down syndrome is approximately 1 in 100 pregnancies. Advanced maternal age is more of a risk factor for having the genetic mutation that causes this condition. Having one child with this condition does not increase the chances that any future children will also have Down syndrome.

153. A: For this patient, overly strenuous exercise may lead to a sickle cell crisis. Before children with sickle cell participate in exercise, they should hydrate well and continue to drink water frequently. Sports drinks and caffeinated energy drinks should be avoided. Of course, if any pain or shortness of breath should develop, they should stop and rest immediately.

154. A: Studies have shown that maintaining a higher serum magnesium level can help to reduce the incidence of neurological developmental delay. It has been found to be helpful with advancing brain development in premature infants, and to some degree, in term infants who have suffered from asphyxia during labor and delivery. It is thought that magnesium can serve a neuroprotective role in early brain development.

155. B: Infants with galactosemia are not able to be breastfed at all and must be bottle-fed with a galactose-free formula. Galactosemia is a hereditary condition in which the infant is deficient in the enzyme that breaks down galactose, the sugar found in milk. Those infants affected will begin with vomiting and diarrhea shortly after ingesting any milk containing this sugar. It can go on to affect the brain, eyes, liver, and kidneys.

156. C: Fetal macrosomia occurs in up to 45% of infants of diabetic mothers. They are large babies that weigh more than 4000 g at term birth. These infants are puffy, fat, ruddy, and often hypotonic. These infants are also more likely to have periods of hypoglycemia shortly after birth and during the first few days of life.

157. C: An autosomal recessive disease is one that requires 2 copies of the gene in order for the disease or trait to occur. For example, both the mother and father of an infant would need to pass on a copy of the gene for cystic fibrosis in order for their child to develop the disease. Down syndrome and Edward's syndrome are both genetic mutations that occur during fetal development and are not genetically inherited conditions.

158. B: An autosomal dominant disorder only requires one parent to pass on the gene for a disease to occur. Examples of autosomal dominant conditions including Huntington's disease, polycystic kidney disease, and neurofibromatosis. Often, one of the parents will have the disease and can pass it onto their children.

159. A: DiGeorge syndrome occurs when there is a mutation to chromosome 22 during fetal development. It results in an immunodeficiency disorder that affects the thymus gland and the production of T-lymphocyte cells. This results in frequent infections, congenital heart defects, and hypocalcemia. This syndrome also causes characteristic facial features with an underdeveloped chin, heavy eyelids, ears that are rotated back, and small upper ear lobes.

160. C: Turner's syndrome is seen in female newborns only, because this condition only affects females. It occurs as a result of a genetic mutation in which the female receives only one X chromosome. This results in females who are short in stature, have delayed puberty, often suffer from infertility problems, and may have learning disabilities. In some cases, it may cause heart defects. Women who want to become pregnant will need to take hormone treatments, but are often unsuccessful at conceiving.

161. C: Bilateral choanal atresia occurs when the backs of the nasal passages are blocked, preventing a newborn from being able to breathe. This occurs due to a bony or soft tissue abnormality during development in utero. The back of the nasal passages fails to open, resulting in the inability to pass air. Infants are obligatory nasal breathers and immediate airway assistance is usually necessary at birth. This condition can be surgically corrected, but may require additional surgeries to widen the opening as the child matures.

162. C: Retinopathy of prematurity was a leading cause of blindness in children in the 1940s and 1950s due to high levels of oxygen given to premature infants in incubators. This condition occurs in premature infants, usually those at less than 31 weeks gestation. The eye, optic nerve, and blood vessels begin to develop around the 16th week of pregnancy. The last 12 weeks of pregnancy sees a rapid development in the blood vessels. Children before that gestation time often do not fully develop the blood vessels to the retina, causing retinopathy and possibly blindness.

163. A: Tracheomalacia is a softening of the cartilage in the trachea. It results in partial or total collapse of the airway during expiration, often resulting in expiratory stridor. Depending upon the severity of the condition, mechanical ventilation, CPAP, or BiPAP therapy may be necessary. In severe cases, surgical correction may be necessary to reinforce the airway so that it can remain open.

164. B: A subgaleal hemorrhage can be massive and may lead to hypovolemic shock. This condition occurs when there is bleeding in the loose connective tissue of the subgaleal space. The subgaleal space is composed of loose connective tissue that allows the scalp to slide easily on the cranium. There is an increased risk of a subgaleal hemorrhage with vacuum and forceps use during delivery. The trauma to the scalp results in rupture of the blood vessels in this space. This usually develops over several hours to several days with the first clinical sign being an increase in head circumference.

165. B: Polyhydramnios is an abnormal finding on ultrasound that may indicate the presence of an esophageal atresia. During normal development, the esophagus and trachea form side by side. An abnormality in development in utero may result in the esophagus not fully developing all the way to the stomach. This results in a closed-ended esophagus. The fetus drinks amniotic fluid while in the womb, so if they are not able to do this, polyhydramnios, or an increased volume of amniotic fluid, can occur. Occasionally, a fistula may form between the esophagus and the trachea, resulting in any intake of liquids being bypassed directly into the trachea and lungs.

166. A: The CCHD screening identifies those infants who may have a critical congenital heart defect that requires early surgical intervention. This screening is performed using pulse oximetry in the newborn nursery to measure the oxygen saturation in the blood of infants. This screening decreases the risk of overlooking a critical congenital heart defect that may require early intervention.

167. B: Tracheostomy care can be taught to caregivers so this can be performed at home without having a Respiratory Therapist come to the home each day. The trach tube can be reused at home once it has been cleaned with soap and water and once mucus inside the tube has been cleaned out. In the hospital setting, trach care is done using aseptic technique to prevent contamination, but it is done under "clean" conditions at home.

168. C: Though not the first choice for an IV site, the scalp is used once other sites in the hands and feet have already been used. The scalp is a good site because there is very little fat under the skin so the veins are easily visible.

169. B: The Teach-Back system is a method used to improve patient and family understanding of the plan of care. After teaching a patient and/or family about an illness or treatment, they are then asked to repeat or demonstrate what was reviewed. This ensures that there is full understanding of the treatment plan, which improves patient compliance and decreases potential complications.

170. C: Whenever possible, have an interpreter present in these types of situations who has undergone some training in medical terminology. Using a family member is not ensuring that any medical training or terms will be correctly translated. Online software may not be accurate and there is no way to verify that the terms and concepts are being interpreted appropriately.

171. A: Beneficence is acting in a kind and thoughtful way in order to help someone. In nursing, this can be expressed through helping a patient with their ADLs when they are not able to do them on their own. There are many different examples of beneficence played out in nursing from providing pain medications to keep someone comfortable, to performing the nursing duties that aide in helping someone recover from an illness. The ethical principle that addresses treating patients fairly and equally regardless of background is justice. The principle ensuring that no harm is done is referred to as nonmaleficence.

172. B: Nonmaleficence is performing actions to reach a beneficial outcome, but doing so in a manner that will cause the least amount of harm possible. For example, a patient will benefit by having wound care performed to help heal, but ensuring they have had pain medication beforehand will make the procedure less uncomfortable for them. This is often confused with beneficence, which is the act of helping someone. Truth and honesty refer to the ethical principle of justice.

173. A: Medical negligence is any action that results in a bad outcome for a patient as a result of carelessness or medical error. This is not an intentional act, but occurs as a result of the actions of the healthcare provider. On the other hand, medical malpractice occurs when the standard norms or accepted standards of practice are not followed, resulting in an injury or bad outcome for the patient.

174. C: Quality improvement is instrumental in improving the way healthcare services are provided, while continually measuring the effect those changes have on the health status of the patients served. This is often measured through patient satisfaction information.

175. C: HIPAA regulations prohibit the release of any patient information to someone who has not been authorized to receive this information. In this case, the child's parents would need to give written permission indicating the child's grandmother is someone who can receive this

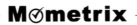

information. The best response would be to let the parents know so they can contact their family member.

NICU Nurse Practice Tests #2 and #3

To take these additional NICU Nurse practice tests, visit our bonus page:
mometrix.com/bonus948/nicnurse

How to Overcome Test Anxiety

Just the thought of taking a test is enough to make most people a little nervous. A test is an important event that can have a long-term impact on your future, so it's important to take it seriously and it's natural to feel anxious about performing well. But just because anxiety is normal, that doesn't mean that it's helpful in test taking, or that you should simply accept it as part of your life. Anxiety can have a variety of effects. These effects can be mild, like making you feel slightly nervous, or severe, like blocking your ability to focus or remember even a simple detail.

If you experience test anxiety—whether severe or mild—it's important to know how to beat it. To discover this, first you need to understand what causes test anxiety.

Causes of Test Anxiety

While we often think of anxiety as an uncontrollable emotional state, it can actually be caused by simple, practical things. One of the most common causes of test anxiety is that a person does not feel adequately prepared for their test. This feeling can be the result of many different issues such as poor study habits or lack of organization, but the most common culprit is time management. Starting to study too late, failing to organize your study time to cover all of the material, or being distracted while you study will mean that you're not well prepared for the test. This may lead to cramming the night before, which will cause you to be physically and mentally exhausted for the test. Poor time management also contributes to feelings of stress, fear, and hopelessness as you realize you are not well prepared but don't know what to do about it.

Other times, test anxiety is not related to your preparation for the test but comes from unresolved fear. This may be a past failure on a test, or poor performance on tests in general. It may come from comparing yourself to others who seem to be performing better or from the stress of living up to expectations. Anxiety may be driven by fears of the future—how failure on this test would affect your educational and career goals. These fears are often completely irrational, but they can still negatively impact your test performance.

> **Review Video: 3 Reasons You Have Test Anxiety**
> Visit mometrix.com/academy and enter code: 428468

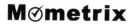

Elements of Test Anxiety

As mentioned earlier, test anxiety is considered to be an emotional state, but it has physical and mental components as well. Sometimes you may not even realize that you are suffering from test anxiety until you notice the physical symptoms. These can include trembling hands, rapid heartbeat, sweating, nausea, and tense muscles. Extreme anxiety may lead to fainting or vomiting. Obviously, any of these symptoms can have a negative impact on testing. It is important to recognize them as soon as they begin to occur so that you can address the problem before it damages your performance.

> **Review Video: 3 Ways to Tell You Have Test Anxiety**
> Visit mometrix.com/academy and enter code: 927847

The mental components of test anxiety include trouble focusing and inability to remember learned information. During a test, your mind is on high alert, which can help you recall information and stay focused for an extended period of time. However, anxiety interferes with your mind's natural processes, causing you to blank out, even on the questions you know well. The strain of testing during anxiety makes it difficult to stay focused, especially on a test that may take several hours. Extreme anxiety can take a huge mental toll, making it difficult not only to recall test information but even to understand the test questions or pull your thoughts together.

> **Review Video: How Test Anxiety Affects Memory**
> Visit mometrix.com/academy and enter code: 609003

Effects of Test Anxiety

Test anxiety is like a disease—if left untreated, it will get progressively worse. Anxiety leads to poor performance, and this reinforces the feelings of fear and failure, which in turn lead to poor performances on subsequent tests. It can grow from a mild nervousness to a crippling condition. If allowed to progress, test anxiety can have a big impact on your schooling, and consequently on your future.

Test anxiety can spread to other parts of your life. Anxiety on tests can become anxiety in any stressful situation, and blanking on a test can turn into panicking in a job situation. But fortunately, you don't have to let anxiety rule your testing and determine your grades. There are a number of relatively simple steps you can take to move past anxiety and function normally on a test and in the rest of life.

> **Review Video: How Test Anxiety Impacts Your Grades**
> Visit mometrix.com/academy and enter code: 939819

Physical Steps for Beating Test Anxiety

While test anxiety is a serious problem, the good news is that it can be overcome. It doesn't have to control your ability to think and remember information. While it may take time, you can begin taking steps today to beat anxiety.

Just as your first hint that you may be struggling with anxiety comes from the physical symptoms, the first step to treating it is also physical. Rest is crucial for having a clear, strong mind. If you are tired, it is much easier to give in to anxiety. But if you establish good sleep habits, your body and mind will be ready to perform optimally, without the strain of exhaustion. Additionally, sleeping well helps you to retain information better, so you're more likely to recall the answers when you see the test questions.

Getting good sleep means more than going to bed on time. It's important to allow your brain time to relax. Take study breaks from time to time so it doesn't get overworked, and don't study right before bed. Take time to rest your mind before trying to rest your body, or you may find it difficult to fall asleep.

> **Review Video: The Importance of Sleep for Your Brain**
> Visit mometrix.com/academy and enter code: 319338

Along with sleep, other aspects of physical health are important in preparing for a test. Good nutrition is vital for good brain function. Sugary foods and drinks may give a burst of energy but this burst is followed by a crash, both physically and emotionally. Instead, fuel your body with protein and vitamin-rich foods.

Also, drink plenty of water. Dehydration can lead to headaches and exhaustion, especially if your brain is already under stress from the rigors of the test. Particularly if your test is a long one, drink water during the breaks. And if possible, take an energy-boosting snack to eat between sections.

> **Review Video: How Diet Can Affect your Mood**
> Visit mometrix.com/academy and enter code: 624317

Along with sleep and diet, a third important part of physical health is exercise. Maintaining a steady workout schedule is helpful, but even taking 5-minute study breaks to walk can help get your blood pumping faster and clear your head. Exercise also releases endorphins, which contribute to a positive feeling and can help combat test anxiety.

When you nurture your physical health, you are also contributing to your mental health. If your body is healthy, your mind is much more likely to be healthy as well. So take time to rest, nourish your body with healthy food and water, and get moving as much as possible. Taking these physical steps will make you stronger and more able to take the mental steps necessary to overcome test anxiety.

Mental Steps for Beating Test Anxiety

Working on the mental side of test anxiety can be more challenging, but as with the physical side, there are clear steps you can take to overcome it. As mentioned earlier, test anxiety often stems from lack of preparation, so the obvious solution is to prepare for the test. Effective studying may be the most important weapon you have for beating test anxiety, but you can and should employ several other mental tools to combat fear.

First, boost your confidence by reminding yourself of past success—tests or projects that you aced. If you're putting as much effort into preparing for this test as you did for those, there's no reason you should expect to fail here. Work hard to prepare; then trust your preparation.

Second, surround yourself with encouraging people. It can be helpful to find a study group, but be sure that the people you're around will encourage a positive attitude. If you spend time with others who are anxious or cynical, this will only contribute to your own anxiety. Look for others who are motivated to study hard from a desire to succeed, not from a fear of failure.

Third, reward yourself. A test is physically and mentally tiring, even without anxiety, and it can be helpful to have something to look forward to. Plan an activity following the test, regardless of the outcome, such as going to a movie or getting ice cream.

When you are taking the test, if you find yourself beginning to feel anxious, remind yourself that you know the material. Visualize successfully completing the test. Then take a few deep, relaxing breaths and return to it. Work through the questions carefully but with confidence, knowing that you are capable of succeeding.

Developing a healthy mental approach to test taking will also aid in other areas of life. Test anxiety affects more than just the actual test—it can be damaging to your mental health and even contribute to depression. It's important to beat test anxiety before it becomes a problem for more than testing.

Review Video: Test Anxiety and Depression
Visit mometrix.com/academy and enter code: 904704

Study Strategy

Being prepared for the test is necessary to combat anxiety, but what does being prepared look like? You may study for hours on end and still not feel prepared. What you need is a strategy for test prep. The next few pages outline our recommended steps to help you plan out and conquer the challenge of preparation.

STEP 1: SCOPE OUT THE TEST

Learn everything you can about the format (multiple choice, essay, etc.) and what will be on the test. Gather any study materials, course outlines, or sample exams that may be available. Not only will this help you to prepare, but knowing what to expect can help to alleviate test anxiety.

STEP 2: MAP OUT THE MATERIAL

Look through the textbook or study guide and make note of how many chapters or sections it has. Then divide these over the time you have. For example, if a book has 15 chapters and you have five days to study, you need to cover three chapters each day. Even better, if you have the time, leave an extra day at the end for overall review after you have gone through the material in depth.

If time is limited, you may need to prioritize the material. Look through it and make note of which sections you think you already have a good grasp on, and which need review. While you are studying, skim quickly through the familiar sections and take more time on the challenging parts. Write out your plan so you don't get lost as you go. Having a written plan also helps you feel more in control of the study, so anxiety is less likely to arise from feeling overwhelmed at the amount to cover.

STEP 3: GATHER YOUR TOOLS

Decide what study method works best for you. Do you prefer to highlight in the book as you study and then go back over the highlighted portions? Or do you type out notes of the important information? Or is it helpful to make flashcards that you can carry with you? Assemble the pens, index cards, highlighters, post-it notes, and any other materials you may need so you won't be distracted by getting up to find things while you study.

If you're having a hard time retaining the information or organizing your notes, experiment with different methods. For example, try color-coding by subject with colored pens, highlighters, or post-it notes. If you learn better by hearing, try recording yourself reading your notes so you can listen while in the car, working out, or simply sitting at your desk. Ask a friend to quiz you from your flashcards, or try teaching someone the material to solidify it in your mind.

STEP 4: CREATE YOUR ENVIRONMENT

It's important to avoid distractions while you study. This includes both the obvious distractions like visitors and the subtle distractions like an uncomfortable chair (or a too-comfortable couch that makes you want to fall asleep). Set up the best study environment possible: good lighting and a comfortable work area. If background music helps you focus, you may want to turn it on, but otherwise keep the room quiet. If you are using a computer to take notes, be sure you don't have any other windows open, especially applications like social media, games, or anything else that could distract you. Silence your phone and turn off notifications. Be sure to keep water close by so you stay hydrated while you study (but avoid unhealthy drinks and snacks).

Also, take into account the best time of day to study. Are you freshest first thing in the morning? Try to set aside some time then to work through the material. Is your mind clearer in the afternoon or evening? Schedule your study session then. Another method is to study at the same time of day that you will take the test, so that your brain gets used to working on the material at that time and will be ready to focus at test time.

STEP 5: STUDY!

Once you have done all the study preparation, it's time to settle into the actual studying. Sit down, take a few moments to settle your mind so you can focus, and begin to follow your study plan. Don't give in to distractions or let yourself procrastinate. This is your time to prepare so you'll be ready to fearlessly approach the test. Make the most of the time and stay focused.

Of course, you don't want to burn out. If you study too long you may find that you're not retaining the information very well. Take regular study breaks. For example, taking five minutes out of every hour to walk briskly, breathing deeply and swinging your arms, can help your mind stay fresh.

As you get to the end of each chapter or section, it's a good idea to do a quick review. Remind yourself of what you learned and work on any difficult parts. When you feel that you've mastered the material, move on to the next part. At the end of your study session, briefly skim through your notes again.

But while review is helpful, cramming last minute is NOT. If at all possible, work ahead so that you won't need to fit all your study into the last day. Cramming overloads your brain with more information than it can process and retain, and your tired mind may struggle to recall even previously learned information when it is overwhelmed with last-minute study. Also, the urgent nature of cramming and the stress placed on your brain contribute to anxiety. You'll be more likely to go to the test feeling unprepared and having trouble thinking clearly.

So don't cram, and don't stay up late before the test, even just to review your notes at a leisurely pace. Your brain needs rest more than it needs to go over the information again. In fact, plan to finish your studies by noon or early afternoon the day before the test. Give your brain the rest of the day to relax or focus on other things, and get a good night's sleep. Then you will be fresh for the test and better able to recall what you've studied.

STEP 6: TAKE A PRACTICE TEST

Many courses offer sample tests, either online or in the study materials. This is an excellent resource to check whether you have mastered the material, as well as to prepare for the test format and environment.

Check the test format ahead of time: the number of questions, the type (multiple choice, free response, etc.), and the time limit. Then create a plan for working through them. For example, if you have 30 minutes to take a 60-question test, your limit is 30 seconds per question. Spend less time on the questions you know well so that you can take more time on the difficult ones.

If you have time to take several practice tests, take the first one open book, with no time limit. Work through the questions at your own pace and make sure you fully understand them. Gradually work up to taking a test under test conditions: sit at a desk with all study materials put away and set a timer. Pace yourself to make sure you finish the test with time to spare and go back to check your answers if you have time.

After each test, check your answers. On the questions you missed, be sure you understand why you missed them. Did you misread the question (tests can use tricky wording)? Did you forget the information? Or was it something you hadn't learned? Go back and study any shaky areas that the practice tests reveal.

Taking these tests not only helps with your grade, but also aids in combating test anxiety. If you're already used to the test conditions, you're less likely to worry about it, and working through tests until you're scoring well gives you a confidence boost. Go through the practice tests until you feel comfortable, and then you can go into the test knowing that you're ready for it.

Test Tips

On test day, you should be confident, knowing that you've prepared well and are ready to answer the questions. But aside from preparation, there are several test day strategies you can employ to maximize your performance.

First, as stated before, get a good night's sleep the night before the test (and for several nights before that, if possible). Go into the test with a fresh, alert mind rather than staying up late to study.

Try not to change too much about your normal routine on the day of the test. It's important to eat a nutritious breakfast, but if you normally don't eat breakfast at all, consider eating just a protein bar. If you're a coffee drinker, go ahead and have your normal coffee. Just make sure you time it so that the caffeine doesn't wear off right in the middle of your test. Avoid sugary beverages, and drink enough water to stay hydrated but not so much that you need a restroom break 10 minutes into the test. If your test isn't first thing in the morning, consider going for a walk or doing a light workout before the test to get your blood flowing.

Allow yourself enough time to get ready, and leave for the test with plenty of time to spare so you won't have the anxiety of scrambling to arrive in time. Another reason to be early is to select a good seat. It's helpful to sit away from doors and windows, which can be distracting. Find a good seat, get out your supplies, and settle your mind before the test begins.

When the test begins, start by going over the instructions carefully, even if you already know what to expect. Make sure you avoid any careless mistakes by following the directions.

Then begin working through the questions, pacing yourself as you've practiced. If you're not sure on an answer, don't spend too much time on it, and don't let it shake your confidence. Either skip it and come back later, or eliminate as many wrong answers as possible and guess among the remaining ones. Don't dwell on these questions as you continue—put them out of your mind and focus on what lies ahead.

Be sure to read all of the answer choices, even if you're sure the first one is the right answer. Sometimes you'll find a better one if you keep reading. But don't second-guess yourself if you do immediately know the answer. Your gut instinct is usually right. Don't let test anxiety rob you of the information you know.

If you have time at the end of the test (and if the test format allows), go back and review your answers. Be cautious about changing any, since your first instinct tends to be correct, but make sure you didn't misread any of the questions or accidentally mark the wrong answer choice. Look over any you skipped and make an educated guess.

At the end, leave the test feeling confident. You've done your best, so don't waste time worrying about your performance or wishing you could change anything. Instead, celebrate the successful

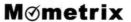

completion of this test. And finally, use this test to learn how to deal with anxiety even better next time.

> **Review Video: 5 Tips to Beat Test Anxiety**
> Visit mometrix.com/academy and enter code: 570656

Important Qualification

Not all anxiety is created equal. If your test anxiety is causing major issues in your life beyond the classroom or testing center, or if you are experiencing troubling physical symptoms related to your anxiety, it may be a sign of a serious physiological or psychological condition. If this sounds like your situation, we strongly encourage you to seek professional help.

Thank You

We at Mometrix would like to extend our heartfelt thanks to you, our friend and patron, for allowing us to play a part in your journey. It is a privilege to serve people from all walks of life who are unified in their commitment to building the best future they can for themselves.

The preparation you devote to these important testing milestones may be the most valuable educational opportunity you have for making a real difference in your life. We encourage you to put your heart into it—that feeling of succeeding, overcoming, and yes, conquering will be well worth the hours you've invested.

We want to hear your story, your struggles and your successes, and if you see any opportunities for us to improve our materials so we can help others even more effectively in the future, please share that with us as well. **The team at Mometrix would be absolutely thrilled to hear from you!** So please, send us an email (support@mometrix.com) and let's stay in touch.

> **If you'd like some additional help, check out these other resources we offer for your exam:**
> **http://mometrixflashcards.com/Neonatal**

306

Additional Bonus Material

Due to our efforts to try to keep this book to a manageable length, we've created a link that will give you access to all of your additional bonus material:

mometrix.com/bonus948/nicnurse